Multiple Sclerosis:
The History of a Disease

Multiple Sclerosis: The History of a Disease

T. Jock Murray

OC, MD, FRCPC, FAAN, MACP, FRCP, LLD, DSc, D. Litt

Professor of Medical Humanities
Director, Dalhousie MS Research Unit

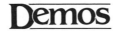

New York

Demos Medical Publishing, 386 Park Avenue South, New York, NY 10016

www.demosmedpub.com

Library of Congress Cataloging-in-Publication Data

Murray, T. J.

  The history of multiple sclerosis / T. Jock Murray.

     p. ; cm.

  Includes bibliographical references and index.

  ISBN 1-888799-80-3 (softcover : alk. paper)

  1. Multiple sclerosis—History.

  [DNLM: 1. Multiple Sclerosis—history. WL 11.1 M984h 2005] I. Title.

  RC377.M88   2005

  616.8'34—dc22

                                                    2004022222

To Janet

Contents

Acknowledgments

I am indebted to many people for their assistance and inspiration in this work. My wife Janet Murray assisted with library searches and referencing at the Wellcome Institute for the History of Medicine, and with all my work is a generous, wise, and understanding critic. Dalhousie University, the Department of Medicine, and my colleagues in the Division of Neurology and the Medical Humanities Program were supportive of my sabbatical leave.

My tireless and efficient assistant Roxy Pelham suffered through many drafts and was able to guide me through the complexities of organizing the manuscript.

I am grateful to the Burrows-Wellcome Foundation for a grant in 1998 to work at the Wellcome Institute for the History and Understanding of Medicine, and to Berlex Canada for an unrestricted education, grant to complete the research and writing at the Wellcome Library in 2000. For one period of writing during a six-month sabbatical in 2000, Janet and I had the luxury of writing and walking the beach at the summer home of Dr. Barrie and Martha Silverman on Sullivan's Island, South Carolina.

I relied heavily on the excellent historical work of my colleagues Alastair Compston, George Ebers, and W. Ian McDonald, each of whom has advanced the understanding of MS in so many ways over the last four decades.

Dr. Andrea Rideout assisted with library searches when working with me as an elective student when I was beginning this project a decade ago. Susan Drain of Mount Saint Vincent University introduced me to the case of Margaret Gatty, Maria Aguayo to William Brown, David Shephard to Will Coffin, Nick LaRocca to Alan Stevenson, and Heather Spears to Margaret Davies.

I have benefited from the helpful staff and the resources of the Wellcome Institute for the History and Understanding of Medicine, The Kellogg Library for the Health Sciences at Dalhousie, the British Library, the National Archives of Canada, the National Hospital, Queen Square, the Harveian Library of the Royal College of Physicians of London, the New York City Library, and the Waring Library of the Medical University of South Carolina. I particularly acknowledge John Simonds of the Wellcome Library, who helped me date the atlases of Carswell and Cruveilhier; Dr. Leslie Hall, who introduced me to the papers of Frederick Parkes Weber, and Professor W. Ian McDonald, who assisted me in viewing all the correspondence and the diaries related to Augustus d'Esté. Dr. David Hopkins assisted in verifying the name of the physician Godfried "Zonderdank" de la Haye. Dr. Hans K. Uhthoff, Emeritus Professor of Surgery at the University of Ottawa, kindly provided photographs of his great uncle, Wilhelm Uhthoff.

I am grateful to Jack S. Burks and Kenneth P. Johnson, editors of *Multiple Sclerosis: Diagnosis, Medical Management, and Rehabilitation* and to Demos Medical Publishing Inc. for allowing me to include material from my chapter in that book, Chapter I: The History of Multiple Sclerosis, which was expanded into this quite different history.

A special thanks to my friends Professor W. Ian McDonald of London, Donald Paty of Vancouver, and George Ebers of Oxford, who were kind enough to read a very rough first draft of the manuscript and offer comments and advice.

I am also honored to have Professor W. Ian McDonald, Harveian Librarian at the Royal College of Physicians of London, write the Foreword. He has contributed to all aspects of multiple sclerosis research in his outstanding career at the Institute of Neurology and the National Hospital, Queen Square, and has always been a kind and supportive friend to me and so many others who work for the cause of MS patients.

Foreword

The social and professional histories of multiple sclerosis are rich in their sources and their detail. Dr. Murray, in this scholarly but at the same time engaging book, brings together a mass of material, some not easily accessible otherwise.

His range is wide. He gives a balanced assessment of the claims for the existence of multiple sclerosis in historical figures and of the accounts of sufferers from MS who have written of their experiences. He charts the evolution of our knowledge of the nature of multiple sclerosis, of the factors involved in its causation, how it affects the nervous system, and of the changing strategies for treatment.

This book is a mine of information. People with multiple sclerosis, physicians, nurses, physiotherapists, and others involved in the care of patients, as well as historians interested in the social context of disease, will be greatly in Dr. Murray's debt.

W. Ian McDonald
Harveian Librarian
Royal College of Physicians, London

1

Terminology and Disease Description

"The story of knowledge of multiple sclerosis is like a history of medicine in miniature."

Tracy J. Putnam, 1938[1]

In earlier centuries, there were people in every community who had symptoms of a slowly increasing paralysis, with episodes of numbness, dizziness, blurred vision, and decreasing ability to get around. They eventually walked with canes and later were unable to walk unassisted. This process often took many years, usually decades.

Such people were said to be ill, but with a palsy, or a paralysis. By the 18th century, they were classified by their physicians into broader groups such as rheumatic disease, a constitutional weakness, or a paraplegia. By the late 18th century, the term paraplegia was used for all people who had a progressive paralysis. Physicians divided the condition into active or passive, functional or organic. A separate group was recognized due to "the pox," syphilis, which could affect the central nervous system (CNS) in many ways. By the beginning of the 19th century, pathological studies were beginning to show differences in the appearance of some of these cases when examined by the naked eye and the feel of the brain and spinal cord under the fingertips.

Robley Dunglison, a Scottish physician and anatomist recruited to the new medical school at the University of Virginia at age 26 by Thomas Jefferson, divided all such cases into *paraplegia* if there was weakness, and *paraplexia* if the paralysis was complete.[2] Later, as forms of neurological disease were being separated, the patient with intermittent and progressive neurological symptoms might be grouped with patients diagnosed as having paraplegia, or inflammation of the nervous system, but might also be included among patients with general paralysis or tabes dorsalis due to syphilis.

In 1824, a young man in France named Charles Prosper Ollivier d'Angers published, at age 28, a remarkable 400-page book on disorders of the spinal cord that helped make some sense out of the various conditions that caused paraplegia. Before him, the spinal cord was given little attention by clinicians, who regarded it simply as a very large nerve. In the next few decades, the pattern of combining the clinical picture in the patient with the pathological findings led to the separation and naming of a number of disorders that had been previously lumped together as paraplegia. In the great clinics of Paris, Vienna, and Berlin, clinicians were differentiating forms of neurological disease such as locomotor ataxia, neurosyphilis, Friedreich's ataxia, and multiple sclerosis by correlating the specific clinical findings with examination of the brain and spinal cord at autopsy.

There are many examples of illnesses, even ones that are common, which were probably always there, but were only recognized when someone conceptualized their features and framed the disease. Others then began to see the disease among their patients, and it seemed as if the disease had suddenly appeared, in an epidemic. Examples are sleep apnea, attention deficit disorder, dyslexia, Alzheimer's disease, and fibromyalgia. Tourette syndrome was thought to be a neurological curiosity until the Shapiros noted that haloperidol was very helpful to these patients, and the presence of a therapy sparked a wave of recognition. Repeatedly, clinicians wonder what patients were regarded as having before such disorders were named and framed.

One of the physicians who classified and separated the great variety of sick, elderly, and frail inmates of the great Salpêtrière hospital in Paris was Jean-Martin Charcot. He and his colleague Edmé Vulpian contemplated the tremors of patients and attempted to differentiate a condition of younger people from the paralysis agitans described by James Parkinson in 1817. Charcot did not like the term *paralysis agitans,* as he did not feel that paralysis was characteristic of the disease. He and Vulpian noted a pattern that earlier clinicians had also seen and described—a condition occurring in younger adults with tremor and paralysis, who at autopsy were noted to have grey patches (plaques) scattered throughout the spinal cord, brain stem, and brain. To separate this type of tremor from that of Parkinson's disease, they presented three cases to a hospital rounds in 1866, and later Charcot gave a series of lectures on the features of this disease, which he called *sclérose en plaque disseminée.*

As had occurred with Parkinson's description of paralysis agitans, once Charcot defined and framed this disease and gave it a name, others could then recognize it. Over the next 150 years, medical knowledge of the disease would build on these early descriptions, adding to its understanding and, recently, to the development of new therapies. As this is being written, there are efforts to further subdivide and classify different types of multiple sclerosis (MS) by their clinical characteristics and course, their magnetic resonance imaging (MRI) features, and the differing pathological findings.

I will discuss some of the people who suffered with a progressive neurological disorder that resembled what we would now call multiple sclerosis, but who lived in the centuries before the disease was named, and examine how they were regarded and treated. I will survey the many early reports of this disease in the medical literature before Charcot gave his famous lectures. The progress in knowledge of MS over the following century will occupy the largest part of the book, followed by a more cursory sweep of the developments of the last 25 years.

> *"The early history of MS is somewhat easier to put into context and perspective than that of the last 50 years."*
> George Ebers, 1998[3]

Paradoxically, most of the research on MS has been in the last quarter century, but this research is the most difficult to put into a historical context. Recent work is still in evolution and the players are still busy with this exciting work in their clinics and laboratories. They may be disappointed to see their recent work with T-cells, cytokines, macrophages, gene probes, and diffusion-weighted MRI given only cursory attention. It will be left for some medical historian in the future to put much of the current work into historical perspective.

MS is a recurrent demyelinating disease of the white matter in the CNS, which usually becomes progressive. Thought to be a neurological curiosity in the mid-19th century worthy of single case reports in the journals of the day, by the turn of the 20th century, it was recognized as one of the most common causes of admission to neurology wards—"an epidemic of recognition rather than the effect of altered biological factors," said Alistair Compston.[4] Even Charcot, in his early descriptions of the disease, said that it seemed rare, but the disease would be more frequently diagnosed when the variations (*forme frustes*) were better understood. At the turn of the 21st century, MS is recognized as the most common serious neurological disease in young adults living in temperate climates.

MS has also become well known to the general public because it *is* common (most people know someone with the disease), because it has been a major focus in neuroscience research, and because the MS societies have increased public awareness. Public attention has also been captured by the personal stories of well-known personalities who have MS and who have discussed their struggle with the disease. The development of new therapies in the past decade has increased public interest and created an air of hopeful expectation.

Although the "discovery" of MS is often credited to Charcot, when he stepped onto the lecture stage at the Salpêtrière in 1868 to give his regular Friday Leçon on the clinical and pathological features of the disorder we now know as MS, he was taking one further step in a process of defining the disease that had begun in the previous century. Even as he spoke, he acknowledged many individuals who had discussed this condition before him, and who contributed to the knowledge that he was summarizing. His gift and his contribution was a unique and brilliant manner of assimilating information from diverse observations and visualizing a unitary concept. He was, as many observed, a *visuel*, one who sees.

It would be easy to trivialize Charcot's contribution by noting that many knew of this disease and its features before him. But his clear description, derived from only a few well-observed patients, gave other clinicians a picture they could then recognize in their patients. Over the next century and a half, reports of the disease increased, each observer adding observations and speculations upon which the next could build. The knowledge grew and the questions expanded, but the answers in most cases remained tantalizingly out of view.

In the 1940s and 1950s, interest in the disease increased as therapeutic advances increased, not only for MS, but in other fields. As therapies for other diseases developed, they were applied to MS. Although most would prove to be of little help, there was a move from an atmosphere of therapeutic nihilism to one of hopeful polypharmacy. Although clinicians in the 19th and 20th centuries stated flatly in print that therapy was hopeless, all employed a long list of agents and procedures in the hopes that something might help their individual patients. In the 1930s, Brickner listed 29 pages of therapies that had been applied to MS, and Putnam believed that half of them improved the patients.

By the 1950s, a dramatic change occurred with the development of the MS societies, founded by Sylvia Lawry, a young woman in New York distressed by the lack of information and helpful treatments for her brother Bernard, whose MS was worsening. There was now a lay interest in fostering research, in seeking public support for the funding needed, and a serious effort at patient and public education about MS. The "rare curiosity" of the mid-19th century was now becoming one of the foremost areas of neuroscience interest, and research on the disease became a major focus of the new National Institute of Neurological Disease and Blindness (NINDB), which had a close link with the new but very active National MS Society (NMSS). Advances in other areas of medicine, new technologies, and discoveries in other fields led to a "spillover effect" that increased the capacity to address the questions in MS.

The theories about what causes MS changed as the major advances in medical science changed. In the era of Pasteur and Koch, it seemed to be an infectious disease; in the era of environmental illnesses, it seemed a disease due to some toxin; when epidemiological techniques improved, interest centered on mysterious demographic and environmental factors; as immunology flourished, it became an immunological disease, and in this age of genetics, gene probes, and the human genome, there is great interest in a genetic factor. With advances in virology, slow virus infections, and now prions, it is again being considered an infectious disease, with the virus perhaps acting as a trigger in a genetically predisposed individual. One might well ask if the theories of MS just follow the current interests in science, but it is evident that each stage provided important building blocks for the next. As a new theory in MS developed, it did not become an either/or conflict with previous theories. When a new therapy arose, it was included in a new overarching concept. This umbrella concept included a new theory to explain some clues and features, while retaining older theories for which there was still some evidence, and placed it within a framework.

There *does* seem to be a genetic predisposition to the disease, but it is not the result of a simple genetic defect. Some trigger is likely to determine if someone with the predisposition actually gets the disease and the most likely agent is a virus. Many viruses have been accused but not yet found guilty, including the usual suspects: measles virus, herpes simplex 6, Epstein-Barr virus, or the C. pneumonia agent. Whatever the trigger, it likely causes episodic breakdown in the *blood–brain barrier*, allowing immunologically active cells to enter the CNS and damage myelin, initiating an immunological reaction that involves nitrous oxide and cytokines and that continues the process. *Scavenger cells* have a number of roles in the demyelination, and later a thinner myelin re-forms. Eventually, repeated and widespread patches of myelin damage occur with increasing damage as well to the central axon, which cannot regenerate, and progression of the disease becomes evident. There is evidence that the axonal damage may be more widespread than the scattered lesions seen on MRI scans, and that this damage occurs earlier in the disease than the first symptoms would suggest. Even in this simplistic construct, we can incorporate most of the prominent theories of etiology, many of them first enunciated in the 19th century.

TERMS USED FOR MULTIPLE SCLEROSIS

"A peculiar disease state."

Robert Carswell, 1838[5]

Multiple sclerosis has been known by many names over the last century and a half. Carswell, in one of the earliest illustrations of the disease, referred to it simply as a "peculiar disease state"[5] and in the same period Cruveilhier commented on "gray degeneration of the cord" without giving it a name.[6] Charcot was impressed by the sclerosis in the scattered lesions and called it *sclérose en plaque disseminée*.[7] Shortly after, Moxon in England was impressed by the characteristic islets of change (the plaques) and preferred the name *insular sclerosis*, which was then favored by the English and their Commonwealth partners.[8] Sachs, in his 1895 textbook, uses the three terms *multiple sclerosis, insular sclerosis*, and *disseminated sclerosis* interchangeably.[9] In their 1899 textbook, Church and Peterson would use the term *multiple cerebrospinal sclerosis,* but indicate that *multiple sclerosis, insular sclerosis, sclérose en plaque, cerebro-spinal disseminated sclerosis, multilocular sclerosis*, and *spinal sclerosis* were all terms in use.[10] Some of these terms suggested they were different conditions, but most felt it was all one.

Some of the old terms persisted, and the World Health Organization used the term *cerebral sclerosis* up to the 1950s. *Disseminated sclerosis* (DS) was a common term in England during the first half of the 20th century, while *multiple sclerosis* was widely used in the United States. Physicians in Canada, characteristically finding themselves somewhere in the middle, used both terms. William Osler in Montreal used the term *insular sclerosis* in his 1880 paper. Fisher in Ontario in 1926 used both terms interchangeably in the same article. Although Risien Russel in his excellent 1899 review used a slightly shortened "disseminate sclerosis," in a footnote his lenient editor, Sir Thomas Clifford Allbutt, commented that "it would be better to use the term insular sclerosis; for, even docked of a syllable, disseminate sclerosis is too long."[11]

At a major meeting on MS of the Association for Research in Nervous and Mental Diseases (1921), both *Multiple Sclerosis* and *Disseminated Sclerosis* were used in the title of their publication (1922).[12]

The French still use the term *sclérose en plaque* (SP). The term *multiple sclerosis* is derived from the German term "multiplen sklerose," and became generally accepted by the 1950s when it was adopted by the newly formed MS societies, and by its use in the now classic book on MS by McAlpine, Compston, and Lumsden in 1955.[13] By 1965, the term used in virtually all English publications was *multiple sclerosis*.

In this brief review of the history of the disease, I use the term *multiple sclerosis* for clarity and consistency, even when discussing the work of contributors who may themselves have used one of the other terms in their publications. Thus, I refer to the contributions to the understanding of MS by Jean-Martin Charcot, William Gowers, William Osler, Kinnier Wilson, and others, although they did not use that term.

Earlier Terms for Multiple Sclerosis

Sclérose en tache ou en îsles

Sclérose en îles

Îsles de substance blanche

Grise masses disseminée

Multiplen Sklerose

Hirnsklerose

Multiple Sklerose

Inselförmige sklerose

Multiple Sklerose des
    Nervensystems

La Sclérose en plaques disseminée

La sclérose multiloculaire

La sclérose generalisée

Sclérose en plaque

Sclerosi in plache

Insular sclerosis

Multilocular sclerosis

Multiple cerebral sclerosis

Cerebral sclerosis

Spinal sclerosis

Disseminate sclerosis

Lobular and diffuse sclerosis

Multiple cerebral spinal sclerosis

Disseminated cerebral spinal
    sclerosis

Cerebro-spinal sclerosis

Polysclerosis

Polynesic sclerosis

Sclerosis multiplex

Dissemineret sklerose

Multiple inselförmige Sklerose

Disseminated sclerosis

Lobular sclerosis

Cerebrospinal disseminated
    sclerosis

A Brief Summary of the Disease

Multiple sclerosis is a common neurological disease, which usually affects young adults, most often beginning with episodic attacks of neurological symptoms, but entering a progressive phase some years later. It usually begins between the ages of 15 and 50 (average age 30), and occurs in about 1 in 500 individuals of European ancestry living in temperate climates. There appears to be a complex interaction between a genetic predisposition and an environmental "trigger" that initiates the disease.

The disease may have a number of different courses after the onset of symptoms, such as a *relapsing-remitting* course (85 percent), with attacks and remissions of symptoms. Many patients will later make the transition to a *secondary-progressive* course. Or, they may begin with a *primary-progressive* course (15 percent), with slow progression without attacks. Recently, there has been an attempt to separate the small number of patients whose cases begin as progressive, but who later have one or more acute relapses, and to call this *progressive-relapsing* type of disease. After many years, it may be evident that some of the cases have had a very long mild course, and can be called *benign*. The benign type, which represents 10 percent of cases, is more difficult to define and can only be recognized after many years have passed.

Symptoms may occur in any area served by the myelinated nerves of the central white matter of the brain, brain stem, and spinal cord. Thus, the person may have weakness or sensory changes in the limbs, particularly the legs; unsteadiness; difficulty with bladder control; visual changes because of involvement of the optic nerve; vertigo; facial numbness or weakness; or double vision.

MS affects the myelinated nerves of the CNS, but not the peripheral nerves. The optic nerve is affected, as it is an extension of the brain and contains central CNS myelinated nerves, not peripheral nerves. The clinician can often find signs on the neurological examination that verify the presence and location of the abnormality experienced by the patient. Sometimes the symptoms are subjective, experienced by the patient, but little can be found by the examining physician. Also, remission may have begun by the time the patient sees the physician and the signs may have cleared or disappeared. It is common to hear that the patient has had vague symptoms off and on for many years before it is evident that MS is the cause.

Overall, there is little effect on life expectancy, but there is a significant effect on the person's quality of life, even early in the disease, and there is often serious disability in the later years. People with MS usually learn to cope with the difficulties the disease brings, but it has a major effect on their life plans, employment, and hopes for the future, as they are mostly young adults who are just beginning to develop their families and careers. Another stressful aspect of the disease is the uncertainty about the future, and even how they will feel next week. Just when they may have adapted to the disability left by previous attacks, another attack brings still more limitations and requires yet another period of adaptation and life change.

Although the cause is uncertain, MS appears to involve an immune-mediated inflammatory process in the CNS characterized by breakdown in the myelin that surrounds the nerve axon. Myelin is necessary for the rapid (saltatory) conduction in myelinated nerves. There appears to be a breakdown in the blood–brain barrier, allowing immunologically active cells in the blood to enter the brain and cause patchy damage to myelin. These scattered circumscribed lesions, or *plaques*, cause the symptoms of MS by slowing or disrupting conduction in the nerve axons. The plaques are characterized by inflammation, demyelination, and scarring (gliosis). The axons may remyelinate again, which explains to some extent how remissions may occur after a relapse (attack). The remyelinated axons may appear to be functioning normally, as the symptoms may have cleared, but electrophysiological measurements (evoked potential studies) may show that conduction is slower than normal. Perhaps more important in the long-term is the amount of damage that occurs to the axons.

The immune reaction in the nervous system is accompanied by inflammation and gliosis, which are evident on MRI scans and which may also cause increased antibodies in the spinal fluid. The MRI appearance of many lesions in characteristic areas, and the spinal fluid tests (elevated gamma globulin and oligoclonal banding), are helpful in confirming that MS is present, but do not correlate well with specific symptoms. For this reason, they are not usually used to follow the course of the disease once it has been confirmed. Although these tests can help confirm the suspicion of MS, they do not by themselves make the diagnosis, because similar changes can occur in other conditions. Confirmation of the clinical diagnosis requires correlation with the clinical picture, the presence of characteristic changes on the MRI, evoked potential studies, and spinal fluid analyses.

MS occurs two to three times more often in women and is more common in temperate climates. The reasons are unclear. Perhaps the genetic predisposition is one that is primarily in those of European stock, and those people tended to migrate to more temperate climates during the last centuries.

The earliest investigators recognized that this disease was difficult to treat, especially when the cause was unclear. This is still the case, but drugs are now available that can modify the acute attacks and reduce many of the symptoms. More importantly, for the first time, there are new agents that can reduce the number and severity of the attacks and perhaps slow the progression of the disease.

Tracy Putnam said in 1938 that the history of MS was like the history of medicine in miniature, but added that neither is yet complete. This book will chronicle the early part of the MS story.

For those interested in a fuller review of current knowledge of MS, I recommend the overview by John Noseworthy and colleagues[14] or the comprehensive text by Donald Paty and George Ebers[15] and the classic *McAlpines's Multiple Sclerosis*.[16]

REFERENCES

1. Putnam TJ. The Centenary of Multiple Sclerosis. *Arch Neurol Psych*. 1938;40(4):806-813.
2. Dunglison R. *A Dictionary of Medical Sciences*. Philadelphia: Henry C. Lea; 1868.
3. Ebers G. A Historical Overview. In: Paty D, and Ebers G, eds. *Multiple Sclerosis*. Philadelphia: FA Davis; 1998:1-4.
4. Compston A, ed. *McAlpine's Multiple Sclerosis*. London: Churchill Livingstone; 1998:3.
5. Carswell R. *Pathological Anatomy: Illustrations of the Elementary Forms of the Disease*. London: Longman, Orme, Brown, Green and Longman; 1838.
6. Cruveilhier J. *Anatomie pathologique du corps humain*. Paris: JB Baillière; 1829-1842. (Individual livraisons in this work appeared separately but Livraisons 32 and 38, both of which deal with MS, also can be found in Volume 2, published in 1842. In the

Wellcome Library a number of copies can be found, bound differently. In Copy 2, the two illustrations of MS are found in Planches V, Anatomie de l'appareil des sensations et l'innervation.)

7. Charcot JM. Histologie de la sclérose en plaques. *Gaz Hôp Civils Milit (Paris)*. 1868; 41:554-558.

8. Moxon W. Eight cases of insular sclerosis of the brain and spinal cord. *Guy Hosp Rep*. 1875;20:437-478.

9. Sachs B. *A Treatise on the Nervous Diseases of Children*. New York: William Wood; 1895:345-356.

10. Church A, Peterson F. *Nervous and Mental Diseases*. London: Rebman Publishing Company Ltd.; 1899:434-442.

11. Russell JSR. Disseminated Sclerosis. In: Albutt TC, ed. *A System of Medicine*. London: Macmillan & Co.; 1899:50-94.

12. Association for Research in Nervous and Mental Disease. *Multiple Sclerosis (Disseminated Sclerosis)*. New York: Paul B Hoeber; 1922.

13. McAlpine D, Compston ND, Lumsden CE. *Multiple Sclerosis*. Edinburgh: E&S Livingston; 1955.

14. Noseworthy JH, Lucchinetti C, Rodriguez M, Weinshenker BG. Multiple Sclerosis. *NEJM*. 2000;343:938-952.

15. Paty DW, Ebers GC, eds. *Multiple Sclerosis*. Philadelphia: FA Davis; 1998.

16. Compston A, ed. *McAlpine's Multiple Sclerosis*. London: Churchill Livingstone; 1998.

2

The Framing of
Multiple Sclerosis

"Medicine, an often-quoted Hippocratic teaching explains, consists in many things—the disease, the patient, and the physician. ... But disease is an elusive entity. It is not simply a less than optimum physiological state. The reality is obviously a good deal more complex; disease is at once a biological event, a generation-specific repertoire of verbal constructs reflecting medicine's intellectual and institutional history, an occasion of and potential legitimization for public policy, an aspect of social and individual—intrapsychic—identity, a sanction for cultural values, and a structuring element in doctor and patient interactions. In some ways disease does not exist until we have agreed that it does, by perceiving, naming and responding to it."

Charles E. Rosenberg
Framing Disease, 1992[1]

The medical historian Charles Rosenberg indicated that in one aspect, disease is a biological event unrelated to its social context. Just as disease occurs in an animal, which suffers unassociated with a social construct for the pain and dysfunction, in our culture, a disease exists only when it is named. And the complex social, psychological, medical, political, and personal aspects that surround the biological change go to make up the experience, or the disease.

We can construct "disease" out of a behavior or complaints that were not previously regarded as disease, such as alcoholism, hyperactivity, personality disorder, premenstrual syndrome, seasonal affective disorder, gambling addiction, and chronic fatigue. Once named, it is experienced differently and the reaction of family, friends, and health professionals is different.

Access to the health care system and therapy may depend on having a disease that is named and thus accepted as existing. Conversely, many patients suffer not only their symptoms, but the rejection and perhaps derision of the health care system and society if there is no name and thus no diagnosis for their problems. This reminds me of the cartoon of the physician saying to a patient, "Our tests show that whatever you have doesn't exist."

The naming and acceptance of existence of a disease is heavily influenced by many cultural and social factors.[2] It is also characterized by specificity and having a logical mechanism and concept for the disorder. The reductionist approach that can outline the specific nature of a disease will give it legitimacy and acceptance. But it should be emphasized that the defining and naming of a disease have many consequences in the lives of those suffering those symptoms. It also can alter public policy, how the health care system responds to them, and how they are regarded by others, including their friends and family. For instance, chronic pain without an evident physical abnormality to explain the pain has lacked the specificity and logical explanation that would allow its acceptance as a disease. For this reason, physicians, workers' compensation agencies, and insurance companies, as well as fellow workers and friends, are often reluctant to recognize that the person has a legitimate condition.[3] People with multiple sclerosis (MS) who complained of their symptoms for many years before being diagnosed often show relief when they find they have MS because they now have an understanding of their problem, and now know it is not imaginary or "all in my head." Having a name for their disease has made their suffering legitimate. They can now be given a diagnosis, an explanation for the problem, a therapeutic regime, and a prognosis. This process is central to the role of a physician and the patient–physician process.[4]

Rosenberg[5] indicated that ways of seeing the disease and explanations for the patients' symptoms altered over the centuries. Initially, there were references to cooking as explanations for how the body worked and disease produced symptoms, and we now do it with descriptions of hormonal feedback loops and alterations of physiology, immune mechanisms, or the delayed effects of viral infections. If the understanding of a disease was in terms of altered balance of humors, then purging, bloodletting, and diuresis were a logical therapeutic approach, but if the problem is seen as an overactive or deranged immune system, the approach might be a drug known to suppress or alter immune function. The framing not only allows differentiation of the disease from others, but permits a construct that determines the understanding of how the disease affects the body, and how it might be eradicated or modified.

Rosenberg also makes the interesting point, well understood by many people diagnosed with a disease, that the framing of the disease can then frame the person with the disease. In other words, they may perceive that they have *become* the disease, not only have it. For instance, the person *is* an epileptic, a tubercular, a schizophrenic, a sexual deviant, a migraineur, not only to the insensitive physician who refers to "the liver case in bed number seven," but also to the community and the people who now define themselves by their disease. Their diagnosis has implications for their present, but also for their future, and may redefine how they see their past.[6] They are part of a dynamic narrative that changes if the disease is redefined and reframed. This is why Rosenberg says a disease can be viewed as existing only when it is named—before that the experience would have been quite different.[7]

The naming and classification of disease, *nosology*, also changes. Charcot may have been remarkably complete in his definition of the characteristics of the disease and its patterns, but MS has been repeatedly redefined since then, and there are currently a number of separate committees redefining and reclassifying the types and patterns of the disease in order to better comply with concepts of pathophysiology, clinical types and courses, and responses to therapies. At the turn of the 20th century, a person might be diagnosed simply as having MS, but at the turn of the 21st century, another patient may be diagnosed as having primary progressive MS with evidence of widespread MS lesions in the brain and spinal cord, some cerebral atrophy, and an Expanded Disability Status Score (EDDS) of 6.0, all of which will govern how he or she is regarded and what therapies, services, and opportunities for clinical trials and experimental therapies will be offered.

There have been differing views on the historical existence of MS. It might have been present in the population for many centuries, relatively similar in prevalence, but more evident recently because of increased recognition of the disease. There have been increasingly refined criteria and greater awareness of clinical variations, coupled with remarkable tools that can diagnose MS in mildly involved patients who would not have been diagnosed at this stage in the past. On the other hand, MS may be a new disease (only a few centuries old and increasing), defined in the early and mid-19th century because that is when it began to appear in increasing numbers. Or perhaps it was always there, blending into many diagnostic categories as they developed, changed, and became more focused. People with MS may have been residing in the categories of conditions known as paraplegia, apoplexy, flying gout, creeping paralysis, hysteria, rheumatic disease, myelitis, paralysis agitans, general paresis, tabes dorsalis, muscular dystrophy, Fredreich's ataxia, locomotor ataxia, chorea, and more general categories that included people with a slowly progressive debility and infirmity.

As I will outline, cases of MS, by our current definitions, have existed for centuries, but were framed differently in different eras. Thomas Willis would have included a patient with MS under the classification of a Habitual Palsy, which he felt should be treated with bleeding and chylification, purging, and the use of salt of vitriol, sulphur of antimony, crocus metallorum, mercury, and a long list of other herbal preparations and drugs that took up many pages of his book, *The London Practice of Physick* (1685).[8] People could just be regarded as having a condition that caused chronic lameness and was unresponsive to treatments, as was Margaret Davis in the late 1600s. Or they might be regarded as having a palsy that should be treated with the wide array of therapies that could be applied to any disease of the nervous system, the opinion of Augustus d'Éstés and many physicians in the early 18th century. Or the condition could be classified as due to some action of the patient herself, such as gardening excessively and using tools in the manner of a man, as Margaret Gatty's physician wrote in *The Lancet* in 1860.

The concept of MS was becoming clear in the early 19th century. The clinico-pathological approach of defining diseases was developing and cases of progressive paralysis characterized by grey patches of degeneration in the brain and spinal cord were being examined by Frerichs, Türck, Rokitansky, and others many years before Charcot's lecture. Frerichs could diagnose the disease in patients in life, as he was aware of its clinical features as well as its pathological ones. The framing of the disease came from many influences, crowned, but not completely, by Charcot when he stepped into the lecture stage at the Salpêtrière. We continue today to try and fill in the picture enclosed in the current frame, aware that the picture and the frame may be quite different in the future.

REFERENCES

1. Rosenberg CE, Golden J, eds. *Framing Disease: Studies in Cultural History*. New Brunswick, NJ: Rutgers University Press; 1992.
2. Ibid, p. xiii.
3. Murray TJ. *Chronic Pain*. Report to Workers Compensation Board of Nova Scotia. 1996.
4. Rosenberg CE, Golden J. *Framing Disease*: p. xiii–xxvi.
5. Ibid, p. xv.
6. Ibid, p. xvi.
7. Ibid, p. xvii.
8. Willis T. *The London Practice of Physick*. London: Thomas Basset; 1685.

3

The Palsy without a Name: Suffering with Paraplegia 1395–1868

"Believe me, there is no cure for this illness; it comes directly from God."

Godfried de la Haye, Dutch court physician, 1396

WHAT IS A DISEASE BEFORE IT GETS A NAME?

Since people suffered with a relapsing and progressive neurological disease in the centuries before Charcot gave that disease a name, it is instructive to see how such people were regarded, how they and their physicians regarded the disorder, and what therapies were offered.

Lidwina of Schiedam, Holland, had features of a recurrent and progressive disorder over 37 years. She took joy from her misery, believing that she was sent to accept suffering for the sins of others. Her plight brought attention from the community and from prominent officials, and a cult developed around her even before her death. Not all were impressed by the physical nature of her disorder, but some modern writers have suggested that she suffered from the illness we now recognize as multiple sclerosis (MS).

Other disease reports, too brief to be convincing exist, but the case of Margaret Davies of the Parish of Myddle is certainly suggestive. She also had a 20-year progressive lameness that a prominent surgeon recognized as a slow progressive disorder that would not respond to the many remedies she sought from the apothecary. She eventually became bedridden, her limbs paralyzed and contracted.

There is no doubt that Augustus d'Esté, grandson of George III, had MS. His condition was documented in poignant detail in his diaries and notebooks over the 26 years of his disease. This documentation helps us understand how the disease of someone with access to the best medical care and the outstanding consultants of his age was managed.

Heinrich Heine, the German poet, also had a chronic progressive disease that probably was MS. Though he had access to all available medical services, he progressed to death in two decades, aware to the end of the loss of physical ability, but still able to compose great poetry. He is another that we will list as having "possible MS."

Mrs. Margaret Gatty, a talented early Victorian children's writer and naturalist, came late to her literary career, just as she was developing the early signs of a recurrent and progressive neurological disease. She also saw many prominent physicians, and, unbeknownst to her, was described in *The Lancet* by her physician as someone who had developed a neurological disorder from overexertion.

It is evident that the biological process of MS has been with us for many centuries. We are not sure if it is increasing, or if its patterns are changing. Examination of the earliest cases that resemble MS can be instructive, revealing how chronic neurological disease was viewed and managed in an era when illness had a systemic rather than a focused pathological concept. Many of the cases suggested in the medical literature as early examples of MS can only be regarded as possible cases because of sketchy details; they are worth mentioning because they are so frequently raised in discussions of the history of the disease.

Lidwina the Virgin

One of the early but uncertain reports, often put forward as the earliest recorded case of MS, relates to the "strange disease of the Virgin Lidwina." Although confounding issues of religious fervor characterize her symptoms, aspects of her case led some to consider that she might have been suffering from MS in the four decades prior to her death in 1433.[1]

Lidwina was born on April 18, 1380 in Schiedam, Holland, the daughter of a laborer, and one of nine children. She was healthy and active as a child and teenager, but in the winter of 1395–96 developed an acute illness from which she gradually recovered. On February 2, 1396, she was feeling better and her friends encouraged her to go skating on a frozen canal. She fell while skating and broke ribs on the right side. Healing was slow and it was thought she had an internal abscess in the area of the fracture. She had difficulty walking and used furniture for support. She was described as having violent lancinating pain in her teeth, which may have been trigeminal neuralgia.

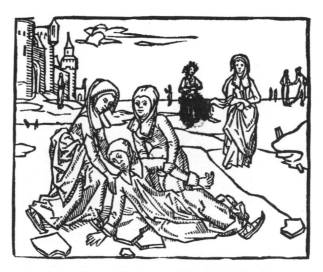

Figure 3.1(a)   The virgin Lidwina of Schiedam (1380–1433) fell while skating at age 16. She had an illness over the next 37 years that had many of the features we would now identify as multiple sclerosis, but the diagnosis must remain as "possible MS." She is the patron saint of figure skaters. (Woodcut from "Vita alme virginis Lidwine" by Jan Brugman, 1498. Original book is in the "Koninklijke Bibliotheeks' Gravenhage, The Hague, Netherlands.) (Courtesy of Dr. Robert Medaer.)

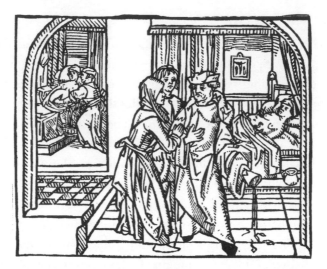

Figure 3.1(b) Dr. Godfreid Zonderdank, physician to the Count of Holland, tells the parents of the poor prognosis of Lidwina's condition. She is lying in bed with leeches over her abdomen as a form of therapy. The physician is pouring the urine sample that was viewed to assess the prognosis and this gesture indicates he has concluded the prognosis is grave. He advised against attempting a lot of therapies for such a condition, as it would be of little help and just impoverish the father. It was an illness that comes from the hand of God. (Woodcut from "Vita alme virginis Lidwine" by Jan Brugman, 1498. Original book is in the Koninklijke Mibliotheeks' Gravenhage, the Hague, The Netherlands.) (Courtesy of Dr. Robert Medaer.)

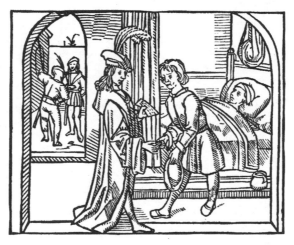

Figure 3.1(c) Instead of medical treatments, the physician advised that the Count of Holland instead provide the parents with two golden guilders to provide her for support and care. (Woodcut from "Vita alme virginis Lidwine" by Jan Brugman, 1498. Original book is in the Koninklijke Mibliotheeks' Gravenhage, the Hague, The Netherlands.) (Courtesy of Dr. Robert Medaer.)

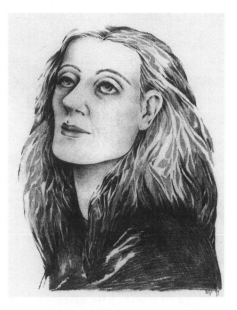

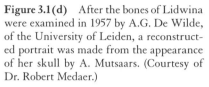

Figure 3.1(d) After the bones of Lidwina were examined in 1957 by A.G. De Wilde, of the University of Leiden, a reconstructed portrait was made from the appearance of her skull by A. Mutsaars. (Courtesy of Dr. Robert Medaer.)

Her parish priest, Father John Pott, visited regularly and suggested she join her suffering with that of the Lord.[2] Some three years later, she realized that she was called to be a victim for the sins of others. Her suffering would be her joy, and she even took steps to increase her discomfort, such as sleeping on planks instead of her feather bed. She said she would reject recovery even if it could be achieved by praying one Hail Mary.

She became blind in one eye, the other became sensitive to light, and she spent much of her time in bed, able to move only her left arm as she suffered with an "unbearable neuritis" in her right shoulder. By the time she was 19, her condition had improved, but she could walk only with difficulty; she developed paralysis in her right arm as well as more sporadic pains. There is mention of a split face and hanging lip, which may refer to facial weakness, but some of the descriptions suggest a deep cut down the bridge of her nose, which could have been due to self-mutilation. Soon she was unable to walk and had to be carried. She also had some loss of sensation and eventually developed sores, which may have been pressure sores (decubitus ulcers).

Her pious suffering gained public attention, and many physicians were consulted, including the prominent Andrew of Delft. Word of her plight reached William VI, Count of Holland and his wife Margaret of

Burgundy, who sent their own physician, Godfreid de la Haye,[*3] who reported that this disease was incurable because it came directly from God. Any attempts to cure her would just impoverish her father, and would do no good; even Hippocrates and Galen would be helpless in this situation. Butler's *Lives of the Saints* (1990) ascribes this statement to Andrew of Delft, and it indicates the sense of hopelessness this disease produced, in an age when prognostication was the most prized talent of physicians, and when the initial classification of conditions separated those that could be cured from those that could not.[4]

Lidwina's illness continued and her pious acceptance of worsening symptoms impressed everyone. Over the years, she had increasing pain and weakness and had difficulty swallowing, first solid food and, later, liquids. The disease progressed slowly with occasional periods of improvement.

Beginning in 1407, she experienced supernatural visits, ecstasies, and visions in which she participated in the Passion of Christ, saw purgatory and heaven, and visited with saints. During these "ecstasies," she had improvement in her sight and was more mobile. Although a cult grew around her when she was alive, not all were so impressed. Fr. Pot was eventually replaced by a new priest, a skeptical newcomer who felt she was a hypocrite. He refused to give her communion and asked the parishioners to pray that she be delivered from her diabolical hallucinations. Only intervention by the local magistrates prevented him from being run out of the parish. An ecclesiastical inquiry declared Lidwina to be of good faith, and she was again permitted communion. Further trials came to her as many members of her family died while she was lingering in her quiet, dimly lit room.

As a mythology was growing around her, townspeople said her putrefying body gave off a fragrant perfume, and the room, always dark, emitted such a glow that some raised the alarm of a fire. In the last years of her life, she was going blind; she was said to take little sustenance except communion, and to sleep little. Both stories are difficult to credit

---

*He is sometimes called Godfreid Zonderdank, or Sonderdank, but *zonderdank* is a nickname that means, "don't mention it," which he repeatedly said to the many poor who thanked him in the streets for curing them without charge, "as did Sts. Cosmas and Damian."

in their extremes. For example, it was said that she had only communion as sustenance for the last 19 years of her life and did not sleep for the last seven years. Enthusiastic, exaggerated reports and myth building by those who revered her saintliness make interpretation of her condition difficult for the historian. For instance, the official document prepared by the municipality of Schiedam in 1421, 12 years before she died, declared that at that time, she had not had anything to drink for seven years.

Her condition worsened further and she died on April 14, 1433 after 37 years of suffering. A year later, a chapel was built over her grave. Through the efforts of the son of Godfreid "Zonderdank," a hospital was built on the site of her home.[5] A cult developed around her memory and she was eventually beatified by the church. An ecclesiastical commission declared her experiences to be valid, and she was said to be a "prodigy of human suffering and heroic patience."[6,7]

Lidwina's bones were found in 1947 and a 1957 analysis at the Laboratory of Anatomy and Embryology of the University of Leiden indicated changes in keeping with paralysis of the legs, and probably of the right arm.[8]

The first document commenting on Lidwina was an official document dated August 4, 1421 in which Jan van Beieren, Count of Holland, acknowledged a letter from the Schiedam local authorities about her disease and stated that he had seen the young woman.[9] Details of her illness came from her biographer, the Franciscan Priest Johannes Brugman (1400–1473), who acquired information from relatives, her priest and confessor, local clerics, and other "reliable persons." Another biographer, Thomas à Kempis, wrote *Vita Lidewigis Virginis* some 15 years after her death, based on the information published by Brugman. An incunabulum of 1497, *T'Leven van Liedwy die Maghet van Scyedam*, was written by a relative of Lidwina, who lived with her for two years. There is also a biography of her in Hubert Muffel's *Les Saints* (1925).

Dr. Robert Maeder considered her case according to current diagnostic criteria for MS and concluded that the diagnosis is definite. He pointed out that she seemed to have abnormalities in the central nervous system, symptoms and signs characteristic of MS (paralysis of legs and her right arm, facial weakness, blindness of different degrees in both eyes, sensory change, and later swallowing difficulty); a variable but progressive disease course over 37 years; he noted no other evident way to explain the disorder. The violent lancinating pain in her face was probably trigeminal neuralgia, a condition that almost always means MS in a young adult. Even the onset after her fall on the ice could be explained. If it was an abscess, Maeder argues the infection may have precipitated the attack of MS that paralyzed her legs. Another possibility is that this was a fall due to leg weakness, and the painful chest and subsequent paralysis were due to a transverse myelitis with band-like pain in the chest, interpreted as an internal abscess because of the local pain.

Although it is often said that the plight of Lidwina is the first known case of MS, I am convinced that the evidence suggests elements of marked religiosity, mysticism, histrionic behavior, and even self-mutilation. Although there may have been an underlying neurological disease, the diagnosis must be left open.

Saint Lidwina (variously spelled Lydwyna, Ludwyna, Liedwy, Lidewigis, and Ludwine) was canonized by Pope Leo XIII in 1890. She is listed in *Lives of the Saints*, with "saint day," April 14. *Online Saints* lists her as the patron saint of sickness, and because of her fall while skating, she is also the patron saint of figure skating. The United States Figure Skating Association has a medal featuring a picture of Lidwina.

Halla, the Drummer Bock, and Will Coffin

A less credible case, because of the paucity of information, is the case of Halla in the Icelandic saga of Thorlakr.[10] This information was found by Dr. Margaret Cormack. A woman named Halla developed an acute illness with loss of the sight of both eyes, and on the next day, she lost her speech. She made a vow to God and to the Bishop Thorlakr for intercession; if cured, she would walk to Skalholt, fasting and saying prayers. On the third day, a candle wick was put around her head and she began to experience a return of sight; she had recovery of speech on the feast of St. Michael. The miracle is said to have occurred somewhere between 1293 and 1323, but no other information is available. This is scanty evidence for MS in an era when powerful emotions were associated with religious belief, but I mention it because it appears in the literature of MS.[11]

Another case with incomplete information is that of "the drummer Bock," described in a paper by C.J.T. de Meza in 1810 and discussed by Stenager, who suggested he might have had MS.[12] When describing the beneficial effects of electricity on seven conditions, de Meza outlined the course of illness in a young drummer named Bock. Beginning in 1789, he had "arthritic seizures," and paralysis of the right arm and leg. His subsequent recovery over six weeks is ascribed to electrical therapy. Stenager also refers briefly to a Danish report of a case of a "peculiar, ordinary paralysis" in a person who had accompanying mental changes.

Another possible case of MS comes from the detailed casebooks of Dr. John MacKieson of Prince Edward Island, Canada. (Personal communication, Dr. David Saunders.) In 1837, he documented Will Coffin, a 37-year-old who had persistent dimness of vision associated with some head pain and falling. Coffin had experienced similar visual symptoms three years before, as well as double vision and unsteady gait. When MacKieson saw him, his vision was improving, but he had tinnitus. He had more visual difficulty when he looked to the side, suggesting an ocular paresis or an intranuclear ophthalmoplegia. He was treated with

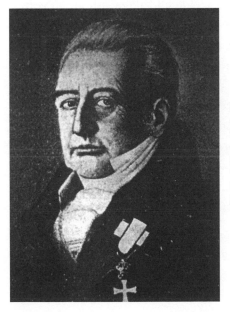

Figure 3.2 C.J.T. de Meza described the case of "the drummer Bock," a young man who had a transient paralysis of the arm and leg who recovered after a course of electricity. (From: Stenager, Egon. A Note on the Treatment of Drummer Brock: An Early Danish Account of Multiple Sclerosis? *J Hist Neurosci*, 1996; 5(2)198.)

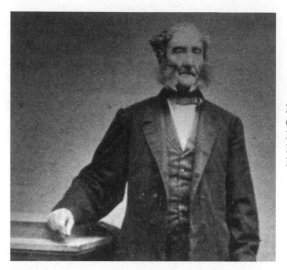

Figure 3.3 Dr. John MacKieson. (Courtesy of Prince Edward Island Public Archives and Records Office, No. 2398-8d and Dr. David Shepard.)

venesection, blisters, purgatives, cold cloths to the head, and warmth to the feet. Two and a half months later, he had recovered from this second episode of neurological symptoms.

Margaret of Myddle

The delightful *Antiquityes and Memoyres of the Parish of Myddle* was written by Richard Gough (1634–1723) between 1700 and 1706, although the date on his hand-drawn cover is 1700, the year he began his project.[13] This is one of the most interesting typographical and geneological books ever written, but it remained unpublished for over a century, and the first printing was from an imperfect copy; an accurate copy did not appear until 1875.

The author, Richard Gough, an elderly man of the parish of Myddle, described the parish and the objects of interest in his village. In a unique approach to local history, he then proceeded to discuss the occupants of each pew in the church. In pew 7, sat the family Davis, of the tenement of Vicar Gittens. Thomas Davis, a weaver, had a wife, Margaret, who had a lameness that progressed over 20 years. Gough says:

> *"When hee removed to Myddle, Thomas Davis, a weaver who now lives att the Wood Lesows by Myddle Wood, came to bee tenant to it. Of him I have spoken before, but somewhat I must say of his wife; Margaret the wife of Thomas Davis dyed on the 17th of this instant,*

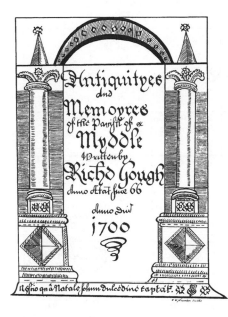

Figure 3.4   Front cover of *Antiquityes and Memoyres of the Parish of Myddle* by Richard Gough. *County of Salop, 1700*. Shrewsbury. Adnitt and Naunton, 1875. He drew the cover when he started to work in 1700, accounting for the date, but it was completed in 1706.

January, 1701. Shee tooke cold in childe-bearing, above twenty yeares before her death; shee was seized therby with paine and lameness in her limbs, and made use of severall remedyes for curing therof, butt all proved ineffectual. At last, as shee was in an Apothecary's shop buying ointments and ingredients for fomentations my uncle, Mr. Richard Baddley, an able chirurgeon, saw her and asked her how shee gott her lamenesse: shee sayd by taking could in child-birth. Then says hee spare this charges and labour, for all the Doctors and Surgeons in England cannot cure it. Thou mayest live long, butt thy strength will still decay. After this shee went to lytle more charges, only when King James II, came his progresse to Shrewsbury, shee was admitted by the King's Doctors to goe to His Majesty for the Touch, which did her noe good. Shee was forced to use crootches almost 20 yeares agoe, and I thinke it is now 10 yeares since shee grew so weake that shee was faine to bee carryed in persons' armes. About two years-and-an-halfe before her death, shee kept her bedde continually; shee was bowed soe togeather, that her knees lay cloase to her brest; ther was nothing but the skin and bones upon her thighs and legges. About a yeare-and-a-halfe past, her thigh bones broake as shee lay in bedde, and one of them burst through

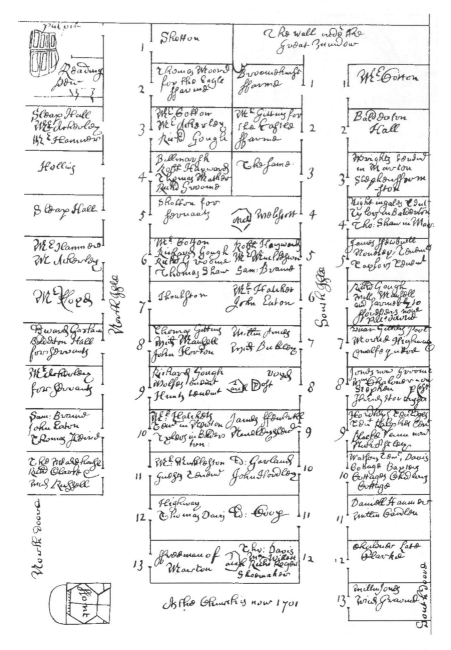

Figure 3.5 The drawing of the pews in the church in Myddle. Thomas Davis and his family sat in pew 7, on the South (right) wall, in the pew for the tenants of Vicar Gittens' tenement. From *Antiquityes and Memoyres of the Parish of Myddle* by Richard Gough. *County of Salop, 1700.* Shrewsbury. Adnitt and Naunton, 1875.

the skin and stood out about an inch, like a dry hollow sticke, but there
was noe flesh to bleed or corrupt; shee could stir noe part of her body
save her head and one of her hands a lytle. When shee was dead they
did not endeavor to draw her body straite, butt made a wide coffin and
putt her in as shee was. I heard one say that was present att laying her
in her coffin, that as they layd her downe one of her legge bones broke
and gave a cracke, like a rotten sticke; and it is not to bee forgotten that
the Vicar Gittens, seeing that Thomas Davis had a great charge of chil-
dren, and his wife lame upon his hands, did give him his house and gar-
den rent free while hee lived in itt:"

"Habet in adversis auxilia in secundis commodat
Non est donum quod pauperi datur sed foenus"

Gough does not relate whether two pigeons came to roost on the house two weeks before death and then left, as locals sometimes noted; which he "had knowe them doe three severall times."

Margaret Davis developed a progressive lameness recognized by her doctor as one that would last a long time and be incurable; this progressed to paralysis of her legs and then her arms, with later contractures and pressure sores, and death after two decades, suggesting the diagnosis of "possible" MS.

William Brown, Hudson's Bay Trader

A plausible case for the diagnosis of MS can be made in the case of William Brown, a 19th-century Hudson's Bay trader. Born in Ayrshire, Scotland in 1790, he was sent by the Hudson's Bay Company to be company trader at York Factory, on the shores of Hudson's Bay. In 1811, at age 21, he began to experience weakness in his legs and some visual problems. He found it increasingly difficult to carry out his duties. When he felt he was too weak to withstand the rigors of a long survey assignment, he sent a replacement in his stead. For this he was censured by Governor Simpson, who felt Brown was neglecting his responsibilities. He had an intermittent and progressive disorder with visual symptoms, weakness, and gait difficulty. His symptoms progressed and he was eventually relieved of his post and returned to Scotland to be cared for by his family. He died a few years later. In a differential diagnosis for the condition in this young man, MS would lead the list.

Augustus d'Esté

There is no doubt of the cause of the relapsing and remitting neurological symptoms and progressive disease of Augustus d'Esté (1794–1848), the grandson of George III and cousin of Queen Victoria.[14,15] His disorder was documented in his diary between 1822 and 1848 and in an almanac of 1847–1848.

King George III was very unhappy when he learned of the clandestine marriage of his son, Prince Augustus Frederick, Duke of Sussex, to Lady Augusta Murray, which took place in the Hotel Sarmiento in Rome, later repeated in a London ceremony. When word of the marriage came to the king, he had the marriage annulled, a power he possessed since the marriage of a royal heir to the crown required the monarch's consent, and he had not given it. He then ordered the son to leave for the Continent. By this time, however, there was a child of the marriage, young Augustus, who was made illegitimate by the annul-

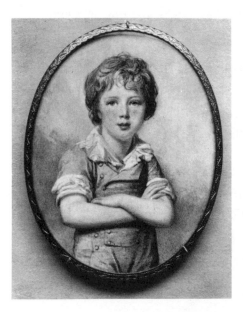

Figure 3.6 Augustus d'Esté (1794-1848). This portrait by the famous miniature painter Richard Cosway, is signed and dated 1799, when d'Esté would have been five years old. Although it is not certain that this is d'Esté, it has long been said to be him, and the age of the child seems correct. (Courtesy of the Royal College of Physicians, London.)

ment. The young boy was raised in England by his mother, abandoned by his royal father.

While attending Harrow, Augustus contracted measles at age 14, late for childhood measles, an observation that would be of interest a century and a half later. He was vaccinated against smallpox by the method of Lady Mary Wortley Montague a few years before Jenner published his method. He later served with the VIIth Royal Fusiliers. His military career was marked by disinterest, immaturity, and arrogance, says his biographer, but he managed to attain the rank of lieutenant-colonel.*[16] He served in America and was present at the defeat of the British near New Orleans in 1815.

He was later given a knighthood, but that did not appease him in his unsuccessful appeals to four monarchs, a prime minister, and the House of Lords[17] to establish his links with the royal family as the legitimate son

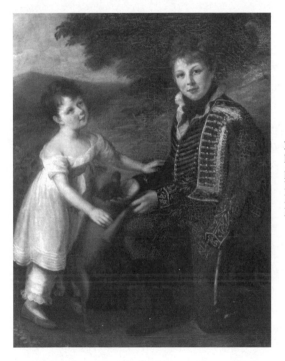

Figure 3.7 Augustus d'Esté with his sister, Emma. The original painting hangs in the Edinburgh Portrait Gallery. (Courtesy of the Royal College of Physicians, London.)

---

*Firth characterized him as extravagant, argumentative, difficult, careless, and selfish, borrowing from the servants and developing "a relationship" with Mary, the housemaid. As we shall see, he was more mature and sensitive as the years went on and he had to deal with his increasing limitations.

of the Duke of Sussex. Even more frustrating, however, was the progressive and puzzling illness that began when he was 28 years old.

Augustus kept a diary beginning in 1822; on the first page of this diary, he described blurring of vision after leaving the funeral of a beloved relative. He felt the blurring was due to his attempts to suppress tears, but his vision deteriorated to the point that others had to read for him. Fortunately, his vision gradually cleared without treatment. Visual blurring recurred twice over the next few years, and he consulted Dr. Henry Alexander, surgeon oculist to the Queen. After his second episode, a year after the initial blurring, he was sent to a spa at Driburg, where he

Augustus d'Esté's Debility

"At Florence I began to suffer from a confusion of sight: - about the 6th of November the malady increased to the extent of my seeing all objects double. Each eye had its separate visions. - Dr. Kissock supposed bile to be the cause: I was twice blooded from the temple by leeches: - purges were administered; One Vomit and twice I lost blood from the arm: one of the times it was with difficulty that the blood was obtained. - The Malady in my eyes abated, again I saw all objects naturally in their single state. I was able to go out and walk. - Now a new disease began to show itself: every day I found gradually (by slow degrees) my strength leaving me: I could clearly perceive each succeeding day that I went up and down the staircase with great difficulty. When I slapped myself sharply on the loins (though only momentarily the effect) yet for the time it increased my strength. - A torpor or numbness and want of sensation became apparent about the end of the Back-bone and the Perinaeum. At length about the 4th of December my strength of legs quite left me, and twice in one day I fell down upon the floor in attempting to go the closed stool without assistance; I was obliged to remain on the floor until my Servant came in and picked me up. I remained in this extreme state of weakness for about 21 days, during which period I fell down about 5 times (never fainting) from my legs not being strong enough to carry my body. I never once fainted or had any sort of fit: - debility, extreme debility was the only cause of my falling."

Augustus d'Esté, October 17, 1827[18]

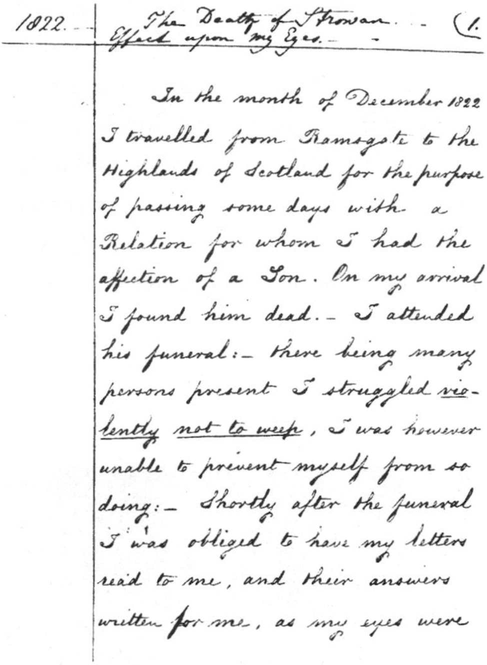
1822. – The Death of Strowan. . . (1.
Effect upon my Eyes. – –

In the month of December 1822
I travelled from Ramsgate to the
Highlands of Scotland for the purpose
of passing some days with a
Relation for whom I had the
affection of a Son. On my arrival
I found him dead. – I attended
his funeral: – there being many
persons present I struggled vio-
lently not to weep, I was however
unable to prevent myself from so
doing: – Shortly after the funeral
I was obliged to have my letters
read to me, and their answers
written for me, as my eyes were

Figure 3.8 Page 1 of d'Esté diary begins in 1822, in which he describes the first episode of visual loss, so that his letters had to be read to him. He believed the visual loss was due to his efforts to suppress tears at the funeral of a relative. (Courtesy of the Royal College of Physicians, London.)

said he "drank steel-water, bathed in it, and douched my Eyes with it:–my Eyes again recovered."

In 1827, he complained that the heat of the country was intolerable and he developed visual loss and double vision. In the next few years, he developed numbness in his legs and difficulty walking. He consulted a Dr. Kent, who did not agree with the previous therapies and recommended that he "eat beef steaks twice a day, drink London Porter and Sherry and Madeira wines." His legs were to be rubbed twice a day with brushes and his back with a liniment made of camphorated alcohol, opium, and Florence oil. He was pleased to write in his diary: "This new system succeeded completely. Every day I found strength returning." This is the hopeful observation of many patients taking a variety of treatments for MS in a disease that waxes and wanes. He continued to have his legs rubbed with flesh brushes, but discontinued the back rubs, substituting slaps on the back by the open hand of a servant. He later took up horseback riding, a common therapy in the 17th and 18th century.

A Milan physician treated him for pain in the area of his kidneys with a counterirritant plaster that aimed at producing an eruption of the skin over the area. This was of no help, so he switched to flannel bandages as hot as he could tolerate. He took baths and a wash of sulphate of zinc and aqua plantaginis. He was treated with herbs and flowers and daily shower baths. He took 20–30 drops of valerian twice a day mixed in the herbs.

On the recommendation of his father, he saw a number of prominent physicians including Sir Astley Cooper,*[19] Dr. W.C. Mattin, physician to the Westminster Hospital, Dr. Kent, and Mr. Pettigrew. He followed

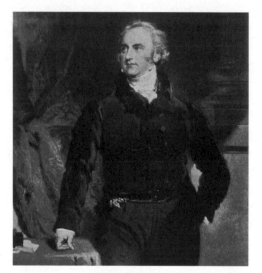

Figure 3.9 Sir Astley Cooper was one of the physicians called in consultation for the paraplegia of Augustus d'Esté. He was a much loved teacher and admired surgeon and consultant. As was the habit in the early 19th century, he was called upon as often for medical consultations as surgical, and tended the King for his gout. Another of d'Esté's physicians, Sir Benjamin Brodie, said Cooper had an income greater than any other physician or surgeon of that day. This portrait is a reproduction of the engraving by cousins after the painting by Sir Thomas Lawrence. The original is in the Council Room at the Royal College of Surgeons. It was subscribed for by his pupils in 1812 when Sir Astley was 46, but was not finished until some years later. (Reproduced with kind permission of the President and Council of the Royal College of Surgeons of England.)

---

*Sir Astley Cooper was a prominent London surgeon and teacher who had few original ideas but was said to be a better teacher and operator than any other, graceful and careful in everything he did. He himself said he had a flair for diagnosis but was not a good operator where delicacy was needed.

their prescriptions and also took up sea bathing. At the seaside, he developed a liaison with a young woman, but noticed that his "acts of Connection" lacked a "wholesome vigor." He consulted a Dr. Courtenay who passed bougies and a metal catheter into his penis and gave him some medicines and pills that proved beneficial. He later underwent a course of electricity, as well as tepid douches to the loins and sacrum. Following this, he was treated with a course of galvanism with disappointing results. He derived more benefit from a trip to Scotland where he was "much braced and invigorated by the Highland air." He found the horseback riding and walks to be helpful, and he continued the waters, warm baths, douches, and the visits to various spas.

By 1840, 18 years after the onset of his disease, he made a note in his diary that he was no longer using any measures for the improvement of his health or for the restoration of his vigor and strength, presumably because of disappointment with previous treatments. At this point, he read a book on hydropathy and decided to visit the celebrated Vincent Priessnitz,[20] who thought his infirmity originated in the nerves. D'Esté was treated five times over two days with the application of wet sheets and friction and walked about wearing a wet cincture around his waist.

He next consulted Sir Benjamin Brodie, and John Scott, a surgeon who prescribed tincture of lyttae or Spanish fly, which seemed to have little effect. Prescriptions over the next few years included zinc sulphate, Spanish fly, strychnine, quinine, silver nitrate, and stramonium. Later he developed vertigo, but other than a little brandy with water, he took no medicines. Scott consulted with his colleague John Farre; they agreed the diagnosis was "paraplegia," a condition that can be active or passive, functional or organic, and can be "very imperceptible." They agreed that d'Esté's paraplegia was of the passive phase, which could remain for a long time in the functional form, and the transition to an organic form had not yet been confirmed. Healing would require improvement in the

---

*Vincent Priessnitz (1799–1851) was said to be the founder of hydrotherapy, although water therapy was an ancient approach to healing. It was said that he "owed his wonderful experience to his ignorance of medical science." Six years younger than d'Esté, he had a hydrotherapy building in Gräfenberg at the time d'Esté consulted him.

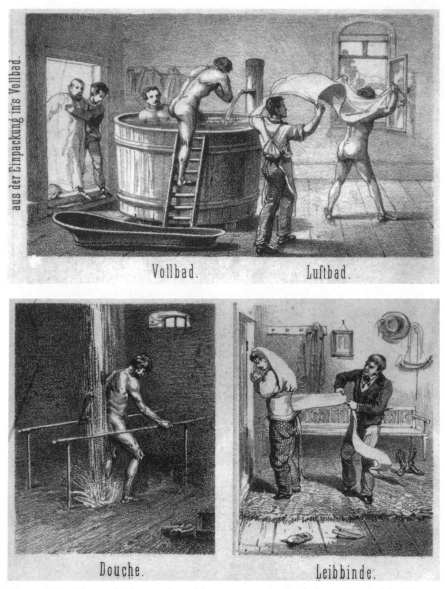

Figure 3.10 The establishment for cold water cures in Gräfenberg, founded by Vincent Priessnitz in 1822. The regime he applied to his patients, including Augustus d'Esté, made no concessions to the gentle or weak. Prints by E. Gaskell. (Courtesy of the Wellcome Library, London.)

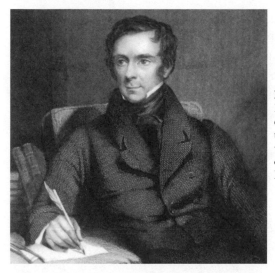

Figure 3.11 Sir Benjamin Collins Brodie also saw Augustus d'Esté in consultation and recommended tincture of Lyttae and Spanish fly, which, unfortunately, had little effect. (Courtesy of the Wellcome Library, London.)

circulation, but because the illness is in the patient, it can frustrate the best medical therapy. They suggested he control his diet, keep his emotions calm, and keep his heart quiet. The therapy would be iron, mercury, and a period of rest in Brighton.

John Scott recommended that d'Esté ride a horse every day as long as he could, and walk as long as possible. Mercury was added to the regimen, and there was another course of electricity, which d'Esté felt was making him worse. He was seen in consultation by Sir Richard Bright in February 1844 and agreed with increasing the amount of iron in his medicine. By this time, he was walking poorly, some days buoyed by how well he was doing, other days anxious and alarmed at how weak he could be. His handwriting became shakier and many of the earlier diary sections are by an amanuensis.

He begin to write in a volume of *Simpson's Gentleman's Almanac and Pocket Journal* for 1847, recording on the left his daily visits, making comments on the weather, and evaluating church sermons he heard. On the right were compulsive recordings of his walks around his rooms, timed to the fraction of a minute by a chronometer that he took pains to keep in repair.

Sept 27 - "I rejoice to write that I have walked in my rooms 50 min."

Sept 29 - "Alas! I only walk in my room for 28 3/4 min."

The diaries reveal that d'Esté was a sensitive man, dealing courageously with his failing strength, and delighting in the visits of friends and family. He worried about the health of a friend with dropsy who was kind enough to come to the door to see him, recognizing that he was unable to negotiate the stairs. He was so concerned with the results of the Irish famine that he sent the proceeds of the sale of his phaeton, which he had been advised to sell. He then got around in a bath chair, but found his leg spasms and fatigue were so marked that he was only comfortable in bed. On the last page of his diary, for Monday, December 17, we sense his positive nature, and his euphoric mood:

"Having received a Present of Indian Moccassins I put them on: - and I walk in them without my Left-Foot, which some time ago always turned outwards at the Ankle joint unless supported by a Steele-Upright, showing any disposition so to do - surely this is a decided Improvement! Thanks to The Almighty!"

Augustus d'Esté died in 1848 and was buried in the d'Esté mausoleum in Ramsgate, whose design he had spent a great deal of time supervising. On the mausoleum is a tablet outlining the details of his parent's marriage, and the sad consequences of the Royal Marriage Act that would not allow his legitimacy.*[21]

There is adequate detail in the diary to make a conclusive diagnosis of MS. This was a young man who developed a recurrent and remitting neurological disease characterized by repeated visual loss, diplopia, sensory change, intermittent and progressive paralysis in his legs, bladder difficulty, and impotence. There was a remitting progressive course to death in 26 years—a characteristic picture of MS.

The diary of Augustus d'Esté was found during a 1940 wartime drive for paper at the Letherhead School for the Blind, that had been taken over as a sector hospital.[22,23] Douglas Firth published an outline of the life

---

*The likely reason the marriage was not legitimized was that another royal heir, the Prince Regent, also had a clandestine marriage to a Mrs. Fitzherbert, with two children resulting, but he later married Princess Caroline. If d'Estés parents' marriage was declared legitimate, then so would the clandestine marriage of the heir to the throne, which would give George IV a Catholic wife and a charge of bigamy. And the children of the first marriage would then have more claim to the throne than Queen Victoria.

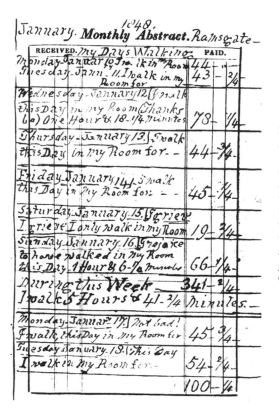

Figure 3.12 A page from the account book that Augustus d'Esté recorded his activities such as the duration he could walk around his apartment, which varied from 19 ¾ minutes to 78 ¼ minutes. His total for the week was 341 ½ minutes. He had a clock to record his walking in fractions of a minute and took pains to have this clock in good repair. (Courtesy of the Royal College of Physicians, London.)

of d'Esté in 1941 and in a monograph in 1948, using available account books, letters, and manuscripts. The diary is now in the collection of the Royal College of Physicians in London, which also has a file on d'Esté compiled by R.R. Hughes of Liverpool.*[24]

The diaries of Augustus d'Esté illustrate a remarkable saga of medicine and therapy as practiced in the early 19th century, and the moving story of a young man trying to understand and cope with a relentless disease.

---

*Although Dr. Firth clearly was rescuing the documents from being pulped in the wartime paper drive, when the masters of Letherhead School for the Blind, where the document was found, were made aware of the diary in the Royal College of Physicians of London, they demanded its return, suggesting it was stolen and inferred that legal action would be taken. A diplomatic lunch, offered to the principal of the school by the Harveian Librarian, and a walk around the new facilities of the College, led to the agreement that the diaries were in better hands there. Many of the papers referred to by Firth are now untraceable and were probably borrowed from members of the Murray family. Why the diary was at the Letherhead School for the Blind is unclear.

Heinrich Heine, the Poet in his Mattress Grave

The works of the German lyrical poet Heinrich Heine (1797–1856) inspired music by Schubert, Schumann, Mendelssohn, Liszt, Berlioz, and Gounod. His poems inspired two of Wagner's operas, the *Flying Dutchman* and *Tannhäuser*, the Oscar Wilde libretto for Richard Strauss' *Salome* and Adams' ballet *Giselle*. His poetry is admired in every language, perhaps even more in France than in his native Germany. Even in England, a country he did not much like, he ranks second only to Goethe in the list of great German poets.[25] His reputation was a subject for heated debate in Germany in recent times and "whipsawed" during the discussion of the German–Jewish question. Interest in Heine is increasing, and although he died nearly a century and a half ago, his grave in Paris is covered with birthday floral tributes each year.

Heine was born in Düsseldorf on December 13, 1797, the oldest of four children of Jewish parents who were initially not able to receive permission to marry. Like his mother, he had frequent migraine headaches. Despite the assistance of a rich uncle, his entree into business as Harry

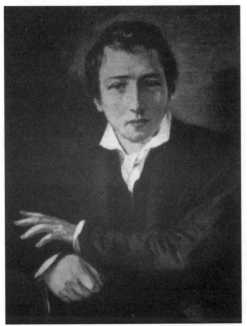

Figure 3.13 Heinrich Heine (1797–1856) as a young man by Horitz Oppenheim, 1831, Deutsher Litteratur in Bilderen. (Courtesy of Heinrich-Heine Institut, Düsseldorf, Landesbildstelle Rheinland.)

Heine and Co. went bankrupt after a year. He then changed careers and studied law. To avoid religious persecution of Jews in Germany at the time, and since he was not a practicing Jew, he accepted baptism in 1925 and took the name Heinrich. He was politically active with a manner that was abrasive and outspoken.[26]

During his 20s, he suffered from severe migraines and recurrent depressions and went to spas for relief. The neurological illness of interest began much later, with a transient "palsy" of two fingers on his left hand in 1832, when he was 35. Dr. Ferdinand Koreff (1783-1851) was consulted. Two years later, Heine had a bout of depression and visual complaints, but recovered.[27] In 1837, his left arm was weaker and he had sudden bilateral loss of vision, beginning in his right eye, which became blind in a few hours, and then in the left, until he could see very little. His condition improved over the next two weeks, but worsened again in three months, before improving again. Six months later, he had an episode of double vision, followed by some worsening of his vision. He then described having giddy turns, which caused objects in his vision to vacillate, and gave them a greyish, partly silver color. The prominent ophthalmologist Dr. J.

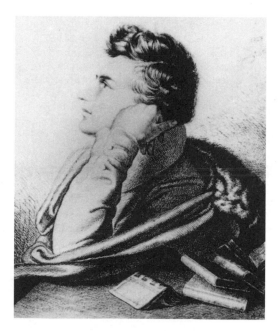

Figure 3.14 Heinrich Heine (1797–1856) as a young poet. He began to have episodic and later progressive neurological symptoms when he was 35 years old, dying 24 years later. Etching by Ludwig Emil Grimm, 1827. (Courtesy of Heinrich-Heine Institut, Düsseldorf, Landesbildstelle Rheinland.)

Sichel applied leeches, which improved his vision. E.H. Jellinek speculated that a fundus picture in Sichel's successful *Traité d'Ophthalmie* showing the optic atrophy in a 45-year-old patient may have been of Heine.[28]

In 1841, his vision worsened and then improved, but he became depressed and developed more neurologic symptoms, including right facial weakness, diplopia, pain in the eye, and numbness down the left side of his body. He complained, "Moreover the left eye is feeble and hurts, does not often agree with the right, and this causes a confusion of sight which is much more intolerable than the darkness of full blindness."[29] It was said that, despite his youthful promiscuity, he became impotent soon after marriage that year to Mathilde, an illegitimate 19-year-old girl.*[30,31]

Much of the information about Heine's illness comes from correspondence with his brother Max, a physician. During the course of his illness, Heine was treated by numerous physicians with a number of therapies including spas, purges, sulphur baths, bloodletting, morphine, leeches, iodine mixtures, laxatives, diets, enemas, and cutaneous oint-

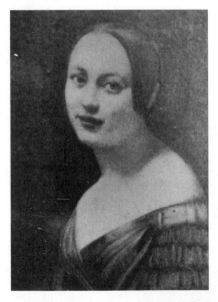

Figure 3.15 Heinrich Heine's wife "beloved Mathilde." Her real name was Crescence Eugénie Mirat Heine. She regularly dismissed physicians to her husband if she didn't agree with their recommendations, and when one criticized her care, she gave him a black eye and then dismissed him. Photograph ca. 1845. (Courtesy of Heinrich-Heine Institut, Düsseldorf, Landesbildstelle Rheinland.)

---

*Mathilde was Heine's name for her, but her name was actually Crescence Eugénie Mirat. Although Critchley gives her name as Grisette Matilde Mirat (Critchley), this is undoubtedly a misnotation from a comment in Aikens biography of Heine (1924) that refers to her as this typical Parisian grisette.

ments applied over an incision that was kept open on the nape of his neck.*[32] Although he complied with their advice, he did not place much faith in the efficacy of his treatments. His wife had even less, and she gave the prominent physician Dr. Leopold Wertheim a black eye and dismissed him for his criticism of her care. In fact, she chased all the physicians away except the Hungarian Dr. David Gruby.†

In 1843, Heine developed ptosis of the left lid, hyperesthesia of the left side of his face, and left facial weakness. In 1844, he had three episodes of deteriorated vision, and was blind for a period of four weeks. In another episode the next year, he became paraparetic and had to stay in bed. He tried spa therapy, but his condition worsened and he then became incontinent. He described the spa bath tubs as a kind of coffin, and his time in the baths as a period of preparation for death.

In 1845, he experienced bilateral ptosis, worsening gait, and further visual deterioration; the next year, he developed numbness around his mouth, loss of taste, and difficulty with swallowing and speech. His gait continued to worsen and he referred to his "paralysis, which like an iron band pressed into the chest," a description of the band-like sensory level of a spinal cord lesion. In 1847, he had right facial paralysis, cramps, and incontinence. On September 20, he wrote to Princess Beliojoso that his feet, legs, and lower torso were paralyzed and that he was unable to walk. He made a moderate recovery, but in 1848, he described his ultimate physical collapse on his last walk, looking at the Venus de Milo in the Louvre. He felt she was looking down on him with wistful sympathy, saying, "Can't you see I have no arms and can't help?"

He felt he was like a fading, drooping flower, not yet completely withered. He was having symptoms of paralysis of his right arm, sensory loss, neuralgical pains, dysarthria, right-sided ptosis, facial weakness,

---

*In the 18th and 19th centuries, it was a common practice to drain off noxious humors by a continuous drainage. A draining incision could be open by inserting into the wound a seton, a small stone, pig hairs, or an inverted skin flap. Such incisions might be kept draining for years, as was the case with Samuel Johnson, the English lexicographer, whose childhood neck incisions for scrofula are visible on his death mask.

†Gruby arrived in Paris from Vienna, where he received his MD and studied anatomical pathology under Rokitansky. He was a prominent microscopist in Paris, but gave up research for private practice.

A Free Mind in a Rotten Body

"...a sick man is always counting on better days. My mind is free, and clear, and even cheerful. My heart is sound, almost sound enough to be eager for and greedy for life, and my body is so paralyzed, so rotten. It is as though I were buried alive. I see no one and talk to no one." (April 25, 1848)

"I have been here in the country for the last twelve days, wretched and beyond all measure unhappy. My illness has increased to a terrible extent. I have been completely paralyzed for the last eight days, so that I can only lie on the sofa or on my bed. My legs are like cotton and I am carried about like a child. I have the most terrible cramps. My right hand is beginning to wither and God knows whether I shall ever be able to write to you again. Dictation is painful because of my paralyzed jaw. My blindness is still the last of my ills."

Heinrich Heine
Letters to Julius Campe, June 7, 1848

altered taste, and trouble swallowing. In addition, he lost weight, was constipated, and had respiratory complications. Visitors noted his thin muscles, deformed feet, and contractures. Rumors that he had died appeared in the American press. From then on he lived in a hospital, in what he called his "mattress grave" (*Matratzengruft*). He said that he read every medical treatise he could find that related to his condition so that when he reached Heaven, he could lecture upon the futility of physicians who tried to deal with spinal disease. Dr. Gruby again took over his treatment in 1849 and was able to bring him some relief of symptoms. Heine was treated periodically by a "Black woman" who cauterized his spine to relieve his distress and pain. Remarkably, he was still writing. He described his state as:

> *"This living death, this unlife ... my lips are paralyzed like my feet, the tools of eating are also paralyzed as well as the channels of excretion. I can neither chew nor shit, and have to be fed like a bird..."*

He had pain and shock-like sensations and was developing pressure sores. He wrote to his mother in July 1851 saying that during hot weath-

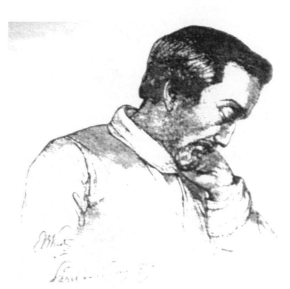

Figure 3.16 Heinrich Heine looking down. Drawing by Ernst Benedict-Kietz, 1851. (Courtesy of Heinrich-Heine Institut, Düsseldorf, Landesbildstelle Rheinland.)

er, his eyes were worse. He had often commented that he was better in cold weather.

Visitors, including Alexandre Dumas, *père*, Béranger, Gautier, Gérard de Nerval, Taillendier, and Berlioz, were distressed by the disintegration of the body of this great poet. Noting later that the German politicians were distancing themselves from the politically outspoken Heine, Dumas said that France would be happy to adopt him.

One frequent visitor was Elise Krinitz, who went by the pen name Camille Seldon. Heine called her his "lotus-flower," and sometimes *La Mouche*, because of the fly on her signet ring. She had a history of a period of paralysis and treatment in a London mental institution, and had answered an advertisement for someone to read to him, a task beyond the abilities of Mathilde. Heine was entranced by her elegance, her fluency in German, her voice, and her intelligence. We know little more about the woman who brought him intellectual stimulation and comfort when he was, in his words, feeling like a withering flower in his mattress grave. She inspired some of his best poems; the last was "für die Mouche."

By this time, he was using morphine and opium often and in large doses for his pain and spasms, but tried to keep his head clear.* Although

---

*One of his poems is called "Morphine."

A Poet's Sense of Loss

"Alas, fame, once sweet as sugared pineapple, and flattery, has for a long time been nauseous to me; it tastes as bitter to me now as wormwood. ... The bowl stands filled before me, but I lack a spoon. What does it avail me that at banquets my health is pledged in choicest wines, and drunk from golden goblets, when I, myself, severed from all that makes life pleasant, may only wet my lips with an insipid potion? What does it avail me that enthusiastic youths and maidens crown my marble bust with laurel wreaths, if meanwhile the shrivelled fingers of an aged nurse press a blister of Spanish flies behind the ears of my actual body? Of what avail is it that all the roses of Shiraz so tenderly glow and bloom for me ... when in the dreary solitude of my sickroom, I have nothing to smell, unless it is the perfume of warm napkins."

Heinrich Heine, 1855
On hearing his poems had been translated into Japanese

the quality of his writing and poems never faltered, he was often under a "desolate narcosis" and in a "doped wilderness." At one point he said, "I have at this moment so much opiate in my body that I hardly know what I am dictating." He often felt despondent, writing, "Sleep is good, death is better—of course, best of all would be never to have been born." In *Aus der Matratzengruft* (from the mattress grave) he wrote: "For seven years now I have been rolling about on the floor with bitter excruciating infirmities, and cannot die!"

Always conscious of his public, he wished them to appreciate his plight but not pity him, and he refused the offer of a public subscription to raise money for his expenses. He could have used the money, but did not want this to be the way he was remembered. A friend asked if he had made his peace with God. He answered: "Don't bother yourself. God will forgive me—that's what He's there for."[33]

He wrote that he had two rooms: "the one I die in, and the grave." He died in 1856 at age 59 of respiratory complications, 24 years after the onset of his illness. His poetry lives on, and his popularity and importance are increasing. There were four new biographies of Heine in 1997, exploring mostly his political influence. Although his lasting fame is as a

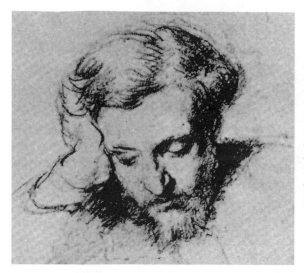

Figure 3.17   Heinrich Heine (1797–1856) during the years of his neurological illness. He was noted to have ptosis and the hand holding his head may also be holding his right eyelid elevated. Pencil portrait of Heine by Marcellin-Gilbert Desboutin, ca. 1853. (Courtesy of Heinrich-Heine Institut, Düsseldorf, Landesbildstelle Rheinland.)

poet, he said he cared little about this, and wished to be buried with a sword and remembered as one who fought for liberty.

Germany has had a hesitant appreciation of Heine, even in his own time, but he was quickly embraced by France and even by England, a country he detested.* Heine indicated in his will that when he died, his body was not to be transported back to Germany, as he did not want to be buried there; his grave is in Montmartre in Paris. Despite his feelings for Germany, the land of his birth, his memory lives on in a university, an institute, and a medical center in Düsseldorf, all named after him.

Stenager[34] suggests that it was unfortunate that Heine did not live long enough to consult Charcot, who gave his great lectures on MS 12 years after Heine's death, but as we will see, Charcot had a negative view of therapy for this disease, so it is unlikely that he would have had much to offer.

Heine's disabling illness baffled historical diagnosticians for 150 years and the arguments have not ended. Putnam[35] and others felt Heine had MS, but still others have suggested he might have had neurosyphilis, amy-

---

*Heine had visited England but even though he was not lacking in ego, he disliked the English for their egotism and their mechanical church-going piety. He said that God would surely prefer a blaspheming Frenchman to a praying Englishman. Despite this, many of the prominent and admiring biographers of Heine are English.

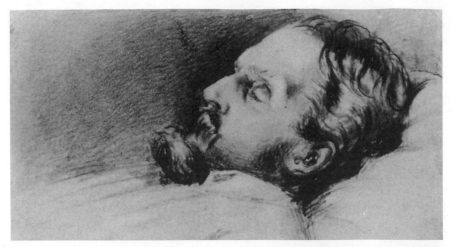

Figure 3.18 Heinrich Heine (1797–1856) on his deathbed. He spent the last years of his life on his "mattress grave." Watercolor and pencil drawing of Heine on his deathbed by Seligmann. (Courtesy of Heinrich-Heine Institut, Düsseldorf, Landesbildstelle Rheinland.)

otrophic lateral sclerosis, sarcoidosis, encephalomyelitis, porphyria, spinal muscular atrophy, chronic polyneuropathy, and spinal tuberculosis.[36] Heine himself thought he had syphilis contracted in his promiscuous youth, and Critchley felt this opinion was about as definite as it could be without serological confirmation.[37] The psychiatrist Nathan Roth reviewed the differential diagnosis, and provided details and psychoanalytical musings about Heine's complex love life, but concluded he had porphyria.[38] Stenager discussed the many differential diagnoses, but leaned toward neurosyphilis, as did many authors in the 19th and early 20th centuries.[39] Certainly Heine's expulsion from school for breaking the rule of chastity, and his frequent use of prostitutes in Paris and London seemed contributing factors to the suspicion of syphilis. Despite all these arguments, the pattern of his recurrent symptoms over 24 years suggested to Schachter,[40] Putnam,[41] Kolle,[42] Stern,[43] Fredrikson,[44] and Jellinek[45] that MS should be strongly considered.

Did Heine have MS? The recurrent nature of the visual loss and the paraplegia, his impotence and incontinence, the recurrent brain stem symptoms, Lhermitte's sign, Uhthoff's phenomenon, heat sensitivity, and the relentless progression due to a constellation of symptoms common to MS occurring over 24 years makes this a plausable diagnosis. One would only hesitate because ptosis is rare in MS, but not undescribed as it is noted in cases described by Charcot, Althaus, Jellinex, Sparks, Zenker, Grauck, Edwards, Osler, and Hammond. Heine's clarity of mind to the end is unusual, but again, not out of the question in someone with symptoms primarily related to the spinal cord, brain stem, and optic nerve. His life and letters have been sifted repeatedly in support of one diagnosis or another, and it is unlikely that other helpful medical details will come to light. Given the evidence, I would conclude that the diagnosis is "probable MS."

Lighthouse Stevenson

One of a remarkable group of Scottish Stevensons, lighthouse keepers for generations in many of the great lighthouses of Scotland and the Hebrides, was Alan Stevenson (1807–1865), an uncle of Robert Louis Stevenson. He was a poet, friend of Wordsworth and Coleridge, fluent in six languages, classical scholar, pioneer in optical technology, and the "architect of one of

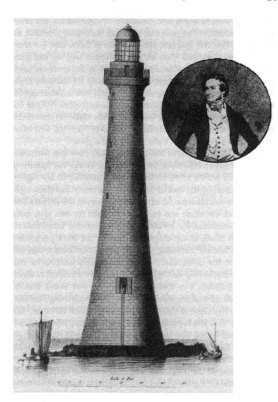

Figure 3.19 Alan Stevenson (inset) in the only known portrait, with the great Skerryvore Light, completed in 1844, said at the time to be one of the great engineering feats of the age. Stevenson was a member of the many generations of "Lighthouse Stevensons," who designed and operated many of the lighthouses of Scotland and England. He began in mid career to develop symptoms of weakness and fatigue and had many episodes of a relapsing and progressive neurological disease that caused his early retirement. He was an uncle of author, Robert Louis Stevenson.

the most exceptional structures ever built."[46] He supervised 35 lighthouses, but began to complain of marked fatigue. Early in his career, he had periods of illness that confined him to bed. Travels to France and examination of Leonor Fresnel's research on lenses suggested to him concepts that eventually changed the lighting methods in Scotland's lighthouses. Alan Stevenson went on to design some of Scotland's most remarkable lighthouses, including Ardnamurchan and Skerryvore.

"I am still grievously afflicted by Drowsiness," he complained in 1844 at age 37. Soon after, he wrote that his suffering was extreme, and described his symptoms as rheumatism. He recovered, but a month later complained that he was again tired and ill. His letters described his symptoms variously as rheumatism, paraplegia, and lumbago. His biographer, Bella Bathurst, felt he was suffering from MS. Lack of improvement forced his return to Edinburgh to seek treatment from his brother-in-law, Dr. Adam Warden. He began to reduce his workload and to frequent various spas. A poet in his free moments, he began to translate the "Ten Hymns of Synesius" from the original Greek, and wrote in the introduction, "it pleased God in 1852 to disable me, by a severe nervous affliction," and said translating the hymns "helped to soothe my pains." As his disease worsened, he was able to do less and less for the many lighthouses he supervised. He had to retire in 1853, and submitted letters from his doctors that indicated he suffered from an unusually severe form of paraplegia. As he continued to worsen, he felt his disease was due to his past sins. Bathurst said, "Alan was aching away the remainder of his life in expensive spa towns, paralyzed by poverty and self-doubt as much as by his own enforced inactivity." He died 21 years after the onset of his relapsing and progressive illness.

Margaret Gatty, Victorian Writer

"Then you see I wage daily warfare with myself when I feel sad at my disablement from even the simplest action."

Margaret Gatty, January 9, 1870

Margaret Gatty (1809–1873), a naturalist and author of popular children's books, probably had MS. Although she lived past the time of Charcot's

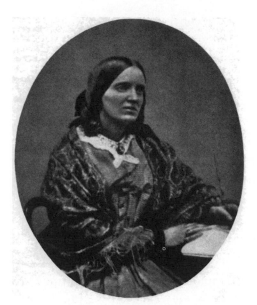

Figure 3.20 Mrs. Margaret Gatty, Victorian novelist. Her successful career as a children's writer and naturalist began at age 41, the year her neurological symptoms first appeared.

lectures, and was published in the medical literature, the end of her life came just at the time of the first English publications on MS as an identifiable entity in *The Lancet*.

Mrs. Gatty was the founder of the popular publication for children, *Aunt Judy's Magazine* and author of a successful five-volume *Parables from Nature*, and also wrote a respected guide to *British Sea-Weeds* (1863).[47] Her writings have survived less well than those of her better-known daughter, Juliana Horatia Ewing (1841–1885).*[48]

Her interest in natural sciences began when she fell ill in Hastings in 1848 and her sympathetic doctor loaned her books that excited her interest in seaweeds. The nature of that illness is unclear, but her daughter reported that in 1849, both her writing career and her first neurological symptoms began. Margaret Gatty's writing career began, at age 41, at the same time she experienced symptoms that she called a nervous disorder affecting her general system. Continuing complaints caused her to consult a physician in London in 1860, but he declared her "organically sound," as she apparently had no obvious outward manifestations of dis-

---

*Her daughter's middle name alludes to the fact that Mrs. Gatty's father was chaplain to Admiral Nelson.

ease. She was clearly uncertain about this conclusion, writing in her diary: "but still one must believe the Drs. know something."

In the next breath, she wondered about the possible benefits of trying homeopathic therapies. Nine months later, she wrote that her hand was tremulous and "losing its cunning." Her illness was at first intermittent, causing her to remain in bed for days due to attacks of "muscular or nervous rheumatism." She repeatedly visited Dr. Thomas King Chambers and was relieved to have him call the cause of her problem, "atrophic degeneration of the muscular fibers from overuse so my troubles have at any rate got a fine name!"

She began to write with her left hand and complained of pain in the paralyzed arm and shoulder. The fourth volume of her *Parables from Nature* was written with her left hand. Doctors said her condition would ultimately recover, even though she had the symptoms for many years. Despite this reassurance, she continued to deteriorate and was referred to a London surgeon, who recommended a leather sling and a splint for her arm. Her left arm weakened though, and in the habit of many MS patients, she assumed this was the result of overuse because of the weakness of her right hand.

Mrs. Gatty seemed unaware that Dr. Chambers had described her condition in a presentation to medical colleagues and later in a publication in *The Lancet* as muscular atrophy due to excessive physical effort.[49]

Chambers concluded that the weakness in her arms was due to overwork, which did not allow renewal of the nerve forces needed by muscles, so that no new store of muscular substance could be laid in and the muscle would degenerate into elastic fiber and finally into pale fatty tissue of low vitality.[50,51] Chambers' use of the term *atrophy* described muscles that were weak and paralyzed, though there was no loss of muscle bulk or obvious thinning.

In the *Renewal of Life*, Chambers outlined his therapeutic approach, "restorative medicine."[52] He expressed little interest in neurological disorders except sciatica and hysteria, but believed in the use of iodides for any diseases of the nervous system, including hysteria, feeling the iodides would renew the nerve sheaths to health. In his Harveian lecture of 1871, he said that all diseases add to the body substances that need to be reduced, opposed, assisted, neutralized, or concentrated.[53]

Lecture XXIX on Muscular Atrophy

"M., age 54, has lived an active literary life, writing much and well. Her vigor of constitution is shown by the menses only lately beginning to grow scanty and irregular. But she has a theory of corporeal discipline not reconcilable with rational physiology. She has thought to compensate for the exhaustion of mental labor by violent physical exertion, and has been in the habit of occupying her leisure by furiously digging her garden with a masculine spade, and mowing her lawns, not with one of the new elegant machines, but an old fashioned scythe. The consequence is that her good right hand has lost its cunning, and a letter she sent to seek my advice was scrawled with the left. The principal atrophy is in the deltoid and triceps muscles (those used in mowing), which are painful when moved, but not when pressed. She cannot raise her arm by independent efforts above the level of her waist, and it 'feels out of joint if she tries to force it.' Friction, brandy and salt, mustard, etc. have only made her worse. Her arm is now by my advice tied up, and she is taking quinine and steel and cod-liver oil in small doses."

Thomas King Chambers
The Lancet, 1864

In 1863, Mrs. Gatty developed a pain in her face she thought was due to dental problems and wished to have her teeth removed. Chambers suggested this course would make her worse rather than better. She persisted and wanted to know if there was not someone who could remove them to relieve the pain using chloroform.*

"In short this affair has made me so like a village old woman that I feel quite one of them when I visit and listen to all their aches & pains & histories of tumbles & sprains & rheumatism with a fellow feeling imagination only never allows one."

Margaret Gatty, November 21, 1863

---

*The pain in her face was probably trigeminal neuralgia, often thought to be dental when it appears in MS patients. Trigeminal neuralgia in a person under age 55 is almost always due to MS.

Dr. Chambers recommended a spa and rest for her weakness, suggesting she go to Bath in the winter. Unable to write and having trouble walking due to weakness and curling of the foot muscles in her right leg, Mrs. Gatty was still reassured by doctors that she might recover. In fact, only her left arm recovered somewhat and the surgeon Mr. Hawthorn felt her condition temporary and due to her "time of life." Mrs. Gatty spent much of her time on a couch, able to walk a little but venturing outside of the house only in an invalid chair.

In 1868, the year of Charcot's lectures on MS, she consulted Dr. Radcliffe, "a paralytic and nervous Dr. who told me there was no doubt whatever about my case: that it was spinal: a want of blood in the spinal cord. And he ridiculed the idea that it was degeneration of the muscles!" Drs. Chambers and Paget ridiculed Dr. Radcliffe, and still spoke hopefully of recovery.

Later, Mrs. Gatty's speech became affected, and she fell more often. Hawthorn noted that cold weather caused her leg muscles to tighten. She had an attack of "liver illness" and her condition deteriorated further. Repeated spasms and jerking of her legs caused great discomfort and her feet began to curl into permanent deformity.

Mrs. Gatty's illness had a variable course, which moved from one arm to the other and then affected her legs. She had a recurrence of a painful "tic" in her face and speech difficulty. After many attacks, "which perfectly disabled me without making me ill," she became progressively worse and confessed she was willing to try anything, even quackery and mesmerism.

Hawthorn now informed her that Dr. Chambers had mentioned her case in his lectures some six years earlier.[54] She was pleased, noting in a letter that "Dr. C. seems to consider it quite a peculiar case," and was buoyed by his confidence in her diagnosis.

In August 1870 she wrote, "You must prepare to see me unable to hold up my head—I tie it up sometimes." Her legs were weaker, although she felt her left arm somewhat improved. A few months later, she noted she was failing despite massage of her spine night and morning.

By January 1871, she noted regretfully that "there was nothing definite except the undeniable fact that I am getting lamer gradually." Her arms felt a little stronger but her hands were weaker, preventing all writing. She saw a notice about the benefits of oxygenating the blood and wrote to Mr. Hawthorn who prescribed a medicine he felt would have the same effect. Her leg and foot spasms got worse. She noticed slowing of movements, such as combing her hair, patting the dog, and brushing her nails, but maintained a positive attitude. She said there was a woman at St. Leonards who was worse afflicted, and could not even swallow. She, on the other hand, could go out in a bath chair: "I am a complete cripple and feel very weak, but not in bad spirits."

Mrs. Gatty had attendants who turned her repeatedly during the night, which distressed her, but she added that although she was sad to have these services, she could afford them, and if she were a poor person, she certainly would be in dire straits. She continued to weaken though "Enry" (Mr. Hawthorn) kept insisting she was better and felt she would improve after her deterioration during a bout of pneumonia. After a further year of complete disability, she developed a respiratory infection and died on October 4, 1873.

Mrs. Gatty originated the idea of financially supporting cots for sick children at the Great Ormond Street Hospital, and over the years, her readers contributed to many cots in that and other hospitals. There was an outpouring of support from her readers in all parts of the world to funnel more beds in her memory. This idea of endowing beds in hospitals was taken up by many institutions, and these cots are a lasting memorial to a magnificent Victorian.

SUMMARY OF THE EARLY CASES

In every era, patients have suffered with conditions not fully understood or effectively treated. Within the concepts and views of their day, physicians proceeded as best they could, and were as confident as we are today dealing with an incompletely understood condition. Multiple sclerosis still has many mysteries, and time will show how similarly we are struggling, as they were, to understand and help our patients.

Therapies did not change much over centuries, even after the disease was framed and named. We will see that the therapies of the 19th century were continued into the 20th century. Although most doctors did not feel the therapies altered the course of the disease, they provided some relief or hope to patients. There was always a desire to offer something to those who suffer.

It is interesting how the illness of many of these early cases lasted 20–40 years, while many later medical writers felt the illness lasts about 8–12 years. This probably indicates that the most serious, advanced, and progressive cases were the experience of the consultants in clinics and hospitals. Those doing well, or with mild disease mostly cared for themselves. Margaret Davies was hardly a mild case, but her condition still lasted two decades, despite disability and pressure sores.

The cases just outlined are examples of disorders of the nervous system that resemble only MS. That only a few are known over a number of centuries should not suggest the disease was rare, or any less common than today. Patients with the disease were regarded differently in different eras and with different nosologies. The concept of disease, particularly of the nervous system, caused patients with many forms of neurological disease to be viewed as having nervous disorders, brain disease, palsy, paralysis, infirmities, or creeping paralysis.

That we can recognize cases before doctors became interested in the disabling disease characterized by scattered lesions throughout the central nervous system just emphasizes that the disease was there. Was it less common in the 15th or 17th century? We cannot tell; MS patients would have been mixed in with those suffering from other disorders. It is hard to find definitive data that the number of cases of MS have increased much in the century and a half since it was recognized. Even correcting for our refined clinical classification, recognition of milder and benign cases, and newer diagnostic tools such as spinal fluid examination, evoked potential tests, and MRI, the apparent stability of the disease suggests it has probably been part of the social fabric for a very long time. As Compston said, it has been more an epidemic of recognition, rather than a epidemic of increasing cases.[55]

REFERENCES

1. Maeder R. Does the history of multiple sclerosis go back as far as the 14th century? *Acta Neurol Scandinav*. 1979;60:189-192.
2. *Butler's Lives of the Saints*. Thurston HJ, Attwatter D, eds. Vol II. Westminister: Christian Classics; 1990:95-98.
3. Ibid, p. 95.
4. Ibid, p. 97.
5. Ibid, p. 98.
6. Delaney JJ. *Dictionary of Saints*. New York: Doubleday and Company Ltd.; 1980.
7. *The Book of Saints*. London: Adams and Charles Black; 1966.
8. Maeder R. Does the history of multiple sclerosis go back as far as the 14th century? *Acta Neurol Scandinav*. 1979;60:189-192.
9. Ibid, p. 189–192.
10. Poser CM. The Dissemination of Multiple Sclerosis: A Viking Saga? A Historical Essay. *Ann Neurol*.1994;36:S231-243.
11. Anonymous. Thorlaks saga. In: *Byskua Sogur*, Editiones Armagnaenae series A, vol 13.2. Copenhagen: John Helgason; 1978.
12. Stenager E. A Note on the Treatment of Drummer Brock: An Early Danish Account of Multiple Sclerosis? *J Hist Neurosci*. 5(2):197-199.
13. Gough R. *Antiquities and Memories of the Parish of Myddle, County of Salop, 1700*. Shrewsbury: Adnitt and Naunton; 1875 (Also Centaur Press, 1968).
14. Firth D. The case of Augustus d'Esté (1794-1848): the first account of disseminated sclerosis. *Proc Royal Soc Med*. 1940–1941;34:499-552.
15. Firth D. *The Case of Augustus d'Esté*. Cambridge: Cambridge University Press; 1948.
16. Ibid, p. 17.
17. d'Esté A. Application to the House of Lords. *The Jurist*, 1844. Vol V(i) II, 793.
18. Firth D. *The Case of Augustus d'Esté*, p. 26-27.
19. Hale-White W. *Great Doctors of the 19th Century*. London: Edward Arnold, 1935.
20. Metcalfe R. *Life of Vincent Priessnitz: Founder of Hydrotherapy*. London: Metcalfe London Hydro Ltd., 1898.
21. Hughes RR. File on Augustus d'Esté. MS 107; 17/1/68, London: Royal College of Physicians.
22. Firth D. The Case of Augustus d'Este (1794-1848): the first account of disseminated sclerosis. *Proc Royal Soc Med*. 1940-41;34:499-52.
23. Firth D. *The Case of Augustus d'Esté*. Cambridge: Cambridge University Press; 1948.
24. Hughes RR. File on Augustus d'Esté. MS 107; 17/1/68, London: Royal College of Physicians.
25. Sammons JL. *Heinrich Heine. A Modern Biography*. Manchester: Carcanet Press; 1979.
26. Reed TJ. Happy Return? Heinrich Heine: the last German poet of the eighteenth and the first of the twentieth century. *Times Literary Supplement*. October 10, 1997;3-4.
27. Stenager E. The Course of Heinrich Heine's Illness: Diagnostic Considerations. *J Med Bio*. 1996;4(1):28-32.
28. Jellinek EH. Heine's illness: the case for multiple sclerosis. *J Roy Soc of Med*. 1990;83:516-519.
29. Ibid, p. 518.
30. Paty DW, Ebers GC, eds. Critchley M. Four illustrious neuroluetics. *Proc R Soc Med*. 1969;62:669-673.
31. Atkens HG. *Heine*. New York: EP Hutton; 1929.
32. Murray TJ. The Medical History of Doctor Samuel Johnson. *The Nova Scotia Medical Bulletin*. 1982; June/August:71-78.
33. Critchley M. Four illustrious neuroluetics. *Proc R Soc Med*. 1969;62:669-673.

34. Stenager E. The course of Heinrich Heine's illness: diagnostic considerations. *J Med Bio*. 1996;4(1):28-32.
35. Putnam TJ. The centenary of multiple sclerosis. *Arch Neurol Psych*. 1938;40(4):806-813.
36. Stenager E. The course of Heinrich Heine's illness, p. 28-32.
37. Critchley M. Four illustrious neuroluetics. *Proc R Soc Med*. 1969;62:669-673.
38. Roth N. The porphyria of Heine. *Prog Psychiat*. 1969;10:90-106.
39. Stenager E. The course of Heinrich Heine's illness, p. 28-32.
40. Schachter M. Un illustre malade: Le poète Henri Heine, *Paris Med*. 1933;(suppl 1):vi-viii.
41. Putnam TJ. The centenary of multiple sclerosis. *Arch Neurol Psych*. 1938;40(4):806-813.
42. Kolle K. Die Krankheit von Heinrich Heine. *Der Hautartz*. 1964;15:162-164.
43. Stern A. Heinrich Heines Krankheit und seine Ärzte. In HeineJahrbuch. Düsseldorf: Heinrich Heine Institute; 1964:63-79.
44. Fredrikson S. Letter to the editor in response to Stenager and Jensen. *Perspect Biol Med*. 1991;32:312.
45. Jellinek EH. Heine's illness: the case for multiple sclerosis. *J Roy Soc Med*. 1990;83:516-519.
46. Bathurst B. *The Lighthouse Stevensons*. New York: Perennial (Harper Collins); 1999.
47. Maxwell C. *Mrs. Gatty and Mrs. Ewing*. London: Constable; 1949.
48. Drain S. Margaret Gatty (1809-1873). In: *Victorian Britain: An Encyclopedia*. Mitchell S, ed. New York: Garland; 1988.
49. Chambers TK. Lecture on muscular atrophy. *Lancet*. 1864;96.
50. Chambers TK. *Lectures: Chiefly Clinical*. London: John Churchill and Sons, 1864.
51. Review of TK Chambers' lectures: chiefly clinical. *Lancet*. 1875;1:545.
52. Chambers TK. *The Renewal of Life: Clinical Lectures Illustrative of a Restorative System of Medicine, Given at St. Mary's Hospital*. London: Churchill; 1863.
53. Chambers TK. *Restorative Medicine: the Harveian Oration 1871*, with two sequels. Philadelphia: Henry C. Lea; 1871.
54. Chambers TK. Lecture on muscular atrophy. *Lancet*. 1864;96.
55. Compston A. The story of multiple sclerosis. *McAlpine's Multiple Sclerosis*. London: Churchill Livingstone; 1998:3-42.

4

The Steps Toward a Discovery: The Early Medical Reports

"... a peculiar diseased state..."

Robert Carswell, 1838

In the late 18th and early 19th centuries, interest in subdividing and classifying medical diseases followed the lead of botanists who had made spectacular advances in organizing the plant and animal kingdoms. William Cullen (1712–1790) and others encouraged the careful classification of all diseases, and although initial attempts mixed diseases and symptoms, the efforts sparked exploration of the specific nature of conditions and how they differed. The development of better clinical examination techniques made classification of diseases easier. The simultaneous increase in medical journals and books, regular meetings, and hospital and medical school case presentations helped spur the movement on. The common pattern of having colleagues name a disease after the person who first brought it to the attention of the medical profession also increased enthusiasm for finding something new to describe. The Viennese, Germans, Scots, and English regularly published the features of new or redefined diseases, but no group was more adept in differentiating neurological disease than the French school of neurology.

Although some, such as Matthew Baillie, John Hunter, James Abercrombie, and John Smyth made advances in anatomical pathology in England, in general, the English school lagged behind in interest in disorders of the nervous system. A medical student at St. Thomas Hospital, London, in 1801–02 wrote to his physician father of the range of illness and diagnoses seen by senior physicians. There was a single category for "nervous disorder."[1] In the Croonian lectures in London on hemiplegia, paraplegia, paralysis partialis, and epilepsy (1819), Dr. John Cooke relied on writings of Galen, with some reference to more recent ideas of Bichet and Legallois, to explain the function and dysfunction of the spinal cord. He noted that different conditions can affect the spinal cord, but did not differentiate the various condition types. Fortunately, these conditions were more interesting to the discerning eyes of the Germans, Viennese, and French, who adapted the botanical classification methods to medicine and used the more enlightened appraisal of Bichat and Cullen coupled with the developing methods of pathological examination, microscopsy, and new staining techniques to help define and classify various diseases further.

This atmosphere of clinical and pathological separation of disease entities demonstrates the evolving view of a peculiar disease of the nervous system that affected young adults and caused a vacillating, eventually progressive, disability. Only later would the disease be fully characterized and given a name so well framed that practicing physicians could recognize the pattern in patients in their clinics. Clinician pathologists in France, Germany, Austria, and England began to recognize the pattern of a neurological disease characterized by grey patches in the nervous system even before it was fully described by Charcot.

CHARLES PROSPER OLLIVIER D'ANGERS (1796–1845)

The first case of multiple sclerosis (MS) to be reported in the medical literature, a case of unmistakable relapsing-remitting MS, can be found in *Maladies de la moelle epiniére* by Charles Prosper Ollivier d'Angers,[2] a large monograph on disorders of the spinal cord in Paris in 1824, when he was just 28 years old. This work of a young practitioner without an academic appointment would be widely quoted for the next half century.

As Spillane points out, the monograph was a splendid work, considering that Ollivier wrote at a time when clinical neurological examination scarcely existed.[3] Without the aid of a microscope, he produced a major work on the anatomy, physiology, and pathology of the spinal cord. He noted that this structure was too often neglected at autopsy, its similarity to a large nerve often much exaggerated.

Ollivier called his monograph merely an "outline" of the diseases of the spinal cord, but it was an impressive review of a large number of disorders of the cord. Many of his observations are original, particularly his description of various congenital malformations. He described the association of hydrocephalus with spina bifida, the cervical cord anomalies in anencephaly, such as bifidity, cyst formation, and absent or fused vertebrae; elongation of the fourth ventricle into the cervical cord, stenosis of the foramen magnum, and faults in the cord itself. He noted cavitation of the cord in spina bifida and gave the earliest and most accurate description of syringomyelia in the third edition of his book. Within this treatise on the spinal cord, there is a case that is probably MS.[4,5]

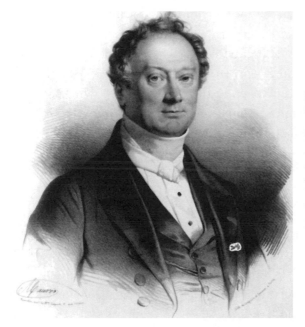

Figure 4.1 Charles Prosper Ollivier d'Angers (1796–1845) gave the first description of a case that we would now regard as multiple sclerosis in his monumental *Maladies de la moelle epiniére*, written when he was 28 years old. Lithograph by N.E. Maurin. (Courtesy of the Wellcome Library, London.)

A 20-year-old man developed a transient weakness of his right foot in 1808. There had been a period of feeling tired and languid at age 17. By age 29, he had weakness of both legs, but this began to improve so that he was able to walk with a cane. He noted that hot waters of a spa induced loss of feeling in his right leg and numbness and clumsiness of his hands when he tried spa therapy at age 30; an early description of the "hot bath test."[6] He had urinary retention, relieved by pressing on his abdomen, and progressive deterioration of his motor function and speech. He found it difficult to write. Sensation was said to be preserved in his legs, but probably was affected, though sensory examination was limited in this era. The young man felt cold water as hot, and when his paretic right hand touched his thigh, he experienced "galvanic shocks." His intellect seemed intact and he retained the "gaiety of his character" despite advanced disability, an effect reminiscent of the surprising cheerfulness of MS patients noted by later authors.

Ollivier said the disease had lasted 29 years and called this disorder a "myelitis," which could be due to an infection, suggesting that the treatment should be bleeding and liberal application of leeches over the thoracic area. The two subsequent editions of his work repeat the clinical features of this young man, without any mention of his later progress or the pathology of his condition.

Ollivier never held an academic post or other position, but devoted his life to his practice, and his private research on the spinal cord and brain. An unusual bust of Ollivier, at the Museé Carnavalet, Paris, was done by Jean-Pierre Dantan.[7] It shows Ollivier arising from a coffin base, a reference to his involvement in the examination of deaths that were medico-legal cases; he was a leading forensic pathologist.

RICHARD BRIGHT
(1789–1858)

Although we know that Richard Bright saw Augustus d'Esté in consultation,[8] and he may have published a case of MS in his extensive case notes, a review of his reports and his great atlas of pathology reveals no case that resembles that of d'Esté.

Bright's notes on a patient with "paralysis with vertigo" describe a bald German of middle stature who had episodes of vertigo ("giddiness") (case CIXXVIII).[9] He began to have cramps that extended to his thighs and throughout his body. While eating dinner, he became hot, developed a rash, and became numb all over. These symptoms persisted, with normal sensation only in his face. He walked with crutches and said he could not feel them. He became weak in all his limbs and dragged his legs when walking with crutches. He complained of tinnitus, some hearing loss, especially in the right side, recurrent vertigo, daily fluctuations in his vision, and photophobia. His vertigo cleared upon treatment with nux vomica,* but his condition was generally unchanged. He left the hospital "very little relieved in his general paralytic condition." This is a doubtful but possible case of MS.

Another case that could be MS is case CCCIII,[10] a woman age 24, with a three-year history of weakness and numbness of the legs, first on

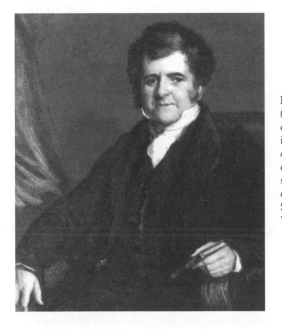

Figure 4.2 Richard Bright (1789–1858) saw Augustus d'Esté in consultation and recommended an increase of iron in his diet. In the case books of Bright, there are two cases that might be multiple sclerosis, but neither are d'Esté. Stipple engraving by H. Cook after F.R. Say, 1860. (Courtesy of the Wellcome Library, London.)

---

*From the nut nux vomica, strychnine and brucine were extracted and used as medicines and poisons. Brucine played a major role as a medicine and a poison in Alexandre Dumas, père's *The Count of Monte Cristo*.

the right and then on the left, and with little change in the hands. She began to improve after two months in the hospital and was eventually able to walk well.

ROBERT CARSWELL
(1793–1857)

Carswell presented the first pathologic demonstration of MS in an atlas of pathologic conditions published in 1838.[11] In the English tradition of Hunter and Thompson, Carswell incorporated the approaches and discoveries of the French school in his observations and illustrations of pathology.[12,13] He also used the visual approach of Hooper, who had produced the first handcolored atlas of neuropathology in 1828.[14]

Robert Carswell was born on February 3, 1793 in Thornliebank, Scotland, and his artistic talent was noted when he was attending Paisley Academy. James Jeffray, professor of Anatomy and Physiology at Glasgow, asked him to illustrate one of his inventions, a machine to propel boats on the Clyde. Jeffray later had Carswell draw anatomical teaching models and encouraged the young man to consider medicine as a career. Carswell's atlas was dedicated to his teacher.*

After his initial medical studies at Glasgow, Edinburgh, Paris, and Lyon, Carswell was commissioned by Dr. John Thompson of Edinburgh to make a collection of drawings of pathology. Thompson was a prominent figure in pathology and surgery in Edinburgh who encouraged his two sons, as well as Carswell, a family friend, to study further in Paris. Thompson wanted the pathological drawings for his teaching. Jacna makes it clear that Carswell had a focused interest in his hospital and dead-house studies, concentrating on the pathology of the cases rather than their clinical background.[15] Jean Cruveilhier, creating his atlas of pathology at the same time, demonstrated an interest in correlating the

---

*Jeffray was a multifaceted dramatic individual involved in body-snatching for his anatomical experiments, and who carried out public dissections on murderers. One of his more dramatic and distasteful displays was to stimulate the body electrically so that it sat up. Then with a flourish, he would cut the neck and the body would fall down. Some observers fainted, and it is not surprising to learn that he was the last to perform such public dissections.

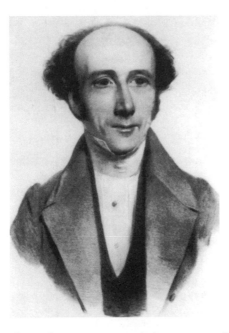

Figure 4.3   Robert Carswell (1793–1857) was a talented Scottish medical student who created a great atlas of illustrations of pathological conditions, one of which is the first illustration of the pathology of multiple sclerosis. (Courtesy of the National Library of Medicine.)

clinical symptoms and the course of the disease with the findings in the autopsy room. Jacna suggests that Carswell had no interest in the patients or the clinical disease because he was focused on the pathological changes, and he foreshadowed the "pure pathologist" of the future.

Carswell spent the years 1822–1823 in Lyon and Paris making drawings in autopsy rooms, and returned to Paris to complete the work after receiving his MD in 1826, remaining there until 1831.[16] He was appointed to the inaugural Chair of Pathology at London University when the prominent anatomist J.F. Meckel turned down the offer, but was allowed to remain in Paris after his appointment, and studied with Pierre Louis while he completed his atlas of drawings.[17] The collection became his *Pathological Anatomy: Illustrations of the Elementary Forms of Disease*, published in 1838. Lithography, invented in Germany in 1790, was ideal for demonstrating the fine features of anatomy and the appearance of tissues. The drawings appeared in 12 separately printed fascicles, each of four plates in its own separately printed wrapper. From 1833 to 1838, 2,361 fascicles were printed, suggesting that 200 of the atlases were produced.[18] The original atlas is at University College Hospital, London. Some drawings were done in Scotland and others in Paris, and although Bourneville

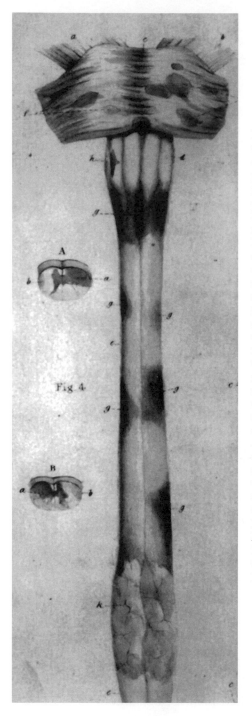

Figure 4.4 The first illustration of multiple sclerosis by Robert Carswell. His description of the cord and pons: "A peculiar disease state of the chord, and pons Varolii, accompanied with atrophy of the discolored portions; A, right crus; B, left crus cerebri; C, pons Varolii; D, medulla oblongata; E,E, medulla spinalis; F,F, isolated points of the pons Varolii, of a yellowish brown colour; G,G,G, patches of the same kind on the spinal chord, all of them occupying the medullary substance, which was very hard, and transparent, and atrophied. The atrophy was more conspicious in some points than others, and is particularly well seen in the figure at H, where it affects a portion of the right olivary body; K, softenings of a portion of the chord. Figure. 4 A and B, represents transverse sections of the chord, to show that the discolouration commences on the surface of the white, and extends inward to the grey substance; A, the brown discolouration which has extended to the grey substance on one side of the chord, a; and is confined to the white substance on the other side, b. Similar appearances are represented in the section B,a,b." Sir Robert Carswell, Pathological anatomy. *Illustrations of the Elementary forms of disease*. London: Longman, 1838. Plate 4, Figure 4. (Courtesy of the Wellcome Library, London.)

and Guerard said the illustration of MS was done in Paris, this is uncertain.[19] The drawings are signed by Carswell and some are annotated as drawn directly on the lithographic stone. Others were done earlier by Haghe, who neglected to reverse the lesions on the surface of the medulla in the illustration of MS.[20]

The earlier plates, including the two plates on MS, have a notation that they were printed by "lithographers to the king," indicating that they were completed before 1836 and printed before June 1837, when Queen Victoria ascended the throne.*[21–23]

Carswell's Plate 4, Figure 4.4, was of the spinal cord, pons, and medulla under the title "Brown transparent discolouration without softening of the spinal chord," demonstrating a condition he described as "a peculiar diseased state of the cord and pons varolii" accompanied by atrophy of the discolored portions, all of them occupying the medullary substance, which was hard, semitransparent, and atrophied, beginning on the surface of the white matter and extending to the grey matter. The patient was paralyzed, but no other clinical details are given and Carswell only saw the patient in the autopsy room. The nervous system was found to have fresh lesions as well as old scars, and Carswell felt these changes were likely due to a deficiency of the blood supply to the cord.[24]

Carswell beautifully illustrated these conditions. He did not think he was describing a new disease, or attempting to separate a disorder from others; he was showing another case of atrophy of the spinal cord, a very general category.

It has been said that Carswell's only contribution was his great atlas, but he did publish a 30-page paper in the *Journal Hebdomadaire de Médicine*, reprinted in the *Edinburgh Medical and Surgical Journal* of 1830, on the changes in the lining of the stomach after death.[25]

Carswell suffered from respiratory problems and after a relatively short career as Professor of Anatomy, he resigned his London post in

---

*For more detailed discussion of the Carswell atlas and its relationship to other great atlases containing prints of MS, see the reviews by Putnam and Compston. The Carswell papers are in the Edinburgh University Library.

Carswell's Case of "A Remarkable Lesion of the Spinal Cord"

"I have met with two cases of a remarkable lesion of the spinal cord accompanied with atrophy. One of the patients was under the care of Mons. Louis, in the Hospîtal of La Pitié, the other under the care of Mons. Chomel at the Hospital of La Charité, both of them affected with paralysis. I did not see either of the patients but I could not ascertain that there was anything in the character of the paralysis or the history of the cases to throw any light on the nature of the lesion found in the region of the spinal cord. I have represented the appearances observed in one case in Plate 4, Fig 4, in which the pons varolii was also affected, and which convey an accurate idea of the physical characters of the lesion. In this case a distinct portion of the cord was affected with softening, which of itself would no doubt have accounted for the paralysis; but in the other case there was no other lesion present than that to which I allude, to which the paralysis could be attributed. The anterior surface of the spinal cord presented a number of spots, from a quarter of an inch to a half an inch in breadth of an irregular form of a yellowish brown colour, smooth, glossy, without vascularity or any alteration in the colour or consistency of the surrounding medullary substance. The medullary substance thus affected was very firm, somewhat transparent, and atrophied. At the root of the medulla oblongata, these changes occupied the whole breadth of both the medullary fasciculi to the extent of half an inch in breadth from above downwards.

Further down, they were confined to distinct spots on each fasciculus, and several of the same kind, but smaller, occupied the pons varolii. The depth to which the medullary substance was affected in this manner varied from half a line to three or four lines, and on dividing the cord, it was seen to penetrate as far as the grey substance."

Robert Carswell, 1838[26]

1840 because of failing health. He changed careers to become physician to King Leopold of Belgium, believing the air of Belgium would be cleaner than the smog and fog of London. He lived at Laeken, near Brussels, and even though he was physician advisor to the king, he also cared for many of the poor. He returned a number of times to London, and on one of these trips was knighted by Queen Victoria for his services in caring for Louis Philippe of France while he was in exile. Carswell died in 1857. Neither the *British Medical Journal* nor *The Lancet* saw fit to recognize his passing with an obituary, but his atlas is a fitting memorial.[27]

William Osler, who owned a copy of Carswell's atlas, said, "These illustrations have, for artistic merit and for fidelity, never been surpassed, while the matter represents the highest point which the science of morbid anatomy had reached before the introduction of the microscope."[28]

JEAN CRUVEILHIER
(1791-1874)

An advertisement in 1828 asked for subscribers to a planned anatomical atlas by Jean Cruveilhier, with lithographs, to begin appearing in 1829.[29] Cruveilhier worked in Paris at the same time as Carswell, and sometimes in the same hospital autopsy rooms, although there is no record of their meeting.* Credit for the first illustration of MS has been given to Carswell, but these were soon followed by similar illustrations by Cruveilhier (1835–1842), who reported four patients in his atlas under the heading "Diseases of the Spinal Cord," all of whom had autopsy findings of grey degeneration in patches though the nervous system. These were well described by Compston.[30]

Jean Cruveilhier was born in Limoges in 1791 and had decided to enter the priesthood, but with his mother's encouragement, he transferred from the College of Limoges to the University of Paris to study medicine under Guillaume Dupuytren, graduating in 1811.[31] His work on anatomical pathology, privately printed during his internship, gave an inkling of things to come. Initially, he wished only for the quiet life of a practicing community physician; he married and returned to Limoges. Things did not go well and he was unsuccessful in two applications to be a surgeon at

---

*Compston notes that there is a striking similarity in the lesions in the pons illustrated by Carswell and Cruveilhier, but Josephine Paget, described by Cruveilhier, was still alive when Carswell's atlas was published, so it could not have been the same case.

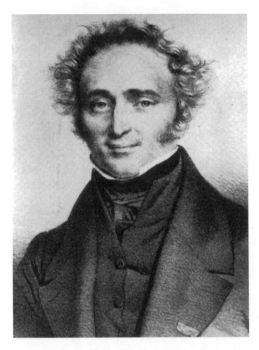

Figure 4.5 Jean Cruveilhier (1791–1874) published his folios of colored lithographs *Anatomie pathologique du corps humain*, dedicated to Dupuytren, which contain cases of multiple sclerosis. They were published after the illustration of Carswell, but with Cruveilhier's illustrations, we have the clinical story, allowing some clinical-pathological correlation. (Courtesy of the National Library of Medicine.)

the City Hospital.* In the meantime, Dupuytren was able to secure for him the offer of the chair of Operative Surgery in Montpellier. He was appointed to the professorship of Anatomy in Paris in 1825. He became the first to hold the chair of Pathology in the Faculty of Medicine, a position secured by a provision in Dupuytren's will, which gave anatomical pathology academic recognition. Access to the deadhouse at the Salpêtrière, the establishment of the Musée Dupuytren, and his role in lecturing on morbid anatomy gave Cruveilhier the opportunity to continue his work on anatomical pathology, which culminated with his serial publication of colored lithographs, in which we find cases of what we now know as MS.

After the siege of Paris, Cruveilhier moved to his country estate at Succac, near Limoges. He died in 1874 at age 83. Although we acknowledge his recognition of the condition characterized by scattered grey patches in the nervous system, his work also made important observations on tumors, infections, and vascular and degenerative disease of the nervous system.[32]

*Cruveilhier eventually had a large private practice, but was not a great clinician.

For many years, there was controversy over which of the illustrators of MS was first. The primacy was accorded to Cruveilhier by Jean-Martin Charcot, who mistakenly gave the publication date as 1835.[33] But Cruveilhier's illustrations were published in separate livraisons between 1835 and 1842, and the illustrations of MS were after 1841. Callison's German bibliography, *Medicinisches Schrifstellar-Lexicon* (1839), has notes on the works of Cruveilhier indicating that livraisons 1–20 were published between 1828 and 1835. By 1837, livraison 27 was available, and in 1838, livraison 28. In 1839, Callison indicated that Carswell had already published his full atlas between 1833 and 1838 in 12 parts, but at that time, livraison 28 of Cruveilhier was the latest available. It is likely that Cruveilhier's livraisons 32 (Plate 2) and 38 (Plate 5) containing the illustrations of MS were published sometime after 1841.*[34-37]

One of the cases in the Cruveilhier atlas had patches in the cerebellar peduncles, optic thalami, corpus callosum, and fornix. The artist had seen this patient daily until her death and noted her progressive disease. Her mental state was said to have been preserved throughout the course of her disease.

In livraison 38 are illustrations of the case of Josephine Paget, who was blind, paraplegic, and had severe proprioceptive sensory loss mimicking locomotor ataxia. She was in bed 16 of St. Joseph Ward at La Charité on May 4, 1840 and died on March 20, 1841 (another clear indication that Carswell's 1836 publication was first). Another patient (who did not have MS) in this livraison was also alive in August 1841. In addition, there is reference to Marshall Hall's *Diseases and Derangements of the Nervous System*,[38] which was published in 1841. There have been many pretenders to the title

---

*On the 150th anniversary of the first depiction of MS by Carswell, Compston clarified further the controversy about whether Cruveilhier or Carswell should be credited with the first published pathological description of MS, although the primacy of Carswell has been declared previously by Putnam. Cruveilhier's atlas was published in two volumes bearing the date 1835 and 1842, respectively. Compston indicates that surviving copies of Cruveilhier's atlas exist with the livraisons bound sequentially by number, a heterogeneous collection of plates and clinical descriptions, or in copies rearranged by subjects, with the plates interleaved in varying order, presumably at the whim of individual collators, or as a separate volume. The separate livraisons began to appear in 1829. Volume I was published in 1835 and contained livraisons 1–20 and volume II contained numbers 21–40. The illustrations of MS are in livraison 32, plate 2 and livraison 38, plate 5, both of which were included in volume II, published after 1841.

of "first" to illustrate MS, and I mention a few. Keppel-Hesselink suggested that the credit should go to the presentation and publication by Marx, who presented a case in a Latin monograph to the Royal Scientific Society in Göttingen in December 1833. This was subsequently published in German in 1838 by Richardson. The patient had a progressive paralysis, but she stayed mentally clear and cheerful until her death. This is difficult to accept as a definite case of MS and Marx himself noted at autopsy that the spinal pathology could be consistent with other diagnoses such as AV malformation or multilocular tumors.[39] Charcot discussed the course of Josephine Paget's illness and described the effects of sensory symptoms resulting from lesions of the posterior columns:

> *"A case, the history of which may be found recorded at length in Cruveilhier's* Atlas d'anatomie pathologique *may be cited as an example of this class [multiple sclerosis]. It is the case of the patient Paget. In order to grasp and use a pin she required to have her eyes open, otherwise the pin dropped from her fingers. On a post-mortem examination, it was found that one of the sclerosed patches occupied a considerable extent of the posterior columns in the cervical enlargement of the cord."[40]*

Due credit must be given to Cruveilhier for giving the first clinico-pathological correlations of MS. While describing cases he felt illustrated the location of sensory and motor functions in the spinal cord and brain, he outlined the history of the cook, Darges, age 37, who had a progressive disease over six years, with increasing gait difficulty, falls in the street, weakness and tremulousness, speech difficulty, visual loss, involuntary laughing and crying, and spasms of the limbs.

He also described a woman of 54, who had a progressive neurological disease for many years before being admitted to the Salpêtrière, where she resided further for 10 years.

> *"There seems to be a very incomplete controlling power of the will over the muscles which seemed to obey imperiously some involuntary cause; and this conflict between the will and some involuntary cause produces incoordinate movements similar to those seen in Chorea. If the patient is carried from bed to bed, the most violent reactions take*

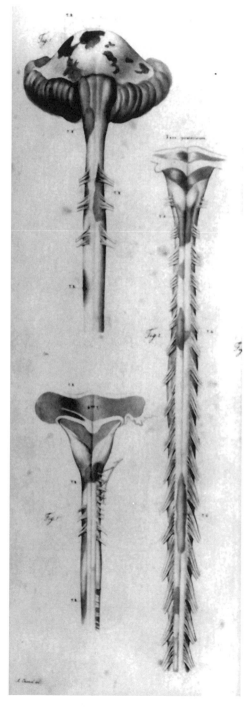

Figure 4.6 Jean Cruveilhier's illustration from *Anatomie pathologique du corps humain, ou descriptions ... des diverses alterations morbides dont le corps humain est succeptible*. Paris: J.B. Balliere (1829-42). Maladies de la moelle epiniere. Plate 2. (Courtesy of the Wellcome Library, London.)

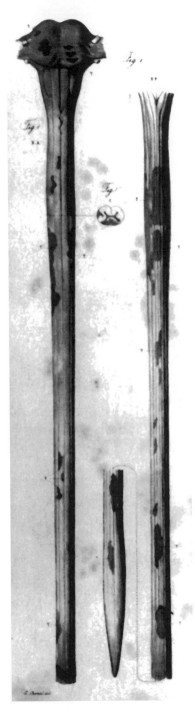

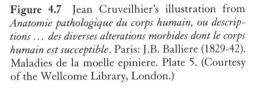

Figure 4.7 Jean Cruveilhier's illustration from *Anatomie pathologique du corps humain, ou descriptions ... des diverses alterations morbides dont le corps humain est succeptible*. Paris: J.B. Balliere (1829-42). Maladies de la moelle epiniere. Plate 5. (Courtesy of the Wellcome Library, London.)

Darges, the Cook

"Darges, a cook age 37 ... had been ill six years without known cause. Six years ago she noticed that the left leg resisted her will to such a degree that she fell in the street. Three months later the right leg was affected like the left. The upper extremities finally became ... tremulous and weak. Sensation was unaffected.... I noticed no spasmodic retraction and no painful spasms of the extremities. ... She gave a complete history, although the articulation of sounds was embarrassed. ... When I spoke to her she became seized with an emotion difficult to describe. She blushed, laughed, and cried; the extremities and trunk became the seat of involuntary movements. ... Swallowing became difficult. ... There was never any headache. She complained of feebleness of vision.

I had made the diagnosis of a lesion of the upper portion of the spinal cord. I was even tempted ... to consider the disease due to compression of the medulla ... by a tumor ... but the complete absence of headache caused me to abandon this idea."

Jean Cruveilhier[41]

place in the legs, and the attendants must exercise care not to be struck by them. These contractions take place when the patient is asked to move the limbs voluntarily. The only thing she can use moderately well is snuff tobacco. To do this she makes a sudden violent effort with the hand in which she holds the snuff, at the same time moving her head towards it; by the sudden combined movement of the head and hand the snuff reaches the nostrils."

He described the woman's toes as "being strongly flexed" and mentioned that she had diminished sensation. I agree with Compston that the other two cases mentioned by Cruveilhier are not convincing for MS.[42,43]

Cruveilhier was able to recognize the essential feature that set this disorder aside from others, the "grey degeneration" in superficial *taches* or *isles*, and that these islands replaced the area of the white matter where they were found. He called the condition "paraplégie par dégénération grise des cordons de la moelle." Cruveilhier felt this condition was caused like the rheumatic diseases, by a general suppression of sweat.*

HOOPER AND ABERCROMBIE

Although the first case of MS in medical literature would seem to be that described by Ollivier, and the first illustration by Carswell, Lawrence McHenry[44] suggested that Robert Hooper might have published an earlier case of MS in his *Morbid Anatomy of the Human Brain*, the first great atlas of pathology,[45] which contains lithographs based on 4,000 necropsies carried out at St. Marylebone Infirmary in London over a 30-year period. McHenry refers to Hooper's Plate 4 as MS, but the description there sounds like Plate 4 from Robert Carswell's work, and a search of Hooper's drawings and lithographs at McGill University by Compston showed no convincing illustrations suggestive of MS.[†]

A suggestion by S.A. Kinnier Wilson that there is a case of MS in John Abercrombie's 1828 *Pathological and Practical Researches on Diseases of the Brain and Spinal Cord*[46] could not be verified.[47] Abercrombie was a pioneer Scottish neuropathologist who increased interest in diseases of the nervous system. The case concerns a young man who had a history of a fall on his sacrum and later developed a transient paralysis and sensory loss. After recovery, he had residual sensory change in one foot. Four years later, he experienced ascending paresis of the legs. Scant detail and lack of further history makes it doubtful, but Abercrombie's case could be considered a "possible case" of MS. Another of his cases might indicate an acute episode of MS with recovery:

> *"A gentleman age 34, of a slender make and very active habits, was affected in the summer of 1815 with numbness and diminished sensibility of all the extremities. In the inferior extremities, it extended to the*

---

*Cruveilhier's name is remembered for his atlas and for the Cruveilhier-Baumgarten syndrome in cirrhosis. Amyotrophic lateral sclerosis (ALS) described by Duchenne and Aran earlier and Charcot later, was described by Cruveilhier in 1853. ALS was once known as Cruveilhier's disease, and later as Charcot's disease.

†The error has been perpetuated in the new *Dictionary of the History of Medicine* by Anton Sebastian, which suggests Hooper first documented MS, followed by Cruveilhier.

tops of the thighs, and sometimes affected the lower parts of the abdomen. In the superior extremities, it never extended above the wrist. There was along with it a diminution of muscular power. He could walk a considerable distance, though he did so with a feeling of insecurity and unsteadiness; but he could not in the smallest degree perform such motions as are required in running, leaping or even very quick walking. He was in other respects in good health. Various remedies were employed, without benefit; evacuations and spare diet seemed rather to be hurtful. He has continued in this state which I have described, for about two months, when he determined to try the effect of violent exercise. For this purpose he walked as hard as he was able, five or six miles in a warm evening, and returned home much fatigued, and considerably heated. Next morning he had severe pains in the calves of his legs, but his other complaints were much diminished, and in a few days disappeared. He has ever since enjoyed very good health."

John Abercrombie, 1838

MARSHALL HALL
(1770–1857)

The confusion in this era between paralysis agitans (Parkinson's disease) and MS, specifically addressed by Vulpian and Charcot, can be demonstrated in the case of Marshall Hall (1770–1857). In his text, *Lectures on the Nervous System and its Diseases* (1836),[48] a case referred to as paralysis agitans is probably MS. The patient manifested what would later be known as Charcot's triad of nystagmus, intention tremor, and scanning speech. This 28-year-old man had weakness of his right arm and leg, and a tremor of his arm that worsened with movement. He had a "peculiar rocking motion of the eyes" and speech difficulty described as stammering and defective articulation.*

---

*Cruveilhier referred to Marshall Hall's text in his atlas, which helped Compston confirm that the MS illustrations were later than Carswell. It is of interest to note that Marshall Hall was on the list of subscribers to the Cruveilhier's atlas when it was advertised in 1828. Hall developed his theory of reflex action in 1832; it was attacked by some as wrong, and by others as right but not new, but was a major contribution to the understanding of the nervous system. Hall's *On the Diseases and Derangement of the Nervous System* referred to by Cruveilhier, was published in 1841.

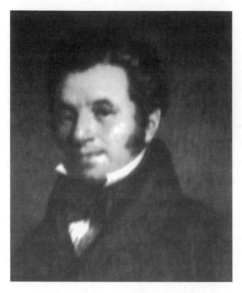

Figure 4.8 Marshall Hall's textbook *Lectures on the Nervous System and its Diseases* demonstrated the confusion between Parkinson's disease and multiple sclerosis in the early 18th century, as his case of a 28-year-old man had Charcot's triad with intention tremor, nystagmus and scanning speech, but was called "paralysis agitans" the term for Parkinson's disease until the 20th century. (Courtesy of the National Library of Medicine.)

THEODORE SCHWANN
(1810–1882)

While Carswell and Cruveilhier were publishing their atlases, Theodore Schwann (1810–1882) was examining the sheath around nerves and described the cell that formed the myelin sheath of the peripheral nerv-

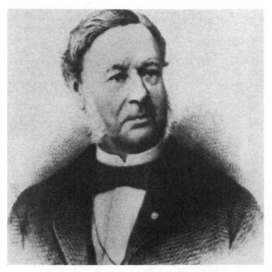

Figure 4.9 Theodore Schwann first observed the myelin sheath.

ous system, now called the Schwann cell (1838). In 1839, he published his classic work on the cell theory, submitting it first to the Bishop of Malines for approval, since he was a devout Catholic who did not want a theory of fundamental body structure to be in conflict with theological teaching. Soon after, clinicians began observing cases with patches of breakdown of the myelin sheath around nerves in the central nervous system, and study of the Schwann cells and myelin in the peripheral nervous system added insights to the changes seen in the central nervous system.

MORITZ HEINRICH ROMBERG
(1795–1873)

Moritz Heinrich Romberg (1795–1873) was professor of neurology in Berlin. His medical thesis was on rickets with a classical description of achondroplasia. He selected the nervous system as his area of interest, and was influenced by Johann Peter Frank (1745–1821), who studied the spinal cord before his interests broadened into public health. Romberg became physician to the poor in Berlin in 1820 and saw over 200 cases per year in a charity hospital. He translated English books into German, especially those of Charles Bell. He published his book on the nervous system between 1840 and 1846, with three editions over the next decade. The Romberg sign appears in the second edition of 1853. Romberg's *Lehrbuch der Nerven Krankheiten* (1846) was the first formal textbook of nervous diseases.[49] His *Textbook on Nervous Disease*[50] (English translation, 1853) contains a case of a young woman with hemiplegia, first on one side and then the other, who was noted on autopsy to have "yellow softenings" about the lateral ventricles. A review of the other cases in his text, such as those with tabes dorsalis, did not reveal other histories suggestive of MS. Although Romberg's sign of proprioceptive sensory loss (reasonable steadiness standing with the feet together and eyes open, but falling when the eyes are closed) is a useful one in the examination of MS patients, it is also useful in tabes dorsalis and many other sensory syndromes, both central and peripheral.

Putnam found no new cases in his review of the pathology collections of Bonet or Morgagni, nor in the treatises of Haslem, Pinel, and Calmeil.[51] Gull wrote about the causes of paraplegia in the Guy's

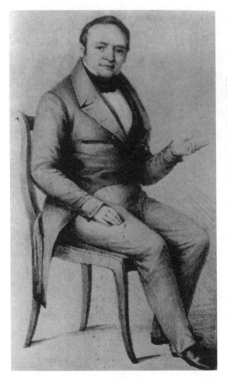

Figure 4.10 Moritz Heinrich Romberg (1795-1873) remembered for *Romberg's Sign*, the instability when patients with sensory loss close their eyes. This sign, also noted by Marshall Hall and Bernardus Brauch in the early 19th century, (American authors referred to the *Romberg-Brauch Sign*) was described as a sign of tabes dorsalis, but later was noted to be related to proprioceptive loss in other conditions such as multiple sclerosis and peripheral neuropathy. Romberg's great textbook, *Lehrbook der Nervenkrankheiten* (1846) was translated into English by Edward Sieveking in 1853. His attention to structural diseases of the nervous system was the basis of modern neurology. (Courtesy of the National Library of Medicine.)

Hospital Reports in 1856 and 1858, and although there has been suggestion that some of the well-described and well-illustrated cases could be MS, my review of these found none that are convincing.

FRIEDRICH THEODOR VON FRERICHS (1819–1895)

In the early 19th century, clinicians in Germany and France often followed their cases to the autopsy room and examined brains and spinal cords to try to understand the nature of the neurological affliction. As the approach of medicine moved from a general concept of illness to an understanding of specific diseases, these observations revealed the different ways the nervous system could be affected. It can be difficult to determine if MS is being reported by early writers who were just beginning to differentiate neurological disorders and their pathology.

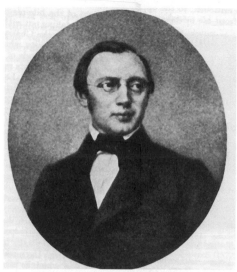

Figure 4.11 Friedrich von Frerichs (1819–1895) was aware of the clinical features, course, and pathology of multiple sclerosis before Charcot gave his famous lecture on the features of the disease and gave it a name. He was the first to diagnose the disease in life and these cases were later confirmed at autopsy by his student, Valentiner. (Courtesy of the National Library of Medicine.)

From German and French writings of the early 19th century, it is clear that clinicians recognized there was a specific progressive neurological disorder of young adults that affected the spinal cord and caused multiple grey patches of softening. In 1849, Friedrich Theodor von Frerichs (1819–1895), a German clinician-pathologist of Breslau, was able to make the first clinical diagnosis in a living patient of the myelitis that would become known as multiple sclerosis, which he called "Hirnsklerose" (1849).[52] His description of a group of these cases was later challenged, and it appears that he includes some patients with features of tabes dorsalis and subacute combined degeneration of the cord.

Frerichs was also the first to note a number of features of MS such as its tendency to occur in young adults, frequent asymmetry of features at the onset, spontaneous remissions and exacerbations, later gradual progression, greater involvement in the legs as time goes on, more motor involvement than sensory involvement, association of mental changes in some cases, and frequent presence of nystagmus. Great interest in differentiating this sclerosis from cases of tabes, paralysis agitans (Parkinson's disease), and syringomyelia arose, but Charcot commented that he suspected some of Frerichs' cases were not MS.[53] In 1856, Frerich's student George Theodor Valentiner published subsequent history and autopsy reports on these cases with pathologic findings, demonstrating "the brilliant correctness of diagnosis" by Frerichs.[54] Valentiner also described two additional patients with a relapsing-remitting pattern of symptoms and cognitive changes.

Frerichs had carefully examined the spinal cords of his patients and noted:

> *"...an abnormal firmness of leathery consistency in irregularly circumscribed parts of the white, rarely involving the gray matter of the cord, with a poverty of blood-vessels. The patches are almost normal in color or milky white, dull and occasionally grayish red. There is a loss of nerve elements."*[55]

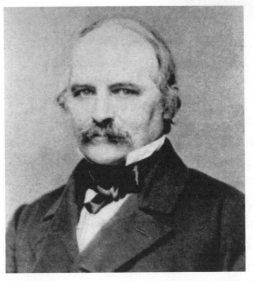

Figure 4.12 Ludwig Türck (1810–1868) was the head of a neurological department in the Allgemeines Krankenhaus in Vienna, and made important contributions to the understanding of the spinal cord, and to secondary degeneration in the nervous system. His book on the spinal cord in 1843 came at a time when there was little interest in the specific anatomy or function of this "large nerve." He showed that the direction of tract degeneration corresponded to the direction of conduction, one of the major discoveries of the 19th century, and he was able to outline six major cord tracts, one of which bears his name (the anterior corticospinal tract). He originated the concept of system disease of the spinal cord, first described the mechanism of the choked optic disc in raised intracranial pressure, and described the cutaneous distribution of the spinal roots. He first described the syndrome now named for Brown-Séquard. Late in his career, after making many other contributions to the understanding of the nervous system, he abandoned neurology and contributed to laryngology, and is thought to have invented the laryngoscope. Photographer: Schultz, Vienna.

It is interesting that Frerichs is not remembered as the person who first described the clinical and pathological features of MS.

Ludwig Türck
(1810–1868)

When referring to those who had described previous cases of MS, Charcot mentioned Ludwig Türck (1810–1868). Türck was a quiet and modest physician who made a number of contributions to neurology and neuro-anatomy and had a particular interest in the spinal cord. He noted that the direction of tract degeneration corresponded to the direction of conduction, which led to a number of clinical observations based on this principle. He outlined six tracts in the spinal cord; the anterior corticospinal tract bears his name. He described the syndrome of hemisection of the cord, now attributed to Brown-Séquard.[56] His observations on the spinal cord have been described as a major medical contribution of the 19th century but were essentially ignored. His last years were devoted to studies of laryngology, and he may have been the inventor of the laryngoscope.[57]

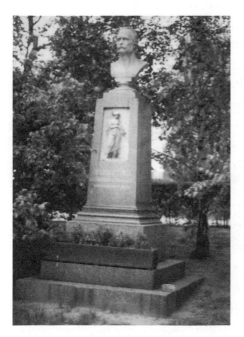

Figure 4.13   Statue to Türck. (Courtesy of Dr. Neil MacIntyre.)

CARL ROKITANSKY
(1804–1878)

Understanding of specific diseases was greatly aided by the use of the microscope and the development of staining techniques. A contributor of important observations was Carl Rokitansky (1804–1878), who carefully investigated the microscopic pathology of neurologic diseases while working at the Institute of Pathology in Vienna. A Bohemian who became professor of pathology, he was also a psychiatrist who worked in mental institutions. He was responsible for Vienna's revival as a medical center because of his enthusiasm for anatomical dissection and pathological anatomy.[58] (He was said to have performed 30,000 to 100,000 autopsy dissections in his career.) He was one of the first to carefully examine MS lesions under the microscope. In 1846, Rokitansky published his *Handbuch der pathologischen anatomie* (trans. 1850),[59] with a description of the connective tissue within the spinal cord, which causes paraplegias. He confused some aspects with tabes dorsalis. He observed in 1857 that there were "fatty corpuscles"

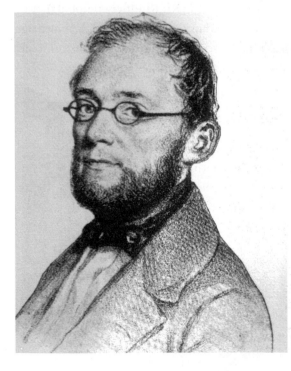

Figure 4.14 Carl Rokitansky (1804–1878) at the Institute of Pathology in Vienna was one of the first to examine the lesions of MS under the microscope. The lenses of microscopes gave poor resolution in those days, so the work was not easy. However, he was able to describe the "fatty corpuscles" in the areas of demyelination. (Courtesy of the National Library of Medicine.)

in the MS lesions, which Charcot later described as "the wreck and detritus resulting from the disintegration of the nerve-tubes."[60]

EDUARD RINDFLEISCH
(1836–1908)

In 1863, Eduard Rindfleisch (1836–1908), a student of Virchow, noted the consistent location of a blood vessel in the center of MS plaques.[61] He showed changes in the blood vessels and nerve elements secondary to inflammation combined with hyperemia. This was an important observation, although it was rejected by Charcot a few years later. Rindfleisch noted perivascular cell infiltrations and fatty changes in the neuroglia. He postulated the need to search for a primary cause of the disease in an alteration of individual blood vessels and their ramifications, where he felt the inflammation originated. The vascular relationship became a focus of attention for the next century. The argument was made that inflammation is the process that initiates a lesion in MS and that argument is important in current discussions of the origin of lesions seen on the MRI. Rindfleisch noted that the disease was more common in women and usually had its onset between ages 20 and 25. He felt the disease could be precipitated by damp and cold, injury, emotional stress, prolonged worry, or an acute illness.

LEYDEN, VON ZENKER, AND FROMMANN

In 1863, E. Leyden summarized the understanding of MS. He collected 34 cases of MS and showed that the condition we now call multiple sclerosis and "chronic myelitis" were the same condition.[62] He confirmed that women were attacked more often than men, and gave the proportion as 2.5 to 1 (25 to 9), about the same ratio seen in today's MS clinics. He also recorded onset as between ages 20 and 25. Leyden also noted that one of his cases was hereditary. He felt that the cause was related to acute illness, exposure to dampness and cold, and concussions of the body, but that psychic effects such as sudden fright or prolonged worry were important in producing the disease. The prognosis seemed to be unfavorable, although in some acute cases, moderate or even complete recovery occurred.

Two others mentioned by Charcot as contributing to the under-standing of MS were Friedrich Albert von Zenker and Carl Frommann. Charcot particularly referred to Frommann, who examined a small sec-tion of the spinal cord and published a rich and remarkably well-illus-trated book in 1864.[63,64]

EDMÉ VULPIAN
(1826–1887)

Edmé Félix Alfred Vulpian (1826–1887) first used the term "sclerose en plaque disseminée" in 1866.[65] He brought three cases before the *Societé Medicale* of the Paris hospitals. Vulpian is listed as the author and carried out most of the discussion, but two of the three cases were presented by Charcot. One of these patients, Mme. V., was "bequeathed" to Charcot, when Vulpian left the Salpêtrière, and Charcot later presented her case in his famous 1868 lesson.

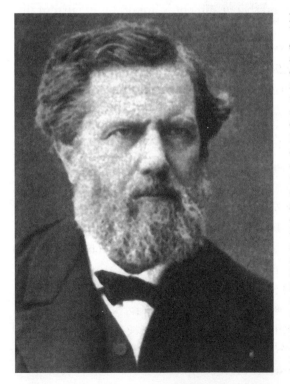

Figure 4.15 Edmé Félix Alfred Vulpian (1826–1887) was appoint-ed to the Salpêtrière the same year as Charcot, and they worked closely together in the early 1860s, making major contributions to the understanding of multiple sclero-sis. Vulpian then succeeded Curveilhier as Professor of Pathological Anatomy, and went on to describe the principles of degeneration and regeneration in the nervous system, the principles of the sudomotor and vasomotor apparatus, the chromaffin system of the superrenals, and the action of curare, strychnine, pilocarpine, anesthetics, and nicotine on the nervous system. He regretted that French medicine was not explor-ing the importance of microscopy as were the Germans, and he made important contributions by experimentation and microscopy. (From the collection of Dr. Maurice Genty, Académe de Medicine, Paris, France.)

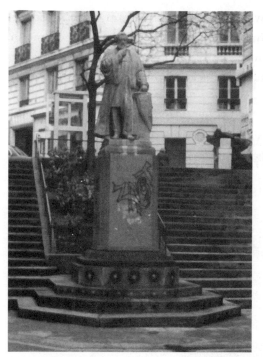

Figure 4.16 Statue of Vulpian, painted each spring by the medical students in blue and red. (Courtesy of Dr. Neil MacIntyre.)

Although the long shadow of Charcot was prominent in French neurology as well as in the history of MS, Charcot himself accorded appropriate credit for elucidating the nature of MS to Vulpian, who was not only a contemporary but a close friend and collaborator. They were appointed the same year to the Salpêtrière. Vulpian replaced Cruveilhier in the chair of Pathological Anatomy, an appointment that was made over violent opposition because of his writings on the higher functions of the brain, which had been criticized by clerics and conservatives.[66] Those who wrote on the function of the brain in the 19th century were at risk of censure (or worse) from the Church.

Vulpian was a careful experimenter and lamented that microscopy was not given as much attention in France as in Germany. He was an influential clinician-scientist who published 225 papers.[67] His stone statue in the rue Antoine Dubois, next to the École de Médecine in Paris notes his contributions, including his work on the description of MS. Vulpian was the intellectual leader of his day, influencing many clinicians and clinical fields, but the broad range of his interests caused him to be eclipsed by those with a more focused view, such as Charcot and Déjerine, who concentrated on the nervous system early in their careers.

J.C. MORRIS AND S. WEIR MITCHELL

The first American report of what is now recognized as MS was presented by J.C. Morris on December 4, 1867 to the College of Physicians of Philadelphia, and published the next year, with pathology carried out by S. Weir Mitchell (1829–1914), who is sometimes referred to as the "father

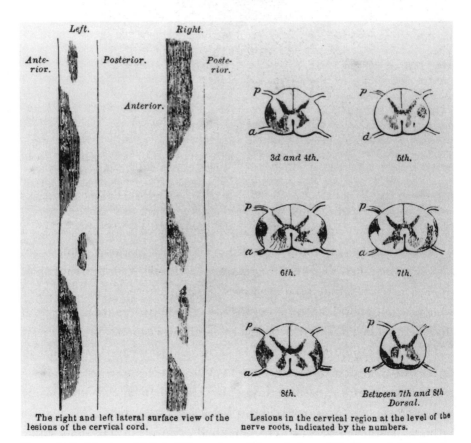

The right and left lateral surface view of the lesions of the cervical cord.

Lesions in the cervical region at the level of the nerve roots, indicated by the numbers.

Figure 4.17 Morris and Mitchell illustrations of the pathology of Dr. Pennock. Morris presented and published the case, with the pathology carried out by S. Weir Mitchell. Views of the left and right lateral surfaces of the cervical portion of the cord show a number of lesions. Views on the right are of horizontal sections of the cervical portions of the spinal cord with the level of the nerve roots numbered, with numerous lesions. This case was published the same year that Charcot gave his famous leçon on the disease. (Morris, 1868)

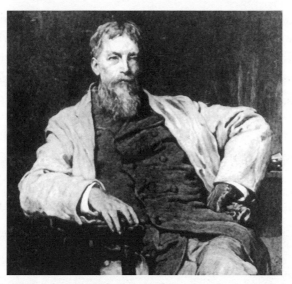

Figure 4.18   Silas Weir Mitchell (1829–1914) is often referred to as the "father of American neurology," and if fame, impact, talent, creativity and productivity are the measure, then this is appropriate. He did the autopsy and detailed neuropathology on Dr. Pennock, who died of a progressive neurological disease. In the year that Charcot presented his lesson on multiple sclerosis, Morris presented the case and later published the appearance of scattered lesions throughout the nervous system. Morris and Mitchell did not name the condition or even speculate on its nature, and were not aware of the description by Charcot. Painted by Frank Hall, engraved by T. Johnson.

of American neurology."[68] The case was that of C.W. Pennock, a Philadelphia physician, graduate of the University of Philadelphia, who later studied in Paris. Dr. Pennock noted symptoms of heaviness and numbness of his left and later right leg in 1843; his weakness progressed so much that he had to cease the practice of medicine in 1849. He noted that his symptoms always worsened when the weather was warm. By 1853, he was unable to walk, he then developed progressive weakness of his left and right arm and hand, to the point that he could not feed himself. He was alert and positive throughout the course of his disease, to the end of his life. He developed urinary retention and died in 1867.

Silas Weir Mitchell noted the irregular grey translucent spots in the cervical and dorsal spinal cord, mainly in the white matter, and particularly in the lateral columns. Under the microscope, he saw a total absence of nerve tubes and nerve cells in these lesions, small globules of fat, and numerous degenerated fibres.

Morris and Mitchell were not aware that they were describing the same disease reported by the French clinicians and classified by Charcot that same year. They suggested no cause for the disease and had no references to other literature on similar conditions. They merely presented the puzzling case, well reported.

REFERENCES

1. Porter D, Porter R. *Patient's Progress: Doctors and Doctoring in Eighteenth-Century England*. Stanford, CA: Stanford University Press; 1989:4.
2. Ollivier CP. *De la Moelle Epiniére et de ses Maladies*. Paris: Crevot; 1824.
3. Spillane JD. *The Doctrine of the Nerves*. Oxford, New York: Oxford University Press; 1981.
4. Ollivier CP. *De la Moelle Epiniére et de ses Maladies*, Paris: Crevot, 1824.
5. Ollivier CP. *Traité de la Moelle Epinière et de ses Maladies, Contenant L'Histoire Anatomique, Physiologique et Pathologique de Centre Nerveau Chez l'Homme*. Paris: Crevot; 1827.
6. Ebers GC. A Historical Overview. In: *Multiple Sclerosis*. Paty DW, and Ebers G, eds. Philadelphia: F.A. Davis; 1998:1-4.
7. Spillane JD. *The Doctrine of the Nerves*, p. 102.
8. Firth D. *The Case of Augustus d'Esté*. Cambridge: Cambridge University Press; 1948:p. 43.
9. Bright R. *Report of Clinical Cases*. London: Longmans; 1831: Case (cixxviii).
10. Ibid, Case ccciii.
11. Carswell R. *Pathological Anatomy: Illustrations of the Elementary Forms of Disease*. London: Longman, Orme, Brown, Green and Longman; 1838.
12. Hannaway C, La Berge A, eds. *Constructing Paris Medicine*. Clio Medica 50. Wellcome Institute Series in the History of Medicine; 1998:143-144.
13. Jacna LS, Carswell R, and Thompson W, at the Hôtel Dieu of Lyon: Scottish views of French Medicine: In: *British Medicine in an Age of Reform*. French R, Wear A, eds. London, New York: Routledge; 1991:110-155.
14. Hooper R. *Illustrated by Colored Engravings of the Most Frequent and Important Organic Diseases to Which that Viscus is the Subject*. London: Longman, Rees, Orme, Brown and Longman; 1828.
15. Jacna LS. Robert Carswell and William Thompson, p. 110-155.
16. Ibid.
17. Cameron GR. Robert Carswell, Pathologist. *Univ Coll Hosp Mag*. 1951;136:10.
18. Hook and Norman 1991, p. 144.
19. Putnam TJ. The centenary of multiple sclerosis. *Arch Neurol Psych*. 1938;40(4):806-813.
20. Compston A. The story of multiple sclerosis. *McAlpine's Multiple Sclerosis*. London: Churchill Livingstone; 1998: p. 3-42.
21. Compston A. *The Story of Multiple Sclerosis*. Chapter 1 in *McAlpine's Multiple Sclerosis*. London: Churchill Livingstone, 1998, p. 3-42.
22. Putnam TJ. The Centenary of Multiple Sclerosis. *Arch Neurol Psych*. 1938;40(4):806-813.
23. Carswell Papers, Edinburgh University Library, MS Gen. 590 and 59.
24. Putnam TJ. Centenary of Multiple Sclerosis. *Arch Neurol Psych*. 1938;40(4):806-813.
25. Carswell R. An inquiry on the chemical solution or digestion of the coats of the stomach after death, with some observation of softening, erosion and perforation of the stomach in man and animals. *Edin Med Surg J*. 1830;34:282-311.

26. Carswell R. *Pathological Anatomy: Illustrations of the Elementary Forms of Disease*. London: Longman, Orme, Brown, Green and Longman; 1838.
27. Spillane JD. *The Doctrine of the Nerves*. Oxford, New York: Oxford University Press; 1981.
28. Osler W. *Bibliotheca Osleriana*. Montreal, London: McGill-Queens Press; 1969:206-207.
29. Cruveilhier J. *Medical Tracts*. 1828. Wellcome Library. 621.4.
30. Compston A. The 150th anniversary of the first depiction of the lesions of multiple sclerosis. *J Neurol Neurosurg Psychiatry* 1988;51:1249-1252.
31. Compston A. The 150th anniversary of the first depiction of the lesions of multiple sclerosis. *J Neurol Neurosurg Psychiatry* 1988;51:1249-1252.
32. Courville CB. Jean Curveilhier. In: *Founders of Neurology*. Webb, H. (Eds). Springfield, IL: Charles C Thomas; 1953:172.
33. Charcot JM. *Lectures on the Diseases of the Nervous System Delivered at la Salpêtrière*. Sigerson G, ed. and trans. London: New Sydenham Society; 1877.
34. Compston A. The 150th anniversary of the first depiction of the lesions of multiple sclerosis. *J Neurol Neurosurg Psychiatry* 1988;51:1249-1252.
35. Putnam TJ. The Centenary of Multiple Sclerosis. *Arch Neurol Psych*. 1938;40(4):806-813.
36. Cruveilhier J. *Anatomie pathologique du corps humain*. Paris: J.B. Baillière; 1829-1842. (Individual livraisons in this work appeared separately but livraisons 32 and 38, both of which deal with MS, also can be found in Volume 2, published in 1842. In the Wellcome Library, a number of copies exist, bound differently. In Copy 2, the two illustrations of MS are found in Planches V, "Anatomie de l'appareil des sensations et l'innervation".)
37. Cruveilhier J. *Anatomie pathologique du corps humain, ou descriptions avec figures lithographiees et coloriées, des diverses altérations morbides dont le corps humain est suceptible*. Vol 2. Paris: J.B. Baillière; 1835-1842.
38. Hall M. *On the Diseases and Derangements of the Nervous System*. London: Baillière; 1841.
39. Keppel-Hesselink JM. Een Monografie van KFH Marx uit, 1938: Mogelijk de eerste Klinisch-Pathologische Beschrijving van Multipele Sclerose. *Ned Tijdschr Geneeskd*. 1991;135:2439-2443.
40. Charcot JM. Lectures on the diseases of the nervous system delivered at Salpêtrière. Sigurdson G. Edition, London, New Sydenham Society 1877.
41. Cruveilhier J. *Anatomie pathologique du corps humain*. Paris: J.B. Baillière, 1829-42. (Individual livraisons in this work appeared separately but Livraisons 32 and 38, both of which deal with MS, also can be found in Volume 2, published in 1842. In the Wellcome Library a number of copies can be found, bound differently. In Copy 2, the two illustrations of MS are found in Planches V, Anatomie de l'appareil des sensations et l'innervation.)
42. Compston A. The 150th anniversary of the first depiction of the lesions of multiple sclerosis. *J Neurol Neurosurg Psychiatry* 1988;51:1249-1252.
43. Compston A. *The Story of Multiple Sclerosis*, p. 1-10.
44. McHenry L. *Garrison's History of Neurology*. Springfield: C.C. Thomas; 1969:253-254.
45. Hooper R. *Illustrated by Colored Engravings of the Most Frequent and Important Organic Diseases to Which that Viscus is the Subject*. London: Longman, Rees, Orme, Brown and Longman; 1828.
46. Abercrombie J. *Pathological and Practical Researches and the Spinal Cord*. Philadelphia: Carey, Lea and Blanchard; 1838:334-335.
47. Compston A. The 150th anniversary, p. 1249-1252.
48. Hall M. *On the Diseases and Derangements of the Nervous System*. London: Baillière; 1841.
49. Romberg MH. *Lehrbuch der Nervenkrankheiten des Menschen*. Berlin: A. Duncker; 1846.
50. Romberg MH. *A Manual of the Nervous Diseases of Man*. Sieveking EH, trans. Vol 1. London: Sydenham Society; 1853.

51. Keppel-Hesselink JM, Koehler PJ. *Romberg's Sign in Neurological Eponyms*. Kochler P, Bruyn G, Pearce J, eds. Oxford: Oxford University Press; 2000:166-171.

52. Frerich FT. Ueber hirnsklerose. *Arch für die Gesamte Medizin*. 1849;10:334-350.

53. Bourneville DM, Guérard I. *De la sclérose en plaques disseminées*. Paris: Delahaye; 1869.

54. Valentiner W. Ueber die Sklerose des Gehirns und Rückenmarks. *Deutsche Klin*. 1856;147-151, 158-162, 167-169.

55. Frerich FT. Ueber Hirnsklerose. *Arch für die Gesamte Medizin*. 1849;10:334-350.

56. Türck is quoted by Kinnier Wilson. *Neurology*. Bruce AN, ed. London: Edward Arnold; 1940:148-178.

57. Haymaker W. *The Founders of Neurology*. Springfield, IL: Charles C. Thomas; 1953:92-95.

58. Rokitansky C. In: *Bericht der Akademie der Wissenschaft zu Wien 24* (1857). (Cited by Charcot 1868, 1877).

59. Rokitansky C. *Hanbuch der pathologischen anatomie*. Braumuller and Seidel; 1846.

60. Rokitansky C. *A Manual of Pathological Anatomy*. Moore, trans. London: The New Sydenham Society; 1850.

61. Rindfleisch E. Histologische Detail zu der Grauen Degeneration von Gehirn and Rückenmark. *Virchow Arch Path Anat Physiol*. 1863;26:474-483.

62. Leyden E. Ueber graue degeneration des Rückenmarks. *Deutsche Klin*. 1863;15:121-128.

63. Charcot JM. *Histologie de la sclérose en plaques*. Paris: Gaz Hôp Civils Milit. 1868;41:554-568.

64. Frommann C. *Untersuchungen über die Gewebsverän-derungen bei der multiplen Sklerose des Cehirns und Rückenmarks*. Jena; 1878.

65. Vulpian EFA. *Note sur la sclérose en plaques de la moelle épinière*. Union Méd 1866;30:459-465, 475-482, 541-548.

66. Haymaker W. *The Founders of Neurology*. Springfield, IL: Charles C. Thomas; 1953.

67. Ibid, p. 158-161.

68. Morris JC. Case of the late Dr. CW Pennock. *Am J Med Sci*. 1868;56:138-144.

C h a p t e r

5

The Building Blocks
of a Discovery

INFLUENCE AND CONSILIENCE

Few, if any, great events or discoveries happen *de novo*—the lone researcher excitedly exiting the laboratory anxious to tell someone of a new finding, discovery, or idea. Most major discoveries in medicine were steps in a regular progression, made by various people. When we examine a "discovery," we frequently find a long history of development of ideas and small advances, with many contributors, from many fields, over many decades or centuries. We often associate the "discovery" with a point in that history, sometimes arbitrarily. We may remember only a few of the many contributors, ascribing the "discovery" to one person at one time, as if it had happened suddenly. Just as often in the growing steps of knowledge building, we recognize someone who came later and made the concept familiar, rather than the person who originated it. We will see all this in the steps to understanding and clarifying the disease of multiple sclerosis (MS).

We may well ask why the concept of a disease like MS becomes defined as a clinical entity at a certain time in the history of medicine. As we will indicate in the history of MS, it is a confluence of influences—increasing interest in separating and classifying diseases and syndromes;

application of anatomical knowledge to the pathology of disease; the professionalization of neurologists; increasing interest in differentiating diseases into specific entities; the post-Revolution development of the Paris school that brought the teaching of medicine into hospitals and to the bedside; the increasing use of microscopes and staining methods to learn about tissue and cellular changes in disease; the refining of clinical and laboratory definitions of disease that further aided the concepts and the framing of diseases; the globalization of medical education, with trainees coming to Paris from America, England, and other countries; and the recognition of leaders and innovators of medical thought. When Charcot gave his eloquent outline of the features of MS in 1868, it was a point in time with roots in these influences.*[1]

The "discovery" of MS is often dated to the series of lectures by Charcot in 1868, but even he gave a respectful nod to people who had contributed to the understanding of MS and had described it previously.† This coming together of knowledge from many people and many fields was called "consilience" (the "jumping" together of knowledge), by E.O. Wilson, and characterizes the growing body of knowledge on multiple sclerosis.[2]

THE STEPS BEFORE CHARCOT'S LEÇON

The process begins with the changes in French, English, and German medicine at the turn of the 18th century. Identifying, separating, and classifying disease occupied Duchenne, Charcot, Vulpian, and the other French clinicians, but this process had been encouraged in the previous century by William Cullen, who pleaded with physicians to use the methods of the botanists in classifying the plant and animal world. Victor McKusick used the terms "lumpers and splitters" in the mid-20th century, but the splitters reached a high point with the French physicians a century earlier and continued to work worldwide for the next century.

---

*Walter Timme (1950) reviewed the history of understanding of the spinal cord and the ideas of paraplegia from Galen in the 3rd century to the views of Bichat and LeGallois in the early years of the 19th century.

†Some have noted that his respectful nod was more in the direction of his countrymen. However, he noted the previous contributions of Cruveilhier, Carswell, Frerichs, Türck, Rokitansky, Rindfleisch, Leyden, and of course his close colleague Vulpian.

In keeping with ideals of the Revolution, there was a dramatic change in French medical education in 1794 that saw the old faculties abolished, and the rise of the three *Écoles de Santé* in Paris, Montpellier, and Strasbourg. Medical teaching moved away from academics and the influence of the Church and into hospitals. A 1790 decree required all patients in large hospitals to be assessed by physicians to determine if they should be freed or confined. The Hôpital Géneral, founded in 1656, held 6,000 people, mostly the poor, insane, prisoners, beggars, and social outcasts. Almost one percent of the population had been in these institutions, which were originally not hospitals, but huge buildings that confined them and confirmed their outcast status. Foucault said communities increasingly became afraid of those who were ill, outcasts, or in some way different and were more comfortable if these people were removed from the community and confined.[3] Initially physicians played no role in these human warehouses, but with the 1790 decree and the work of physician-reformer Phillipe Pinel (1745–1825), this began to change.

Physicians began to play a central role in the admission of patients, classifying them as medically ill or insane, and issuing medical certificates.[4] Now salaried clinical teachers were based in these huge institutions with access to unprecedented numbers of patients for teaching and research. The teaching was in hands-on clinics with real-life problems, taught by physicians caring for them. Following discussions, the physician and his entourage would move to the dead house to see how illnesses in patients previously assessed could be explained by the changes in their organs, and by the tissues under the microscope.

Another change was that surgeons took the same initial training and degree as physicians.[5] Paris medicine rapidly advanced, and the "Paris School" gained a reputation throughout the world, leading the transformation from the confusion of the 18th century toward a more modern scientific medicine based on clinical observation of disease correlated with findings in the autopsy room.* The antecedents of post-Revolution medicine developed in Leyden, Edinburgh, London, and Vienna. A

---

*Although changes in French medicine are identified with physicians, Gelfand wrote that much of the dynamic change actually came from a progressive surgical profession, which was innovative and sparked interest in localism, while the physicians were initially slower to change.

major change in the course of medicine was underway, one that would lead to the classification and framing of the specific condition of the nervous system we now know as MS. Though anatomic pathology and clinico-pathologic correlation characterized the dramatic rise of the Paris School, we should not forget that the process did not begin in Paris, but in Britain after 1750 with the work of Matthew Baillie, James Smyth and the school of John Hunter, Charles Bell, Astley Cooper, Benjamin Brodie, and John Abercrombie.[6] Abercrombie's book on diseases of the brain and spinal cord was widely read in Britain even before the work of Carswell and Hodgkin.[7] The French were influenced by these works, just as the English and others learned from the strong influence of the French in the early part of the 19th century.

The early 19th century was an era when pathology moved from localism in organs, represented by the work of Morgagni, to the 19th-century focus on tissues, fostered by Bichat.[8] It is likely that Bichat's work sprang from ideas first advanced by Smyth, then adopted by Philippe Pinel, who influenced Bichat. Little happens *de novo*, but credit often goes to the person who grasps the concept best, puts it forward, and makes it known.

As the historian Erwin Ackerknecht said, medicine began to pull itself out of the confusion of 18th-century empirical theories and systems, as "the Baron von Münchausen pulled himself out of the swamp by tugging on his own pigtails."[9] Myth-making about the Paris School may have served political and personal agendas,[10] but certainly because of developments in Paris, many factors converged on the day in 1868 when Charcot delivered his lectures that outlined the clinical and pathological characteristics of the disease he called *sclérose en plaque disseminée*.

Various approaches advanced Paris as the center of medical training; leaders included Phillipe Pinel (1745–1826); Xavier Bichat (1771–1826); René Laennec (1781–1821); Jean-Baptise Bouillard (1796–1881); and Pierre Louis (1787–1872). The fame of the Paris School also grew because of the self-promotion of professors. Many physicians from abroad came to study and returned to their countries repeating the message that Paris medicine was superior. Paris afforded the chance to see large numbers of patients on the wards and in the clinics and to follow them to the autop-

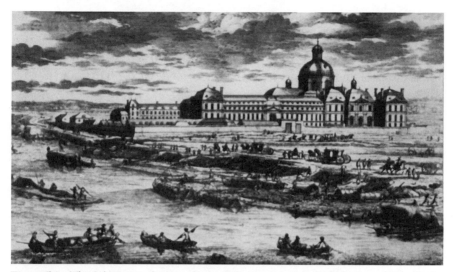

Figure 5.1   The Salpêtrière, the great hospital, became a center for French neurology in the mid-19th century. Originally a munitions factory, when it endangered the neighbors with explosions, it was converted to a prison, then an almshouse, and finally a retreat for old women. When Charcot and Vulpian were appointed to the staff, there were 5,000 souls residing there, and they set about assessing and classifying their disorders. (Courtesy of the Wellcome Library, London.)

sy room, to hear great teachers lecture, while getting hands-on teaching and experience from private instruction available from hospital interns.[11] Great personal and professional cachét was attached to studying in Paris.

Initially the diversity of opinions and innovative professional approaches in Paris caused excitement and stimulated discovery, but soon many pursued their own course, with little collaboration or sharing of ideas, arguing, and forming factions.[12] By the mid-19th century, the rise of German laboratory science rivaled the primacy of French medicine. Paris medicine still attracted physicians from abroad, and had slowly adapted the microscope to the autopsy examination of pathology. In contrast, Charcot made effective collaborations and great use of the microscope to elucidate pathology in the nervous system. Michel Foucault described Paris clinics where the "invisible was made visible,"[13] an art in which Charcot and his contemporaries came to excel.

By the 1850s when Charcot and Vulpian entered medicine, the French began to lose their place as leaders in medical advances to science and laboratory approaches led by the Germans. Slowness in accepting the developing microscopy may have contributed to loss of leadership by the Paris School after 1850; technique with less-than-satisfactory early microscopes and their poor lenses was difficult and seemed to detract from the importance of clinical observation. Even Cruveilhier could not accept the microscope. But there were many scientists enthusiastic about the technique and a number of these would become important in the defining of MS.[14]

Although Ackerknecht suggested that French medicine had maneuvered itself into a dead end by 1848,[15] this was not an abrupt end; some aspects of French medicine continued to flourish. What Ackerknecht called the young Paris School (Paul Broca, Charles Edouard Brown-Séquard, Edmé Félix Vulpian, and Jean-Martin Charcot) were active and influential in the 1850s and 1860s. But German science and laboratory medicine was on the ascendant. Although students still came to Paris, a period of study in that city no longer conferred special distinction. It was now fashionable to study in Berlin or Vienna, where exciting developments in medicine were occurring.[16] Warner points out that students had come to Paris in droves, not just for academic brilliance, but because they had access to patients and clinical resources. English-speaking physicians from Great Britain and North America who might have gone to London, could not find the same access to clinical material there. Consultants carefully managed their private clientele, and the hospitals, unlike the government-supported hospitals of Paris, were private institutions tightly controlled by appointed boards.[17]

The features of the Paris School were focused on: clinical correlation and pathologic anatomy; developments in clinical examination to supplement the history; collection of similar observations on large series of patients; teaching and research in hospitals; and use of statistics.[18] All of these played a role in separating MS from the confusing array of neurologic symptoms that were still mostly undifferentiated and unnamed. Just as the French School was being surpassed by German medicine at the half century, Charcot and his colleagues arrived and continued to make great strides in using clinico-pathologic correlation, to clarify such neurological disorders as MS, amyotrophic lateral sclerosis, muscular dystrophies, locomotor ataxia, and stroke.

Many published their observations on the condition of MS, and some, such as Rindflesich and Leyden, had a clear sense of the clinical and pathologic picture. So why was Charcot able to bring the picture to the fore? The Germans capitalized on the insights brought to pathologic examination, and were all beginning to work with the new stains, such as carmine. Even though many of the French were slow to adopt the microscope, Charcot and Vulpian utilized it fully. Moreover, Charcot had the huge resources of the Salpêtrière to help him explore his neurological interests. This was not the case for the Germans, who tended to have smaller clinics, often private ones, for their work. The 5,000 souls inhabiting the Salpêtrière not only were available for assessment and classification, but were followed by Charcot in a filing system permitting him to keep a record of their condition over a long period. He added notes to the file over the years until the subjects died, and then he could carry out detailed autopsy examination with microscopic examination of the tissues using the new stains, to correlate the clinical picture with the pathology. He called this method the *anatomo-clinique* process, an extension of the process developed by Hunter, Smythe, and Bell, and fostered by earlier French workers. Charcot also focused his efforts on the nervous system after 1868, and was able to make many contributions because of his long-term commitment to assessing patients with neurologic illness. After a medical career initially focused on rheumatologic disease, by 1868, Charcot was a neurologist.

Charcot was fortunate to live in an era when science and the Republic glorified one another, and he was ideally situated geographically in a medical capital imbued with positivism and an unquestioned assumption of progress through science. Charcot was not alone to succeed in this environment, but utilized it to his advantage more perhaps than several other important contemporaries.[19]

REFERENCES

1. Timme W. Multiple Sclerosis: Historical Retrospect. In: ARNMD II (1921). *Multiple Sclerosis*. Paul B Hoeber. Pages 1-8.
2. Wilson EO. *Consilience: The Unity of Knowledge*. New York: Alfred A. Knopf; 1998.
3. Foucault M. *Madness and Civilization*. London: Tavistock Publications: 1969.

4. Hannaway C, La Berge A, eds. *Constructing Paris Medicine*. Clio Medica 50: Wellcome Institute Series in the History of Medicine; 1998:143-144.
5. Gelfand T. Charcot's Brains. *Brain Language*. 1999;69(Aug):31-55.
6. Keel O. Was anatomical and tissue pathology a product of the Paris clinical school or not? In: *Constructing Paris Medicine*. Hannaway C, La Berge A, eds. Clio Medica 50: Wellcome Institute Series in the History of Medicine; 1998:117-184.
7. Ibid, p. 119.
8. Ibid, p. 120-122.
9. Ackernecht E. *Medicine at the Paris Hospitals, 1794-1848*. Baltimore: Johns Hopkins Press; 1967.
10. Hannaway C, La Berge A, eds. *Constructing Paris Medicine*. 1998:143-144.
11. Warner JH. Paradigm Lost or Paradigm Declining? American physicians and the "Dead End" of the Paris clinical school. *Constructing Paris Medicine*. Hannaway C, La Berge A, eds. Clio Medica 50: Wellcome Institute Series in the History of Medicine; 1998:337-384.
12. Ibid, p. 354-367.
13. Foucault M. *Madness and Civilization*. London: Tavistock Publications; 1969.
14. Hannaway C, La Berge A, eds. *Constructing Paris Medicine*. Clio Medica 50: Wellcome Institute Series in the History of Medicine; 1998;143-144.
15. Ackernecht E. *Medicine at the Paris Hospitals, 1794-1848*. Baltimore: Johns Hopkins Press; 1967.
16. Warner JH. *Paradigm Lost or Paradigm Declining?* p. 359-367.
17. Jacna LS. Robert Carswell and William Thompson at the Hôtel Dieu of Lyon: Scottish views of French Medicine. In: *British Medicine in an Age of Reform*. French R, Wear A, eds. London, New York: Routledge; 1991:110-155.
18. Hannaway C, La Berge A, eds. *Constructing Paris Medicine*. Clio Medica 50. Wellcome Institute Series in the History of Medicine; 1998:143-144.
19. Goetz CG, Bonduelle M, Gelfand T. *Charcot: Constructing Neurology*. New York: Oxford University Press;1995:330.

6

The Contribution of J.M. Charcot—1868

"To Dr. Charcot unquestionably belongs the credit of distinguishing this condition from other paralytic disorders and notably from paralysis agitans, of recognizing the pathological features, and tracing its clinical history."

Dr. Meredith Clymer, New York, 1870[1]

"Only within comparatively modern times has the disease been picked out of the medley of spinal paraplegias."

S.A. Kinnear Wilson, 1940[2]

"A disease does not exist as a social phenomenon until we agree that it does—until it is named."

Charles Rosenberg, 1992[3]

Until the 19th century, many manifestations of illness were grouped according to the way they presented—as headache, tremor, blindness, or paralysis, or as more general phenomena, such as dropsy, gout, rheumatism, or inflammation. These were broad classifications that incorporated many forms of illness, and we miss the richness of those diagnoses when we reinterpret them in our much more specific modern classification. For instance, dropsy was not only what we now diagnose as right heart failure, and gout was not only a form of arthritis characterized by uric acid crystals in joints. Gouty disease covered many clinical scenarios and could take on forms such as "flying gout."

As medicine began to become more reductionist in the examination of illness, it also looked more broadly, to see how illness related to society, the environment, social policy, and patterns in population and geographical regions. Virchow had the unusual ability to wear both lenses as he viewed disease, while others focused on one approach or the other.

The Paris physicians adopted the adage of Pierre Cabanis (1757–1808) who said, "read little, see much, do much," and the enthusiasm of Bichat, who wanted to explain the patient's years of symptoms by cutting into the organs at death ("look and see"). They had the unique opportunity to do so because of the huge hospitalized population of as yet unclassified and unexamined individuals. Paris had 20,000 beds, which

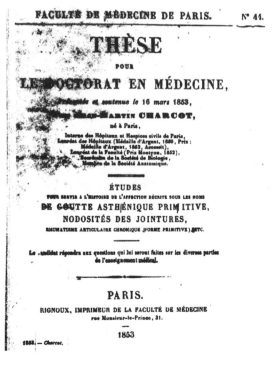

Figure 6.1 Charcot's medical thesis on rheumatological disorders (1853) rated "extrêmement satisfait" by the examiners.

outnumbered the inpatient population of all of England at the time.[4] The Salpêtrière itself, had first 2,000, then 3,000, and later, when Jean-Martin Charcot arrived as a physician, 5,000 souls languishing within its walls.

Jean-Martin Charcot was born in Paris in November 1825, the son of a coach builder. One brother took over the family business, two went into the military, but Jean-Martin wished to pursue medicine. We know little of his childhood except that he preferred to be alone to read and draw pictures.* He was the oldest of four boys and the parents decided the one who performed best in his studies at Lycée Bonaparte should go on for further education. Jean-Martin did best. His brothers agreed with the choice and assisted him in his studies, keeping his study room warm with a hot cannon ball in a bucket of sand. Charcot was educated at the Lycée Bonaparte and the University of Paris. During his medical studies, he was influenced by Professor Rayer, the Dean of Medical Studies and Instructor in Pathology, who taught him that a clinician's skill is only as good as his skill as a pathologist.[5,6]

Charcot's initial attempt in 1847 to secure an internship post, a highly prized and competitive position, failed; but the next year, he was recommended. While completing his four-year internship at the Salpêtrière in 1853, he wrote his doctoral thesis on the differentiation of rheumatoid and gouty arthritis, an early indication of his ability to observe, separate, classify, and characterize clinical conditions.[7] For the next two years, he was a physician in the Faculty of Medicine and then in the municipal hospitals of Paris. He failed in the competitive examinations of the Agrégation for the appointment as Professor Agrége in 1857 as he was nervous during the oral presentation of his thesis on *The Expectations of Medicine*. He was more successful in 1860.

Guillaume Benjamin Armand Duchenne (1806–1875), 19 years senior to the young Charcot, arrived in Paris with no forseeable opportunities, just as Charcot was appointed to the Salpêtrière. Duchenne had studied with Dupuytren, Laënnec, and Magendie. Charcot admired his work, referring to Duchenne as his master in neurology. Duchenne had

---

*Many of his early drawings were donated to the Salpêtrière by his son Jean (1867–1936) who was a reluctant physician, later became an explorer, and lost his life on an exploration.

Why Did Charcot become a Neurologist?

There is little evidence in the early work of Charcot that he had much inter-est in the nervous system, certainly less than in rheumatological disease, where he made original contributions, and in diseases of the aged, pul-monary and thyroid disease. Capildeo suggests his interest was stimulated by the arrival in Paris of a dejected and rejected Armand Duchenne.[8]

settled in Boulogne after his Paris medical studies and became interested in the electrical stimulation of muscles, publishing a book on the subject in 1855. Then his wife died and his in-laws refused to allow him to see his only son. He came to Paris, only to find the hospital closed to him and his electrical studies on muscle ridiculed by clinicians. Charcot, on the other hand, did all he could to help the older physician, providing him with

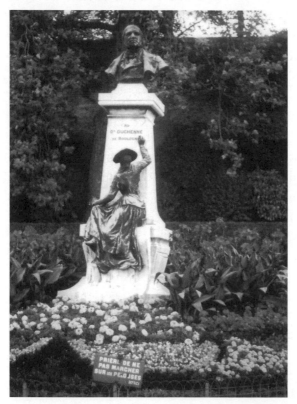

Figure 6.2 Duchenne Statue. (Courtesy of Dr. Neil MacIntyre.)

research facilities and access to his patients to continue work. As so often happens in a close teacher–student relationship, they taught each other, Duchenne teaching Charcot photography and methods to study the nervous system and muscles, and Charcot teaching Duchenne his way of doing clinico-pathologic correlations and histology. Duchenne made many important contributions over the next 13 years before his fatal stroke, and while Charcot always provided support, he never claimed any return or credit for Duchenne's observations. As Capildeo points out, despite their close and mutually supportive work, there is no Duchenne-Charcot disease, or Charcot-Duchenne syndrome.[9]

When Charcot took up his position at the Salpêtrière with his colleague Edmé Vulpian, they looked around and saw an opportunity—to assess and study, follow and classify the sea of human misery. Among the many disorders they began to study and record was the neurological disorder characterized by scattered lesions in the nervous system that had been seen by Carswell, Cruveilhier, Rindfleisch, Türck, Leyden, and others. Initially Charcot had few private patients, but access to a huge number of inmates in the hospital. He began to study patients carefully, keeping notes on them in a file and later following them to the autopsy room when they died, developing his technique of correlating the clinical picture with the pathology at death, a process he called *système anatomo-clinique*. Using an abandoned kitchen for his laboratory and pathology teaching space, he attracted increasing numbers of students and he began the series of free lectures that were later published; these made him known internationally.

One of the diseases he and Vulpian studied was a peculiar disorder that caused tremor; they thought it could be differentiated from the paralysis agitans described by James Parkinson in 1817. Their initial objective was to show that the tremors were different, but over the next few years, Vulpian and Charcot had a few cases that they thought represented a distinct condition. The disease they framed was *sclérose en plaque disseminée*, disseminated sclerosis, later to be called multiple sclerosis (MS). As we have seen, many previous clinicians described and knew features of the disease and its pathology, but to Charcot goes the credit for outlining the clinical and pathological features with great clarity, and for

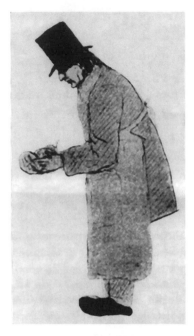

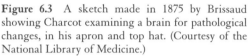

Figure 6.3 A sketch made in 1875 by Brissaud showing Charcot examining a brain for pathological changes, in his apron and top hat. (Courtesy of the National Library of Medicine.)

making the condition known. In the history of medicine and science, the credit usually (and perhaps appropriately) goes to the person who makes a discovery known rather than to the person who may actually have made the discovery first.

According to D.M. Bourneville and I. Guerard, students of Charcot and the authors of the first monograph on MS, Charcot first became aware of the disease in 1855 when he asked a woman who had some motor problems to serve as his housemaid. He thought she had neurosyphilis. She broke many dishes as her condition slowly worsened. Charcot was able to follow the course of disseminated sclerosis by watching her symptoms over the years. When she became too ill to function on her own, he arranged for her to be admitted to the Salpêtrière and when she died, he examined her brain and spinal cord. Although he expected to see the changes of syphilis, he saw instead scattered plaques throughout the nervous system.[10]

On May 9, 1866, Vulpian and Charcot gave a report on the clinical features and autopsy findings of three cases of *sclérose en plaque disseminée* to the Societé Médicale des Hôpitaux. Vulpian described one case and

Charcot presented two. Vulpian managed most of the discussion of these cases. When the presentation was published, Vulpian was listed as the sole author, but indicated that Charcot had presented to the society previously (March 8, 1865)[11] on sclerosis of the lateral columns.[12]

In 1868, Charcot gave a lecture before the Societé de Biologie on the characteristics of disseminated sclerosis; he indicated that it was not usually recognized clinically, but had distinct neurologic and pathologic features. He differentiated the picture from that of Parkinson's disease. He published this lecture and another report on the histology of MS the same year, clearly defining the features of this disorder.[13] Naturally, the patients he described all had advanced signs of the disease, but over the next few years, Charcot was able to study cases earlier in the course of the disease.[14–16]

Although he began pursuing the differentiation of the tremor of this disorder from that of paralysis agitans (Parkinson's disease),*[17] Charcot soon initiated additional studies of the disease, its clinical features, variations, and pathologic features, making his own drawings of the changes he saw under the microscope. He recognized the nature of transient symptoms in the disease and the possibility of remissions. He was able to

Hôpital de Salpêtrière

"This great asylum (of human misery) holds a population of 5,000 persons, among whom are a large number who have been admitted for life as incurables; patients of all ages, affected by chronic diseases of all kinds, but particularly by diseases of the nervous system. There are numerous examples of the clinical types available for study, which enables us to study a specific disease during its entire course, so to speak, since the vacancies that occur in any specific disease are quickly filled in the course of time. We are, in other words, in possession of a sort of museum of living pathology of great resources."

Jean-Martin Charcot

---

*It was Charcot who began to call this disease after James Parkinson, for he objected to the word "paralysis," which he did not think characteristic of the condition. It was only in the 20th century, with the encouragement of a visiting American physician, that the English commonly used the eponym that recognized the contribution of their countryman.

classify the presentations into spinal and cerebral forms and noted the late appearance of amyotrophy. At the time he gave his increasingly popular lectures, Charcot had been a physician at the Salpêtrière for six years.

Early in his career, Charcot was intensely interested in the rheumatic disorders, pulmonary disease, and other medical conditions; when he was appointed a physician at the Salpêtrière in 1862, he had more independence to explore his own directions. With the influence of Duchenne and the collaboration of Vulpian, these studies began to focus on diseases of the nervous system. It had been almost a decade of struggle since his thesis and the appointment to a major hospital position that finally gave him access to a large patient base.

Serious and dispassionate, with a slow pattern of speaking, at this point he was almost indistinguishable from his competitive contemporaries. A methodical, analytical clinician with a capacity to bring others to work with him, Charcot now had access to a huge institution filled with every manner of neurologic and mental disease. The institution was organized to house and care for patients, but Charcot and Vulpian set about assessing, organizing, and classifying the conditions that brought them there. Many of Charcot's publications up to this time were on a variety of medical diseases, but by 1868, he made a major shift to the nervous system in his interest, publications, and lectures.

George Guillain, Charcot's early biographer,[18,19] said that the next eight years at the Salpêtrière were the most important of Charcot's life. During this time, he produced work and ideas that keep his name alive today.*[20] This confusion of mostly undiagnosed diseased humanity was an opportunity for Vulpian and Charcot methodically to assess cases and try to classify each into a recognizable category, bringing order to disarray.[21,22] Most of the inmates were elderly women, and the year Charcot and Vulpian began there, 2,635 of them were regarded as "indigents and non-insane epileptics."[23] The experience of Charcot and Vulpian in

---

*Much of the brilliant neurological description done by Charcot was in the period 1862–1870; his reputation was based on these eight years, after which his work was interrupted by the Franco-Prussian War and the Commune of Paris. He sent his family to live in England and daily crossed the barricades to do his work at the Salpêtrière. During the period 1870–1880, he pursued his interest in cerebral localization and aphasia and after 1880, he concentrated on hysteria. This latter work engendered both admiration and criticism.

La Salpêtrière

The Salpêtrière (from saltpeter, an ingredient in gunpowder) was originally a munitions factory and arsenal. Explosions in the building upset nearby merchants and residents and a petition to King Louis XIII had the arsenal moved to another site, leaving the building to be converted to a hospice for the care of sick women; men were cared for at the Bicêtre. More buildings, eventually a hundred, were added so that the original 800 inhabitants grew to 2,000, then 3,000 and at the time Charcot arrived, 5,000 poor, insane, epileptic, sick, elderly, and demented people who could no longer be accommodated by their families and communities. Philippe Pinel changed the attitude to many of these confined and disturbed women by removing shackles and chains from 49 of them and allowing them to walk in the institution's gardens and courtyards.

rheumatologic, medical, and neurological conditions helped them identify many disorders in those areas. The two began to examine and classify each person, building a file on each case; the file was expanded with later observations and finally with the autopsy.[24] An approach of clinico-pathologic observation was developing, to build the clinical picture and complement it with pathological findings. This differed from the anatomic pathology approach, which focused on the pathology of the disease. Charcot directed his attention to the precise clinical nature of the disease, complementing this with the pathology.

Paris medicine began to pale in comparison against German laboratory science because of the slowness and resistance of Parisian professors to the microscope and laboratory methods, coupled with their tendency to go their own way, not collaborating or cooperating with colleagues. This attitude was not a characteristic of Charcot, who had a close and productive collaboration with Vulpian and many others, including his students. They used the microscope to understand the pathology of the diseases they explored. Charcot's collaboration with Vulpian was so well known, that medical student Mary Putnam Jacobi mentioned in her diary a humorous comment in the medical press that when Charcot's first son was born, there was surprise that this wasn't another Charcot-Vulpian joint production.

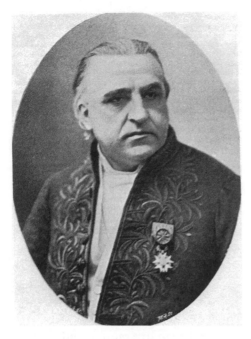

Figure 6.4 Jean-Martin Charcot held the first professorship of neurology, which was created for him at the Salpêtrière in 1882. (Courtesy of the National Library of Medicine.)

In the period between his presentation of cases of MS with Vulpian in 1866, and the lesson on the disease in 1868, Charcot applied for a professorship when two chairs became available. For the first chair, he received no votes against the competitors and for the second post only a few, placing last in the competition.*[25] Vulpian was appointed a professor in 1868, but Charcot waited four more years to be appointed professor of anatomical pathology.

THE LESSONS ON "LA SCLÉROSE EN PLAQUE DISSÉMINÉES"

Perhaps the most important step in addressing any disease is the clear delineation of the disorder, separating it from other similar sounding conditions, so that it can be more clearly recognized, understood,

---

*This was not an unexpected outcome, as he was junior, and these very prestigious posts went to those with seniority, reputations, and political friends. Vulpian fared much better, but he had twice as many publications, an impressive record in physiology, and contributions in many fields, whereas Charcot was concentrating on clinical observations.

researched, and managed, cured, or prevented. Charcot did this for MS in "a strikingly modern account"[26] in his 1868 lessons.

In the lesson 6, Charcot described a disease occurring in three forms: spinal, cephalic or bulbar, and combined cerebro-spinal, which corresponded to the anatomical area involved. The forms had corresponding symptoms and signs.[27–31]

Charcot's Lectures on Multiple Sclerosis: 1868

Lecture VI—Disseminated Sclerosis: pathological anatomy

Lecture VII—Disseminated Sclerosis: its symptomatology

Lecture VIII—Apoplectiform seizures in disseminated sclerosis. Periods and forms. Pathological Physiology. Etiology. Treatment

---

In his second lecture (lesson 7), Charcot discussed the tremor of MS, the cephalic symptoms, lightening pains, and the way the legs were affected by the disease. He mentioned that it was not rare in this disease to find symptoms similar to tabes dorsalis, such as shooting pains. When that occurred, he had often subsequently found characteristic plaques within the posterior columns of the spinal cord. He described the cephalic and bulbar symptoms of nystagmus, diplopia, amblyopia, difficulty with speech, and intellectual change. He noted that memory change may occur, including slowness in forming concepts and blunting of intellectual and emotional faculties. Patients might be indifferent to their circumstances, he said, but they might also demonstrate unexpected laughter or crying for no reason. Charcot recognized that patients could have a posterior column form of ataxia, and experience girdle pain from spinal cord involvement. He outlined the clinical appearance of intention tremor, nystagmus, and scanning speech as three reliable indicators of the disorder (these would later be called the Charcot triad). This was an age that saw the beginning of the artistry of neurologic examination, with refinements in the patient's history, physical examination, and the understanding of the patient's complaints in terms of involvement of specific areas of the nervous system. Charcot's description showed he was a master of this approach.

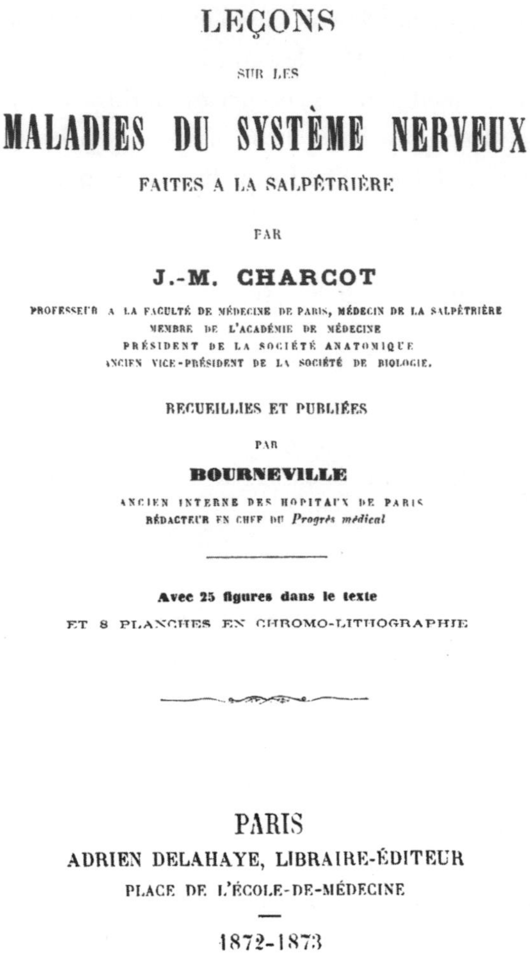

LEÇONS

SUR LES

MALADIES DU SYSTÈME NERVEUX

FAITES A LA SALPÊTRIÈRE

PAR

J.-M. CHARCOT

PROFESSEUR A LA FACULTÉ DE MÉDECINE DE PARIS, MÉDECIN DE LA SALPÊTRIÈRE
MEMBRE DE L'ACADÉMIE DE MÉDECINE
PRÉSIDENT DE LA SOCIÉTÉ ANATOMIQUE
ANCIEN VICE-PRÉSIDENT DE LA SOCIÉTÉ DE BIOLOGIE.

RECUEILLIES ET PUBLIÉES

PAR

BOURNEVILLE

ANCIEN INTERNE DES HOPITAUX DE PARIS
RÉDACTEUR EN CHEF DU *Progrès médical*

Avec 25 figures dans le texte
ET 8 PLANCHES EN CHROMO-LITHOGRAPHIE

Figure 6.5 Frontispiece of Charcot's Maladies du Système Nerveux, lectures collected and published by his student, Bourneville in 1972–1873. It was immediately recognized by those interested in the nervous system throughout the medical world, even before the New Sydenham Society translation into English by George Sigerson in 1881. (Courtesy of the Wellcome Library, London.)

PARIS
ADRIEN DELAHAYE, LIBRAIRE-ÉDITEUR
PLACE DE L'ÉCOLE-DE-MÉDECINE
—
1872-1873

During the 1860s, Charcot and Vulpian had studied the pathology of cases of MS, using a carmine stain to show that myelin was specifically destroyed, with relative preservation of the axons. They noted that the plaques initially looked grey to the naked eye, but in the open air, took on a rosy hue. Charcot did his own drawings of the microscopic anatomy of the plaques and the disruption of myelin. He made drawings of the evidence of fatty corpuscles (macrophages) surrounding an area of inflammation in an MS plaque and removing the breakdown products. He insisted that there was evidence of change in the axis cylinder in the plaques, but felt these alterations did not mean the axons were destroyed.

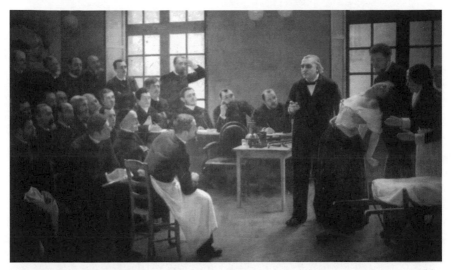

Figure 6.6   Charcot giving one of his famous Tuesday clinical demonstrations, as painted by Louis Brouillet's "A Clinical Lession at the Salpêtrière," displayed at the Paris Salon in 1887. It shows him discussing the hysteric Blance Wittman who is swooning, held by Joseph Babinski. Among the physicians, politicians, medical administrators, writers, and hospital staff are Pierre Marie, Gilles de la Tourette, Charcot's son Jean, D.M. Bournville, H. Perinaud, and A. Goumbault. Many interested members of the public and artistic community, as well as local and visiting physicians would attend these dramatic and carefully planned demonstrations. Other visitors included Guy de Maupassant and Sarah Barnhart. Freud was often said to be in the picture, perhaps because of his resemblance to many of the bearded men. Although he often attended these demonstrations, he is not in the painting. (Erich Lessing/Art Resource, NY.)

This would explain the absence of secondary degeneration, either of an ascending or descending nature in the cortico-spinal tracts. This observation of axonal change became a major focus of attention in the closing years of the 20th century.

In lesson 8, Charcot discussed the possibility of sudden, acute, "apoplectiform" attacks of MS, many in the presence of infection. These were seen in a fifth of the cases in his experience. Although the "fit" might be temporary, there was usually some persistent aggravation of the condition afterwards. He personally observed this in three cases, not associated with fever, which had been seen by Vulpian, Zenker, and Léo. Many physicians believed this to be due to *partial sanguine congestion*, but Charcot, in his usual direct approach to observation, said he followed these cases to autopsy and could find no evidence of vascular congestion

Charcot's Triad

Intention Tremor

"... the tremor ... only manifests itself on the occasion of intentional movements of some extent; it ceases to exist when the muscles are abandoned to complete repose."

Nystagmus

"Nystagmus is a symptom of sufficiently great importance in diagnosis, since it is to be met with in about half the number of cases."

Scanning Speech

"There is a symptom more frequently found than nystagmus ... and this is a peculiar difficulty in enunciation ... The affected person speaks in a slow, drawling manner, and sometimes almost unintelligibly. It seems as if the tongue had become 'too thick', and the delivery recalls that of an individual suffering from incipient intoxication. A closer examination shows that the words are as if measured or scanned; there is a pause after every syllable, and the syllables themselves are pronounced slowly."

Jean-Martin Charcot, 1868[32]

on examination of the tissues. As he said, this was another example where believing a theory did not make it reality.

In lesson 8, Charcot also discussed the three periods of progression, and the pathophysiology, etiology, prognosis, and treatment of the disease. The first period might have only a few of the features of the disease, spinal manifestation being the most common, although cephalic-bulbar symptoms such as dizziness, diplopia, and nystagmus might also occur. Remissions were not uncommon and this gave rise to hope for a decided cure so that the person might resume his or her occupation. The second period had more diverse symptoms and was usually ushered in by leg weakness and "contractures." The patient became paralyzed and even bedbound. In the third stage, the disease manifested as a progressive and debilitated condition with mental changes, even dementia, speech

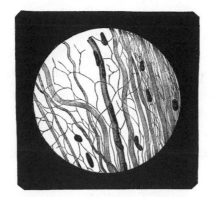

FIG. 9 represents a fresh preparation, taken from the centre of a patch of sclerosis, coloured with carmine, and dilacerated. In the centre is seen a capillary vessel, supporting several nuclei. To the right and left of this are axis-cylinders, some voluminous, others of very small diameter, and all deprived of their medullary sheaths. The capillary vessel and the axis-cylinders were vividly coloured by the carmine ; the axis-cylinders present perfectly smooth borders, without ramification. Between them are seen slender fibrillæ of recent formation, which form on the left and in the centre a sort of network resulting from the entanglement or anastomosis of the fibrils. These are distinguished from the axis-cylinders, 1° by their diameter, which is much smaller ; 2° by the ramifications which they present in their course ; 3° by taking no coloration from carmine. Nuclei are seen scattered about ; some of them appear to be in connection with the connective fibrils ; others have assumed an irregular form, owing to the action of the ammoniacal solution of carmine.

Figure 6.7 This hand-drawn illustration by Charcot is of a carmine stained area in the center of a patch of sclerosis. In the center is a capillary, and around it are demyelinated axons. Connective fibrils can be seen running between the axons. Charcot noted that in the middle of a plaque the axons have diminished and have become thinned, and although he felt the loss of myelin with "persistence" of axons was a unique feature of this disease, he referred to it as "indefinite persistence." From the translation of J-M Charcot's *Lectures on Diseases of the Nervous System (Figure 9)* by the New Sydenham Society, 1881. (Courtesy of the Wellcome Library, London.)

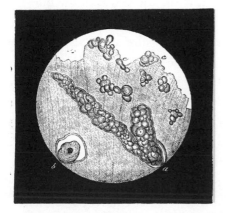

FIG. 10.—Patch of sclerosis in the fresh state: *a*, lymphatic sheath of a vessel distended by voluminous fatty globules ; *b*, a vessel divided transversely. The adventitious coat is separated from the lymphatic sheath by a free space, the fatty globules which distended the sheath having disappeared ; *cc*, fatty globules, gathered into small groups, dispersed here and there over the preparation.

Figure 6.8 Charcot's hand-drawn picture of "voluminous fatty globules" around a vessel, the result of myelin breakdown and eventual removal of the fatty residue of the myelin sheath. (From the translation of J-M Charcot's *Lectures on Diseases of the Nervous System (Figure 10)* by the New Sydenham Society, 1881. (Courtesy of the Wellcome Library, London.)

involvement to the point of unintelligible grunting, sphincter paralysis, bladder inflammation, pressure sores, and death soon after, often brought on by infection.

Charcot then detailed the case history of Josephine Vauthier, a patient of Vulpian's (Mme. V), the subject of the preceding lecture, who succumbed in this fashion. Then he discussed one of his cases, Pauline Bezot, a children's nurse. His lecture contains drawings of the pathology of these cases, showing loss of myelin, diminished numbers of axons in the plaques, and thickening and obstruction of the small blood vessels.

Charcot noted that abortive forms (*forme frustes*) are common in MS, so that there might be only cerebral symptoms, but more commonly, there might be spinal symptoms of the disease, as if the process of advancing sclerosis were fixed in one area. The most common picture encountered in practice, however, was the cerebro-spinal form, with signs of a widespread involvement.

Charcot confined himself to summary points on pathophysiology, etiology, prognosis, and treatment, indicating that knowledge on these subjects was scanty and imperfect. The cause of the disease is unknown, he said, and the suggestion by Rindfleisch that it is due to inflammation in the blood vessels seen in the center of the sclerotic patches only sets the question of cause a little further back. If the cause was in the blood vessels, then what was the cause of the abnormality in the blood vessels? Indeed, from his observations Charcot was unsure of the vascular abnormality. He felt it might be possible to relate the location of the patches to the symptoms in the patient, and gave a suggested locale for various symptoms. He speculated on how the disruption of the medullary sheathing of the axis cylinders (the axons) could still allow conduction along the nerves to continue, even if it did so irregularly, "in a broken or jerky manner," to produce the irregular tremor.

Now that there is so much interest in the role of axonal damage in the progression of MS, many reflect on the fact that Charcot was interested in this question. He realized that the axon had great resistance to the inflammatory damage breaking down the myelin, but also felt that if the axons were finally damaged, the disease would permanently progress:

"Generally one of the lower limbs is first and solely affected. The other limb is seized, sooner or later, in its turn; the paresis advances with extreme slowness ... but at last the day comes when ... they may be

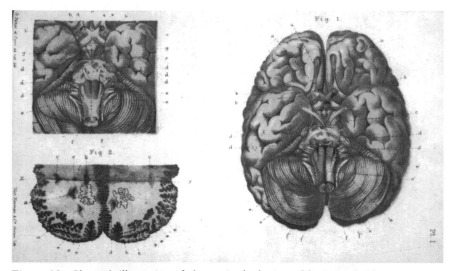

Figure 6.9   Charcot's illustration of plaques in the brain and brain stem. Plaques are seen scattered over the pons and medulla and Circle of Willis and cerebellum showing plaques of demyelination in the base of the brain and in a horizontal section of the cerebellum. From the translation of J-M Charcot's *Lectures on Diseases of the Nervous System (Plate 1)* by the New Sydenham Society, 1881. (Courtesy of the Wellcome Library, London.)

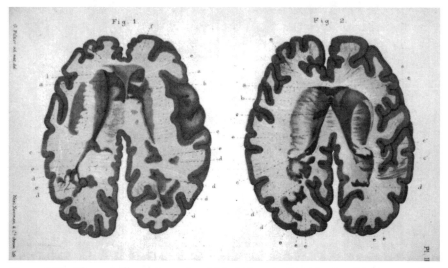

Figure 6.10   Charcot's illustrations of multiple lesions scattered in the white matter of the brain, particularly around the ventricles. From the translation of J-M Charcot's *Lectures on Diseases of the Nervous System (Plate 2)* by the New Sydenham Society, 1881. (Courtesy of the Wellcome Library, London.)

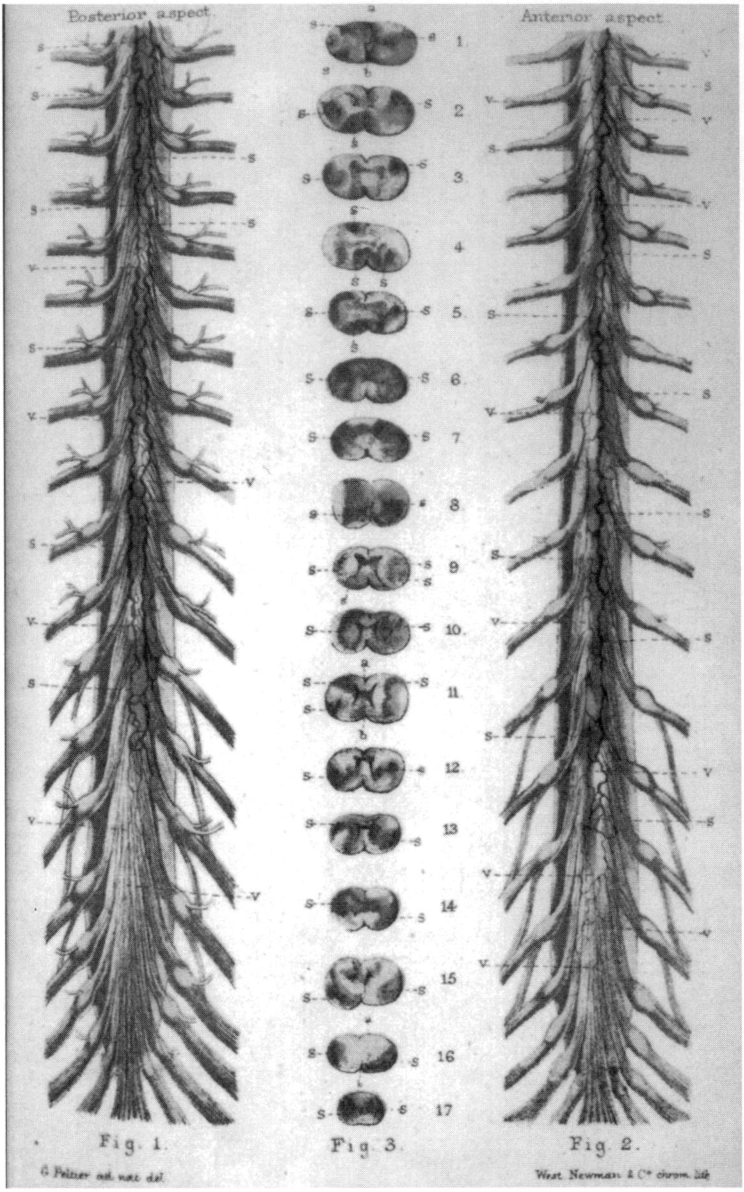

Figure 6.11 Charcot's illustration of plaques in the posterior and anterior spinal cord in his *Lectures on Diseases of the Nervous System*. These are seen as darker patches on the longitudinal views of the cord and in the horizontal sections. From the translation of J-M Charcot's *Lectures on Diseases of the Nervous System (Plate 3)* by the New Sydenham Society, 1881. (Courtesy of the Wellcome Library, London.)

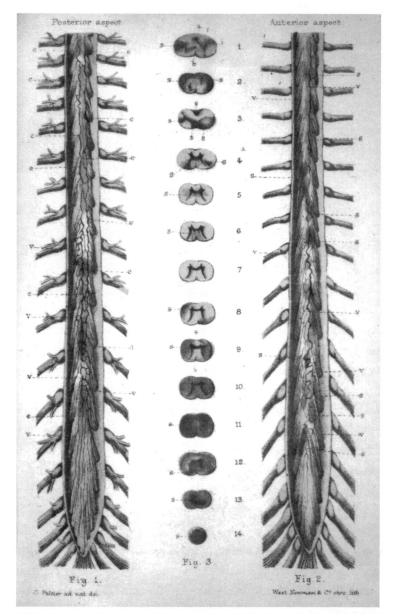

Figure 6.12   Charcot's illustration of plaques in the posterior and anterior spinal cord in his *Lectures on Diseases of the Nervous System*. These are seen as darker patches on the longitudinal views of the cord and in the horizontal sections. From the translation of J-M Charcot's *Lectures on Diseases of the Nervous System (Plate 4)* by the New Sydenham Society, 1881. (Courtesy of the Wellcome Library, London.)

confined to bed. . . . This resistance of the axis cylinders . . . may account for the slowness with which the paretic symptoms advance in disseminated sclerosis and for the long space of time which relapses before they give place to complete paralysis and permanent contracture."

Charcot related the sclerotic lesions in the nervous system to the symptoms experienced, and demonstrated that the features were also distinctive enough to separate *sclérose en plaque* from paralysis agitans, syphylitic disease of the nervous system, Friedreich's ataxia, locomotor ataxia, and chorea. The tremor was different in paralysis agitans. The vertigo present in three-fourths of his sclerosis patients was not usual in paralysis agitans or locomotor ataxia. Sclerotic patients did not have the involuntary jerky sudden movements at rest seen in chorea. Charcot also felt that patients with MS had a particular facial appearance and attitude, with a vague uncertain look, drooping lips, a lethargic look, and emotional lability. Intermittent episodes of symptoms with improvement was a feature of MS. Then there would be progression, spasticity, and spasms with contractures in the terminal stages. Charcot considered the disease a primary form of inflammation affecting the neuroglia, a separate and distinct disease with cerebrospinal, cerebral, and spinal forms, based on the anatomical level most involved in the symptomatology of the patient.

In later writings and lectures, Charcot acknowledged that little was known about the cause of the MS, but that it was most common in females. He said that combining his 18 cases (published in the monograph of Bourneville and Guérard),[34] with 16 new cases, there was a ratio of 25 females to nine males. Multiple sclerosis might develop by age 14, but is most common between 25 and 30 years.* Patients seldom live beyond 40, he thought. As to heredity, he knew of only one suggestive case, an example communicated by Duchenne. Certain infections (typhoid, cholera, smallpox), moist cold, and trauma were related to onset in certain cases.

---

*In a footnote, Charcot referred to a case report in German literature by Leubé (1870) of a girl with onset of multiple sclerosis at age 7, who died at age 14; autopsy confirmed the disease. Childhood reports are common in the early literature of MS due to inclusion of other diseases in the case series.

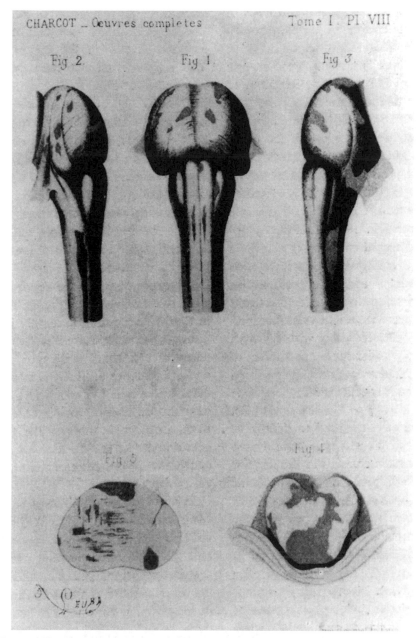

Figure 6.13   Charcot's drawings of three views of the pons showing lesions of multiple sclerosis on the exterior and cross sections of the medulla and pons below. (Bournville, 1892.)

Even though Charcot confessed that he did not know the cause of the disease, patients often referred to issues related to "moral order," such as grief, anger, illicit pregnancy, and the stresses of a false social position. For some reason, he suggested this was especially so in female teachers. In males, MS might relate to loss of caste, having been thrown out of the general social current, and the experience of not being able to cope with the problems of life.

As to outcome, Charcot briefly and somberly concluded: "The prognosis has hitherto been of the gloomiest."

He was no more cheerful on the issue of treatment:

"After what preceded, need I detain you long over the question of treatment? The time has not yet come when such a subject can be seriously considered. I can only tell you of some experiments which I have tried, the results of which, unfortunately, have not been very encouraging."

Charcot stated that little could be done to alter the disease, but therapies were still being applied. In his experience, chloride of gold and phosphate of zinc seemed to aggravate the disease. Strychnine and nitrate of silver had only a transient effect on tremor, and the silver nitrate was contraindicated in advanced spinal involvement, which it might worsen. He noted that hydropathy gave transient benefit in one case, and worsened another. Arsenic, belladonna, ergot of rye, and bromide of potassium, as well as faradic and galvanic stimulation had no effect, although Charcot said it might be necessary to wait for further experience with continuous current before making a firm conclusion on that technique. Although he did not comment on it in his section on therapy, his "suspension apparatus" used at the Salpêtrière, adapted from the inventor Dr. Motchoukowski of Odessa, was later used in cases of ataxia, including MS. Patients thought to have "hysterical signs" were treated with ovarian compression belts.[35]

In lecture 15 on spasmodic tabes dorsalis, Charcot indicated the clinical similarity between spasmodic tabes dorsalis and disseminated sclerosis. He pointed out that MS in its typical widespread form is not difficult to identify, but that "imperfect forms or abortive forms" were a different

question. He mentioned that the legs can become quite involved and contracted, with preservation of the arms, but even if this occurred, there
were often other "cephalic symptoms" such as nystagmus, diplopia,
speech difficulty, vertigo, apoplectiform attacks, and "special disorders of
the mind," which helped in distinguishing the disease. There still
remained some cases in which careful examination did not allow clear
differentiation. Charcot hoped that future clinical observations might
allow clearer demarcation of these neurological diseases.

As a footnote to this discussion, Charcot mentioned that one of the
patients previously exhibited as an example of spasmodic tabes dorsalis
had since died; autopsy did not confirm the diagnosis, "which, had been
given with qualifications." Autopsy showed existence of disseminated
sclerotic patches through the brain, brain stem, and spinal cord including
the posterior columns in the cervical area. Charcot mentioned that the
details of this case (the fourth in the thesis of M. Bétous), would be published later. On reflection, he felt that the history of this patient, the existence of cervical and dorsal lumbar pains, vertigo, an increase of paresis
of the limbs in darkness, and various other points would have indicated
the correct diagnosis of MS if more attention had been given.

After 1869, Charcot called attention to abortive forms of MS, and the
likelihood that instances of the disease would increase as these forms
were recognized, with the expectation that MS would be found to be
much more frequent in neurological practice. It is often said that Charcot
thought this was a rare disease, but we can see otherwise in this quote:

> *"In effect, among the vast array of symptom possibilities, none is
> spared and the picture of multiple sclerosis may be restricted to lower
> extremity contractures with or without rigidity of the upper extremi-
> ties (the spinal form described by Vulpian). In cases of this type, con-
> current or past abnormalities of so-called "cephalic" symptoms are the
> only ways to establish a decisive diagnosis. ... The illness of the spinal
> form is far from rare and beyond a doubt, many cases seen in practice
> and only vaguely categorized under the name "chronic myelitis"
> belong to the domain of multiple sclerosis. Consequently, this disease
> is expanding in incidence as diagnostic accuracy gains in precision."*

Charcot's contributions became even more widely known when his Leçons were published in 1872–1873, and translated in London and Philadelphia in 1877 (under the title *Lectures on the Diseases of the Nervous System*) by George Sigerson for the New Sydenham Society. Sigerson was Dublin's first neurologist and carried out a correspondence with Charcot. The woodcuts from his classic 1868 paper were published into this century and the pathology observations of Charcot served as "the textbooks of a generation." Little was added to them for a further 50 years.[36]

Although Charcot wrote 462 articles on various topics, he did not write much about MS. Many of his views on MS were disseminated through the writings of his pupils Bourneville and Guérard,[37] and by Ordenstein.[38] It was Charcot's habit to develop his notes for a lecture in great detail, and rehearse them to the point where he could dispense with the notes when he gave his lecture. Following the lecture, he would step from the stage and pass drafts for the lecture to an assistant, who was then charged with adapting them for publication.

CHARCOT'S STYLE OF WORK

Charcot's work habits were very organized. He made regular ward rounds, but seldom examined the cases on the wards. Each day, he spent three hours examining cases in his office, a small dark room illuminated by a single window. To add to the somber feeling, the room was painted completely black. On the wall was a single signed portrait of Hughlings Jackson.* The only furniture was a table and a few chairs, and a small wardrobe for his hat, coat, lab coat, and aprons.†[39]

Charcot's way of examining patients reveals much about his manner and method. He would sit silently at his table, listening attentively to the intern's history.

---

*It was Charcot who suggested the term "Jacksonian epilepsy" for the march of seizure involvement seen in this type of epilepsy described by Jackson.

†Fred Hoyle said that great discoveries were often made in rabbit hutches rather than in glass palaces.

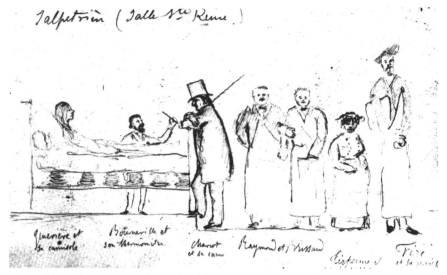

Figure 6.14   Charcot on ward rounds with his entourage, referred to as his charcoterie, a play on the word *charcuterie*, a butcher shop for pork products.

"Then there was a long silence, during which Charcot looked, kept looking at the patient while tapping his hand on the table. His assistants, standing close together, waited anxiously for a word of enlightenment. Charcot continued to remain silent. After a while he would request the patient to make a movement; he would induce him to speak; he would ask that his reflexes be examined and that sensory responses be tested. And then again silence. Finally he would call for a second patient, examine him like the first one, call for a third patient, and always without a word, silently make comparisons between them.

This type of meticulous clinical scrutiny, particularly of a visual type, was at the root of all Charcot's discoveries. The artist in him, who went hand in hand with the physician, played an interesting part in these discoveries."[40]

His students often referred to Charcot's "mysterious silences," during which he observed the patient, thinking, correlating, and seeing. He said:

"It is the mind which is really alive and sees things, yet it hardly sees anything without preliminary instruction."

"In the last analysis, we see only what we are ready to see, what we have been taught to see. We eliminate and ignore everything that is not part of our prejudices."

To his Tuesday clinics and carefully rehearsed Friday lectures, Charcot increasingly attracted admirers and students from abroad, enhancing the reputation of the Salpêtrière and French neurology.[41] Freud said that Charcot was not a great thinker, but had more the characteristics of an artist and was, as Charcot himself said, a "visuel," a man who sees. Despite the drama and excellence of his lectures and demonstrations, Charcot was not a great orator. He spoke slowly and methodically, using no notes, which had been put aside after careful study.

The process of Charcot's assessment of patients in his clinics, evident in how he presented them in his demonstrations, was to arrive at a diagnosis after a careful history, examination of signs on the patients, and observation of how they carried out movements or speech. Then the process would be localized within the nervous system and a demonstration of the pathology he felt to be the basis of the disorder followed. For some patients, assessment and recording of subsequent progress was kept in a file of notes that might extend over a prolonged period of observation in the hospital, and eventually to the autopsy room.

Charcot presented two or three cases in his Tuesday clinics, using a small stage in a miniature theater, complete with footlights and paraphernalia to create a dramatic effect. He gave marvelous displays of clinical skill and knowledge using numerous visual methods, including colored chalk drawings, photographs, slide projections, and plaster casts.[47,48] When the case had been presented, Charcot would project the pathologic and histologic features of the disease onto a screen at the back of the stage. With Albert Londe, he created a photographic studio that was annexed to the Anatomy and Pathology Museum.[42]

Charcot's lectures were attended by students, colleagues, visiting physicians, administrators, journalists, prominent Parisians, and businessmen. Guy de Maupassant (1850–1893) attended the lectures between 1884 and 1886 and in an article in "Une femme" in the periodical *Gil Blas*, commented that Charcot seemed to be "creating hysteria.* Maupassant wrote a novel, "La Horla," describing the intimate life of madness, from material he gathered listening to the medical presentations. Jane Aveil (1868–1943), a dancer at the Moulin Rouge, immortalized by Toulouse-Lautrec, was a patient on Charcot's service in 1892–1884 when he was involved in his studies and lectures on hysteria. Bonduelle and Gelfand said she was there to protect her from her mother's abuse. She later wrote about her time with the hysterics at the Salpêtrière.

Charcot's day was very structured. He was at his desk in his study early in the morning. At 9:00 a carriage took him to the Salpêtrière where he stayed until noon, when the carriage returned him home for an afternoon seeing private patients in his study. His consultation fee was 40 francs. The setting for his private patients in his opulent rooms was a major contrast to the plain black-walled room where he saw patients at the Salpêtrière.

CHARCOT THE MAN

Charcot married Augustine-Victoire Durvis, a young and wealthy widow who continually supported Charcot and protected her husband's privacy by fending off students and visitors who continually sought him out. His character is viewed differently by different individuals. Some said he affected the demeanor of an English country gentleman. Léon Daudet considered him timid and emotional,[43] but others saw him as solemn and withdrawn. Perhaps the most negative portrait is by Axel Munthe, who spent time at the Salpêtrière and described Charcot as domineering, with never a kind or encouraging word for students or

---

*The criticism that Charcot was "creating hysterics" was made by others as well, who suggested that his demonstrations of hysterical features in women who were repeatedly brought to his teaching sessions were inducing the phenomenon by suggestion. Blanche Whitman was the most famous of his patients used in demonstrations. She is the swooning woman in the famous painting of Charcot's teaching, and was said to be the "Reine dés hysteriques," the queen of hysterics. She would perform at demonstrations of hysteria at the Salpêtrière, where she was rude and disdainful of the staff. She later was admitted to the Hotel Dieu under Jules Janet and there was Blanche II, much more pleasant and compliant. She later returned to the Salpêtrière, but to work in the new photography department, and later in radiology, where she developed cancer, and after repeated amputations, died.

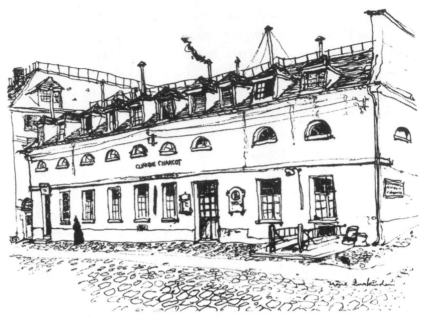

Figure 6.15 The Clinique Charcot at the Salpêtrière. (Courtesy of the National Library of Medicine.)

assistants, sensitive to criticism, and insensitive to the suffering of his patients. Munthe said Charcot had little interest in his patients in the period between diagnosis and the autopsy room, and although a phenomenal diagnostician in his heyday, he was too abrupt and brief in his assessments at the end of his career.[44,45]

Others were more impressed with Charcot. When writing to Martha Bernays, Sigmund Freud said about Charcot, "What I do know is that no other human being has ever affected me in the same way" and indicated that the brilliance of Charcot exhausted his mind, making him feel his attempts to understand phenomena were very small in comparison. Even though Charcot would occasionally rebuff Freud's approaches, Freud translated Charcot's writings on hysteria.[46] Freud wrote that Charcot was a very impressive, visual clinician, although "not a great man." He may have meant that Charcot was not an original deep thinker, but a brilliant observer.

CHARCOT'S LEGACY

Charcot's approach was the epitomé of the elegant combination of clinical science and pathologic correlation. He added to the understanding of MS, hyperthyroidism, hereditary amyloidosis, amyotrophic lateral sclerosis, intermittent claudication, diabetic gangrene, diseases characteristic in the elderly, and localization of cortical functions. With Bouchard, he published early papers on aphasia and important though controversial contributions to the understanding of hysteria. Capildeo says the reason Charcot's reputation came under a cloud was the hysteria controversy, which continued long after his death in arguments by his pupils and a new generation of psychoanalysts.[47] Perhaps that is why no Charcot biography was written until George Guillain's book in 1955, translated into English by Pearce Baillie in 1959.[48]

Charcot's dominance in the faculty also threatened Charles Bouchard, his former student and collaborator. When Bouchard became a professor, Charcot was senior and not well. Both were examiners for the Agrégation examinations and Charcot wanted his favorite student, Joseph Babinski, to succeed. Bouchard determined Babinski would not,

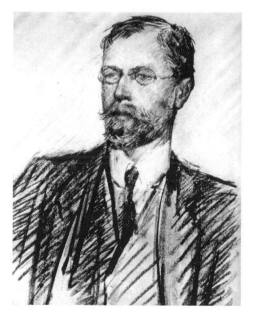

Figure 6.16 Axel Munthe was a young physician at the Salpêtrière who was banished from the hospital by Charcot for taking a young woman to his room. A fashionable physician, Munthe always called himself a neurologist. Munthe, in his hugely popular autobiography *The Story of San Michele*, says he was trying to return the woman to her family so that Charcot would not convert her into one of his hysterics. (Courtesy of the National Library of Medicine.)

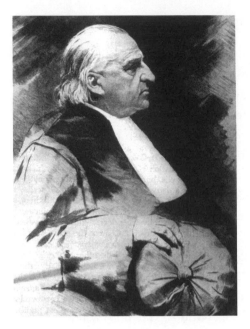

Figure 6.17 Jean-Martin Charcot (1825–1893) was admired as the first among French neurologists and physicians in an era that held physicians in much higher regard that in most countries. His great contribution was to have brilliantly "framed" the disease of multiple sclerosis, clearly outlining its clinical features, course, and pathology so that others could now diagnose it. With Vulpian, he was able to bring order to the assessment of the thousands of souls warehoused in the Salpêtrière. Even he would acknowledge that he was not the first to describe multiple sclerosis, but the credit should go to the man who makes it known. (From the collection of Dr. Maurice Genty, Académie de Médicine, Paris.)

and as a result, Babinski never achieved an academic appointment.* Charcot was hurt by the antagonism of Bouchard, but never spoke of it.

Although Charcot did not lead a scientific revolution as Pasteur did, or make the fundamental discoveries of Claude Bernard, he was internationally famous.[49] Goetz and others noted he was fortunate to live in a time when science and the Republic glorified each other. Not only was Charcot well situated to take advantage of this, but he did so better than his contemporaries.[50]

AFTER THE 1868 LECTURES

Over the decade following his lectures on MS, sporadic cases of MS appeared in the medical press in England, Australia, the United States, and Canada. These indicated the condition was now being more widely recognized and diagnosed. An early abbreviated translation of Charcot's work was produced by Thomas Oliver of Preston, with Charcot's per-

---

*This collaboration is remembered today by the interest in Charcot-Bouchard aneurysms as a basis for hypertensive hemorrhages.

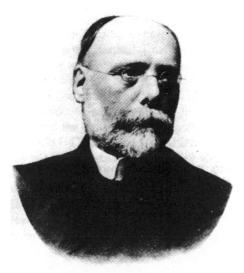

Figure 6.18 Charles Bouchard (1837–1915) studied under and later collaborated with Charcot, but when made a professor, he challenged the dominance of his teacher at the Salpêtrière. Bouchard prevented Babinski, Charcot's favored pupil, from being successful in the Aggrégation examination, a slight Charcot bore in silence. Babinski never received an academic appointment as a result. (Courtesy of the National Library of Medicine.)

mission, and published in *The Edinburgh Medical Journal*, 1875–1876, in two parts.[51] It was not a good translation but did convey Charcot's views to a wider English-speaking audience. Oliver said, "It is surprising that it has existed such a time without being noticed." He commented that the condition was not known in England, even though by the time of this translation, Moxon, in the Guy's *Hospital Reports* of that same year, had published cases anonymously, calling the disease "insular sclerosis."[52] Oliver abbreviated Charcot's lesson in many areas, including Charcot's introduction that stated he would differentiate two kinds of tremor. His translation begins with Charcot's historical note on Cruveilhier, giving him primacy in first depicting the disease.

Although physicians and neurologists from other countries spent time in France, and knew of Charcot's writings, the lessons became further known through a translation by George Sigerson for The New Sydenham Society in 1877.[53] Sigerson noted that his English translation was being published prior to the second French edition of Charcot's work and that publications that had appeared in the four years since the lectures were published included works by Timal,[54] Schüle,[55] Baldwin,[56] Buzzard,[57,58] and Moxon.[59]

In 1881, the French parliament established for Charcot a chair in diseases of the nervous system with a stipend of 200,000 francs. Charcot's

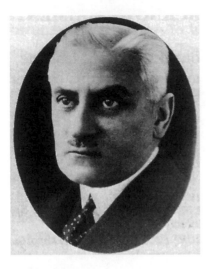

Figure 6.19 George Guillain (1876–1961) was the first biographer of Charcot. It is surprising that no biography appeared about this giant of the 19th century neurology until Guillain's book in 1955, translated into English by Pearce Baillie in 1959. (Courtesy of the National Library of Medicine.)

inaugural address made it clear that he and others had had difficulty getting space and support for their work from the university; it was this political support that gave them the ability to succeed with a neuropathologic institute.

An 1881 version of Sigerson's translation was republished in 1962 by the New York Academy of Medicine[60] with an introduction by Walther Riese. This edition contained four plates omitted from the earlier translation. This was the second series and did not contain lecture four on MS, but did contain the plates. Julius Althaus, senior physician to the Hospital for Epilepsy and Paralysis, Regent's Park, attempted to name the disease after Charcot, an eponym that did not hold.[61,62] Charcot continues to be identified with MS, and the term "Charcot's disease" was used up to 1921, but the eponym is more often used for amyotrophic lateral sclerosis, which he described in 1874.*

Charcot worked constantly, but still took time to enjoy life and his cigars, good food and wine, art, music, and theatre. He died of pulmonary complications of a heart ailment in 1893, mourned by his country and profession. A

---

*Eponymous syndromes always engender argument over who was "first." Many knew and wrote of multiple sclerosis before Charcot gave it a clear description. Amyotrophic lateral sclerosis (ALS), called Charcot's disease by some in the 19th century, was described earlier by Duchenne (1849), Aran (1850), and Cruveilhier (1853). ALS was also called Cruveilhier's disease, and the pattern with primarily muscle wasting, Aran-Duchenne type.

bronze statue of Charcot erected by students and colleagues at the entrance to the Salpêtrière, was melted down by the Germans in their occupation of Paris during World War II.

> *"[Charcot] was heard to say that the greatest satisfaction man can experience is to see something new, that is, to recognize it as new, and he constantly returned with the repeated observations to the subject of the difficulties and the value of such "seeing." He wondered how it happened that in the practice of medicine men could only see what they had already been taught to see; he described how wonderful it was suddenly to see new things—new diseases—though they were probably as old as the human race; he said that he often had to admit that he could now see many a thing which for thirty years in his wards he had ignored."*
>
> Sigmund Freud

> *"Let someone say of a doctor that he really knows his physiology or anatomy, that he is dynamic—these are not real compliments; but if you say he is an observer, a man who knows how to see, this is perhaps the greatest compliment one can make."*
>
> Jean-Martin Charcot

REFERENCES

1. Clymer M. Notes on the Physiology and Pathology of the Nervous System, with Reference to Clinical Medicine. *New York Med J*. 1870;60:225-260;410-423.
2. Wilson SAK. *Neurol*. Bruce AN, ed. London: Edward Arnold; 1940:148-178.
3. Rosenberg CE, Golden J, eds. *Framing Disease: Studies in Cultural History*. New Brunswick, NJ: Rutgers University Press; 1992:xiii-xxvi.
4. Porter R. *The Greatest Benefit to Mankind*. New York: WW Norton; 1997:495-497.
5. Guillain GJM. *Charcot (1825–1893): sa vie—son oeuvre*. Paris: Masson; 1955.
6. Guillain GJM. *Charcot 1825–1893. His life—his work*. Bailey P, ed-trans. London: Pitman Medical; 1959.
7. Lellouch A. Charcot, Découvreur de maladies. *Rev Neurol*. 1994;150:506-510.
8. Capildeo R. Charcot in the 80s. In: *Historical Aspects of the Neurosciences: A festschrift for MacDonald Critchley*. New York: Raven Press; 1982:383-396.
9. Capildeo R. Charcot in the 80s. In: *Historical Aspects of the Neurosciences: A festschrift for MacDonald Critchley*. New York: Raven Press; 1982:383-396.
10. Bourneville DM, Guérard I. *De la sclérose en plaques disséminées*. Paris: Delahaye; 1869.
11. Compston A. The Story of Multiple Sclerosis. *McAlpine's Multiple Sclerosis*. London: Churchill Livingstone; 1998:3-42.

12. Vulpian EFA. Note sur la sclérose en plaques de la moelle épinière. *Union Méd* 1866;30:459-465, 475-482, 541-548.
13. Charcot M. Histologie de le sclérose en plaques. *Gaz Hôp Paris*. 1868;141:554-555, 557-558.
14. Charcot JM. Diagnostic des formes frustes de la sclérose en plaques. *Prog Méd*. 1879;7:97-99.
15. Charcot JM. *Lectures on the diseases of the nervous system*. Delivered at la Salpêtrière. Vol II, Sigerson G, ed-trans. London: New Sydenham Society; 1881.
16. Charcot JM. Séance du 14 mars: Un cas de sclérose en plaques généralisée du cerveau et de la moelle épinière. *Comp Rend Soc Biol*. 1986;20:13-14.
17. Bonduelle M. Portrait de Jean-Martin Charcot. *Bull Acad Natle Méd*. 1993;6:865-875.
18. Guillain GJM. *Charcot (1825–1893): sa vie—son oeuvre*. Paris: Masson; 1955.
19. Guillain GJM. *Charcot 1825–1893. His life—his work*. Bailey P, ed-trans. London: Pitman Medical; 1959.
20. Capildeo R. Charcot in the 80s. In: *Historical Aspects of the Neurosciences: A festschrift for MacDonald Critchley*. New York: Raven Press; 1982:383-396.
21. *Charcot, the Clinician: the Tuesday Lessons*: excerpts from nine case presentations on general neurology delivered at the Salpêtrière Hospital in 1887–88 by Jean-Martin Charcot. Trans. and commen. Goetz CG. New York: Raven Press; 1987.
22. Capildeo R. Charcot in the 80s. In: *Historical Aspects of the Neurosciences: A festschrift for MacDonald Critchley*. New York: Raven Press; 1982:383-396.
23. Goetz CG, Bonduelle M, Gelfand T. *Charcot: Constructing Neurology*. New York: Oxford University Press; 1995:20.
24. Goetz CG, Bonduelle M, Gelfand T. *Charcot: Constructing Neurology*. New York: Oxford University Press; 1995.
25. Ibid, p. 48-50.
26. Charcot JM. *Lectures on the diseases of the nervous system*. Delivered at la Salpêtrière. Vol II. Sigerson G, ed-trans. London: New Sydenham Society; 1881.
27. Charcot JM. *Lectures on diseases of the nervous system*. Sigerson G, trans. Vol I. London: The New Sydenham Society; 1877:158-222.
28. Charcot JM. *Clinical Lectures on Diseases of the Nervous System*. Delivered at the Infirmary of La Salpêtrière by Professor JM Charcot. Savill T, trans. Vol III. London: New Sydenham Society; 1889.
29. Charcot JM. *Lectures on the diseases of the nervous system*. Delivered at la Salpêtrière. Risse W, ed-trans. introd. New York Academy of Medicine; 1962.
30. Sigerson G. *Charcot the Clinician: The Tuesday Lessons by Jean-Martin Charcot*. Goetz CG, trans. New York: Raven Press; 1887.
31. Goetz CG. *Charcot, the Clinician: the Tuesday Lessons*: p. 113-120.
32. Guillain GJM. *Charcot 1825–1893. His life—his work*. Bailey P, ed-trans. London: Pitman Medical; 1959.
33. Charcot JM. *Lectures on diseases of the nervous system*; I:221.
34. Bourneville DM, Guérard I. *De la sclérose en plaques disseminées*. Paris: Delahaye; 1869.
35. Koehler PJ. Book Review of Goetz C et al. Charcot: Constructing Neurology. *J Hist Neurosci*. 1997;6:211-213.
36. Putnam TJ. The Centenary of Multiple Sclerosis. *Arch Neurol Psych*. 1938;40(4):806-813.
37. Bourneville DM, Guérard I. *De la sclérose en plaques disseminées*. Paris: Delahaye; 1869.
38. Ordenstein M. *Sur la paralysie agitante et la sclérose en plaques generalisee*. Paris: A Delahaye, 1868.
39. Goetz CG, Bonduelle M. Charcot as therapeutic interventionist and treating neurologist. *Neurol*. 1995;45:2102-2106.
40. Goetz CG, Bonduelle M, Gelfand T. *Charcot: Constructing Neurology*: p. 137.
41. Goetz CG. *Charcot, the Clinician: the Tuesday Lessons*: p.146-147.

42. Londe A. *Le service photographique de la Salpêtrière*. Paris: Doin; 1892.
43. Didi-Huberman G. *Invention de l'hystérie: Charcot et l'iconographie photographique de la Salpêtrière*. Paris: Editions Macula; 1982.
44. Munthe A. *The Story of San Michele*. New York: E.P. Dutton; 1929.
45. Munthe G, Uexhüll G. *The Story of Axel Munthe*. New York: EP Dutton; 1953.
46. Freud S. *Charcot; Collected Papers*. London: Hogarth Press; 1948:10-11.
47. Capildeo R. Charcot in the 80s. In: *Historical Aspects of the Neurosciences: A festschrift for MacDonald Critchley*. New York: Raven Press; 1982:383-396.
48. Guillain GJM. *Charcot (1825–1893): sa vie—son oeuvre*. Paris: Masson; 1955.
49. Ibid, p. 9.
50. Goetz CG, Bonduelle M, Gelfand T. *Charcot: Constructing Neurology*. New York: Oxford University Press; 1995.
51. Oliver T. The Lessons of Charcot. *Edinburgh Med J*. 1875-1876;21:720-726; 1010-1020.
52. Moxon W. Eight cases of insular sclerosis of the brain and spinal cord. *Guy Hosp Rep*. 1875;20:437-478.
53. Charcot JM. *Lectures on the diseases of the nervous system*. Delivered at la Salpêtrière. Vol II. Sigerson G, ed-trans. London: New Sydenham Society; 1881.
54. Timal H. *Etude sur quelque complications de la sclérose en plaques dissemininées*. Paris: Theses de Paris, 1875.
55. Schüle Hans. Beitrag zur multiplen Sklerose de Ghirns und Ruckenmarks. *Deutsches Archives für Klinische Medicine*. 1870;vii:259.
56. Baldwin G. A case of diffused cerebral sclerosis. *Am J Insanity*, 1872; xxviii. Republished in *J Mental Sci*. 1873;July:304-305.
57. Buzzard T. Case presentation, Clinical Society of London. *Lancet*. 1875;i:545.
58. Buzzard T. Disseminated cerebrospinal sclerosis. *Lancet*. 1875;i:304.
59. Moxon W. Eight cases of insular sclerosis of the brain and spinal cord. *Guy Hosp Rep*. 1875;20:437-478.
60. Charcot JM. *Lectures on the diseases of the nervous system*. Delivered at la Salpêtrière. Sigerson G, ed-trans. Risse W, intro. New York: New York Academy of Medicine; 1962.
61. Althaus J. Two lectures on sclerosis of the spinal cord. *BMJ* 1884;i:893-985.
62. Althaus J. *On Sclerosis of the Spinal Cord*. London: Longmans; 1885.

7

Medical Reports
After Charcot

*It is interesting to follow the stages in the recognition of a new disease.
Very rarely does it happen that at all points the description is so complete as at once to gain universal acceptance ... First a case here and
there is reported as something unusual; in a year or two someone col-
lects them and emphasizes the clinical features and perhaps names the
disease. Then in rapid succession new cases are reported and we are
surprised to find that it is by no means uncommon.*

William Osler, 1908[1]

Although Charcot did not publish a lot on multiple sclerosis (MS),
perhaps only 34 cases,[2] his description of the disease was acknowledged by all who later published on the disease. Ebers[3] pointed out that
Charcot probably had additional thoughts and views on the disease,
which were expressed through the writings of his pupils Bourneville and
Guérard,[4] and in the first monograph on MS by another student,

---

*Désiré Magloire Bourneville (1840–1909) was a Paris neurologist and a student of Charcot's
who coauthored the monograph on multiple sclerosis with Guérard that contained many of
the views of Charcot on multiple sclerosis. Bourneville also described adenoma sebaceum coupled with seizures and mental deficiency (1880), which became known as Bourneville's disease, now called tuberous sclerosis. He founded the Progrès Médical in 1873 and established
the first school in France for medically defective children.

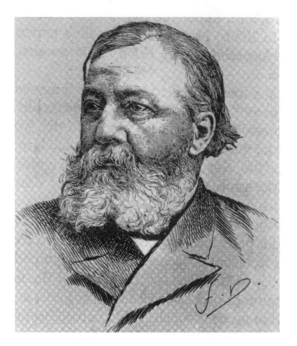

Figure 7.1 Désiré Magloire Bourneville (1840–1909), remembered for his description of tuberous sclerosis (Bourneville's disease), made contributions to many aspects of neurology, and especially to the humane understanding of mentally challenged children. His greatest impact may have been his 1872 editing of Charcot's *Leçons sur les maladies du système nerveux faites à la Salpêtrière*. His career was one characterized by courage, sensitivity, intellect, humanity, and action, embodying the French ideal of *un homme des pensées et actions*. (Portrait by H. Bianchon.)

Ordenstein.[5]* These early monographs contain Charcot's beautiful woodcuts showing pathological changes and his descriptions of the pathology in MS. They were described by Putnam as "the textbooks of a generation to which the next 70 years added little."[6]

Ordenstein published the first monograph on MS as an aggregation thesis in 1867.[7] Following the interest of his teacher, Charcot, the thesis is devoted half to MS and half to Parkinson's disease, continuing the efforts of Charcot and Vulpian to differentiate the conditions. When printed in 1868, it contained the first publication of Charcot's chromolithography of gross MS plaques. Ebers pointed out that the Ordenstein text is repetitious, limited in its critical analysis, erroneous on some facts, and neglectful of previous contributors.[8] Bourneville and Guérard's monograph described more cases and reviewed the previous contributions more fully.[9] This monograph contains the Charcot woodcuts from the 1868 *Gazette Hôpitaux* article as well as clinical descriptions of two of the cases in Cruveilhier's atlas.

Other cases began to appear in French, German, British, American, Australian, and Canadian journals. M. Gonzalez Echeverria's case, published from the notes of his student F.A. Castle in 1869, was, like Morris'

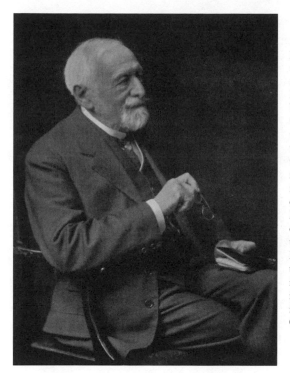

Figure 7.2 Sir Clifford Allbutt was one of the most talented and respected Victorian physicians. He made original observations, but always kept his conclusions to the facts at hand. His textbook was one of the most important of the late 19th century, and contains Risien Russel's chapter on multiple sclerosis. Allbutt was the first to describe acute myelitis and optic neuritis, now known as Devic's disease. He was one of the early advocates of the new ophthalmoscope perfected by von Helmholtz, and wrote one of three early books on the use of the instrument and the eye changes in neurological and general medical diseases. (Photo by J. Palmer Clarke.)

case, later diagnosed as multiple sclerosis.[10] Over the next few decades, reports of cases of MS increased, and although there was refinement of the clinical picture, little was added to Charcot's description of the clinical and pathological picture. Perhaps the most important addition, predicted by Charcot, was the increasing recognition of earlier cases and *forme frustes*, with speculation on possible causes. There was still uncertainty about whether MS was more common in men or women. As reports of large numbers of cases accumulated in clinics in various European countries, it became clear that this was not a rare disease, or a curiosity, but a fairly common disorder in a neurological ward or clinic.

In 1870, Wilhelm Schüle published a detailed 40-page report on *multiplen Sclerose* (a very early use of the German name translated later as multiple sclerosis), giving an account of a 23-year-old patient, with a progressive disease course over four years with autopsy findings.[11]

There were no identifiable cases in Russel Reynolds' 1868 *A System of Medicine*. Sir Clifford Allbutt's 1871 *On the Use of the Ophthalmoscope in*

Diseases of the Nervous System and of the Kidneys has a case: RB (case 103), a patient of Mr. Sedgwick of Boroughbridge, Yorkshire, who had a chronic spinal cord disease with paralysis, altered sensation, loss of bladder control, reduced vision, and pale optic discs.[12]

WILLIAM HAMMOND

S. Weir Mitchell's colleague during the Civil War, William Alexander Hammond (1828–1900), had a remarkable career as Surgeon General of the United States from which he was unjustly court-martialed and dismissed. He became one of America's leading neurologists and was later reinstated to his position. He wrote the first American textbook of neurology, *A Treatise on the Diseases of the Nervous System* (1871),* that contained chapters on "Multiple Cerebral Sclerosis" and "Multiple Cerebro-Spinal Sclerosis," referring to the many French authors on the subject, including Cruveilhier, Carswell, Vulpian, and Charcot.[†13] He suggested that Andral had discussed this condition in 1829, "although his account of it is by no means full or precise." Hammond referred to nine cases he had treated. He commented that "few diseases are so irregular and ununiform in their phenomena as the cerebrospinal form of sclerosis." As to cause, nothing definite was known, but he speculated about excessive "mental application" and trauma. In all editions of his textbook, Hammond separated the cerebral form of multiple sclerosis from the

---

*A reviewer of Hammond's text, borrowing the phrase, said he wished he could be as sure of anything as Dr. Hammond is of everything. Another said, there is not a muddy sentence in it. When he is right, he is clearly right; when he is wrong, he is clearly wrong! Despite these reviews, the book was well-received and regarded as a major advance in neurology, with many prints and editions, edited later by his son.

†Hammond and Mitchell had a long friendship and collaboration that began with an interest and publication on poison arrows and snake venom. After a long career in the military, Hammond resigned to take an academic position but re-entered at the outbreak of the Civil War and became Surgeon General of the United States in 1862. He was instrumental in developing a military medical school arranged for the training of physicians for their role on the battlefield. He established the Army Medical Museum (1862), which became the Armed Forces Institute of Pathology (1949), and was a founder of both the New York Neurological Society (1872) and the American Neurological Association (1875). He made many contributions and was a dramatic teacher and much sought after for consultation and medical expertise, but was always in the center of controversy. His obituary said he came very near to being a great man.

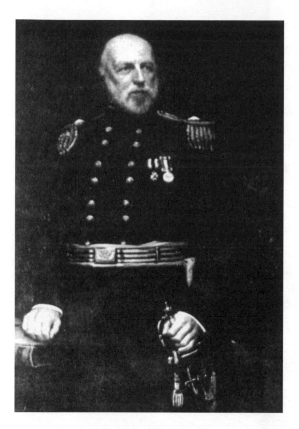

Figure 7.3 William Alexander Hammond (1828–1900) wrote the first American neurology textbook, *A Treatise on Diseases of the Nervous System* (1871), and in it described cases of multiple sclerosis. A large and impressive man, he was Surgeon General of the United States, and when fired from this position became a prominent practitioner with a very high income as well as a professor and a founder of the American Neurological Association. He was later reinstated as Surgeon General. (Courtesy of the National Library of Medicine.)

spinal form, as if they were different conditions, a common approach of other authors of his time.

Despite his remarkable career and writings, Hammond's discussion on multiple sclerosis is a mixture of perception and confusion.[14] Although he said that the diagnosis of multiple sclerosis and Parkinson's disease can be confidently separated, he confused the two in his case discussions. It was said that Hammond based his discussion of multiple sclerosis on Charcot's *Leçons*, but Hammond's textbook appeared a year before Charcot published the *Leçons*.

Hammond described the MS symptom of a vibration in the arm on lying down and also noted that some patients had facial myokymia. It is interesting that he described ptosis as part of the cerebral manifestations, for this was an issue in the question of Heinrich Heine's diagnosis. He commented on electric-like violent pains due to posterior root zone involvement of the lesions.* It is difficult to determine the nature of the epileptic paroxysms Hammond saw in cases of cerebral sclerosis, but they probably reflect sudden acute onset of symptoms, often with infection, called apoplectiform seizures or fits by Charcot. Hammond wrote that the tremor only occurred when there were lesions in the pons or superior ganglia of the brain. He said that there was little pathognomonic about the clinical features to guide diagnosis. The condition could be caused by cold and dampness as well as trauma, such as blows to the spine produced by railroad accidents. He mentioned that Vulpian had a case that occurred after an ankle sprain.

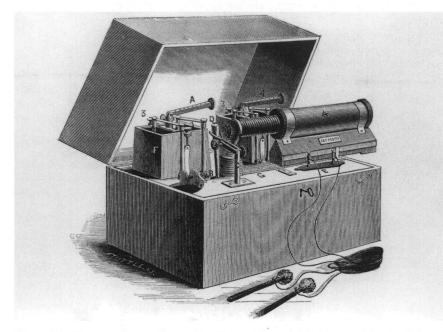

Figure 7.4 Hammond's portable excelsior Electro-Magnetic Machine, made by the Galvano-Faradaic Manufacturing Company "with all the new improvements attached" and used by him for multiple sclerosis, a "powerful adjunct" for his therapy with chloride of barium and tincture of hyoscyamus. He would pass the current antero-posteriorly and laterally to the brain through the skull of the multiple sclerosis patient. (Hammond, 1871.)

---

*Lhermitte described this phenomenon years later, and it has since become known as Lhermitte's sign. As it is a symptom, not a sign, it is more properly termed Lhermitte's phenomenon.

"I am afraid we must await for the scalpel and the microscope to deter-mine with any accuracy the diagnosis of multiple spinal sclerosis."

William Hammond, 1871

In one autopsy case, Hammond found 18 characteristic grey lesions, all in the cerebrum, and none in the brain stem or cord. He felt the like-ly cause of this disease was infection. For the 1876 London edition of his book, he minimized the cerebral epileptiform aspects of the disease. He criticized Charcot and Vulpian for including cases that shared only the features of the pathological lesion (which Compston says is not a bad position).[15] Despite his own confusion of the cases with MS and paralysis agitans, he was critical of Parkinson, Charcot, and Ordenstein for not being careful enough in their diagnosis of paralysis agitans, for he felt that multiple sclerosis was not just a single disease.

Hammond noted that the disease does not directly cause death, but intercurrent infections usually intervene. He found little hope for thera-py preventing the formation of further "islets of inflammation and scle-rosis," and regarded the condition as "unamenable, as far as we know, to medical treatment." This did not stop him from employing the same therapies as others used. His approach was to give repeated courses of chloride of barium, iron, hyoscyamus, strychnine, nitrate of silver, and cod liver oil, in addition to recommending two glasses of wine daily and moderate exercise. He administered hypodermic injections of atropia, which often diminishes the force and frequency of tonic contractions. He also used galvanic stimulation and cautery when these seemed indicated.

Hammond favored the traction machine adapted from the apparatus of Dr. Motchoukowski of Odessa, which Charcot had used in the Salpêtrière for the treatment of ataxia. Hammond felt it helped almost all cases of ataxia except those due to syphilis.

OTHER AMERICAN REPORTS

Meridith Clymer of Philadelphia wrote about multiple sclerosis in 1870 in the *New York Medical Journal* and the *Medical Record*, paying homage to Charcot for making the condition known and separating it from other neurological conditions.[16] He summarized Charcot's understanding and classification of the symptoms, signs, and pathologic findings, and outlined 16 cases to show the various forms of the disease, 15 from published European cases, and one retrospectively diagnosed American case.

Early writers on multiple sclerosis referred to the case presented by G. Baldwin in 1872,[17] but I would question the diagnosis. Baldwin presented a case of diffuse cerebral sclerosis in a "gentleman of rare endowments with extensive requirements" who was charged with offenses unbecoming of his professional status. Even though these charges were unfounded, he "escaped to literary work." Over a year, his disease progressed rapidly, with mental changes and left cerebral lesion, confirmed by a consultation with the visiting Dr. W.A. Hammond. The pathology described seems more like a cystic cerebral tumor, and the course of the illness sounds more like a progressive space-occupying lesion such as a brain tumor, rather than multiple sclerosis. John Cook wrote a paper on multiple sclerosis in 1872 and referred to the description of Hammond.[18] In 1873, Henry B. Noyes, professor of ophthalmology in Philadelphia, described Miss A., who he had diagnosed with a brain tumor, because of her symptoms of diplopia, pale optic discs, paralysis, and intention tremor. No tumor was found at the autopsy, carried out by two experienced pathologists. Furthermore, nothing abnormal in the brain was apparent to the naked eye. Unfortunately, no microscopic examination of the tissues was carried out, but Noyes later believed the woman suffered from the disseminated sclerosis described by Charcot and reviewed by Clymer (1870). C.H. Boardman of St. Paul, Minnesota, referring to the outline by Clymer, reviewed a case in the literature in 1873, but presented nothing new. He wished to make physicians more aware of a condition he felt was more common than many suspected as it was probably confused with other conditions. Stiles Kennedy of Michigan also published a case in 1873, referring to Hammond as his source, but disagreeing with Hammond's separation of the disease into two distinct categories.

THE EARLY ENGLISH REPORTS

"You must know diseases, not as a zoologist knows his species and his genera and his orders, by description of comparative characters, but as a hunter knows his lions and tigers."

William Moxon, 1875

Between 1873 and 1875 in *The Lancet,* there appeared four brief reports of multiple sclerosis, initially under the title "Case of insular sclerosis of the brain and spinal cord."[19-22] These cases were from Guy's Hospital, and although authorship was anonymous, three of the four patients were said to be under the care of Dr. William Moxon. One case was presented to a meeting of the Clinical Society of London by Dr. Thomas Buzzard.[23] These same patients appeared in a later publication by Moxon in 1875, when he reported eight cases, two with autopsy findings.[24]

Moxon's 1875 report is often erroneously claimed as the first major description of MS in the English language.* He referred to his cases as "insular sclerosis," a term he preferred to "disseminated sclerosis," since it better captured the sense of the islets of pathological change. These patients showed the features of paralytic weakness, nystagmus, speech abnormalities, and changes in mental status, including involuntary laughter. Moxon recognized that the disease occurred in the age group 25–45, and it could be mild for five to ten years before progressively worsening. He listed the characteristic findings as:

- Head and limb tremor
- Paralysis of the limbs without sensory change
- Rigidity or contracture of the legs
- Nystagmus
- Late effect on bowels or bladder
- Normal electro-irritability

---

*Moxon's report can be arguably claimed as the first major report in the English language if we regard the earlier reports by Bright, Abercrombie, Morris and Mitchell, Noyes, Baldwin, Boardman, Hammond, and MacLauren as minor. The initial reports by Moxon would be in the same category as the others, but the 1875 discussion of the eight cases with two autopsies could be called the first major report.

- Characteristic abnormal speech
- Some impairment of intellect

Moxon started his discussion by noting surprise that this disease with its "constant and characteristic symptoms, but also a quite peculiar and very remarkable morbid anatomy" is so unrecognized in England. He referred to his two cases with autopsy as the first "on this side of the channel" but admitted that *sclérose en plaque* or *inselförmige sklerose* had been repeatedly verified by autopsy in France and Germany.

Moxon recognized the tendency for multiple sclerosis patients to have a cheerful manner out of keeping with their situation.

"The patients, who, as a rule, are cheerful and thankful for what is done on their behalf, are apt to declare themselves generally rather better, so that the report of the clinical clerk putting down their answers may read like a statement of continual good progress toward recovery. But the general result has been that, after many months' stay

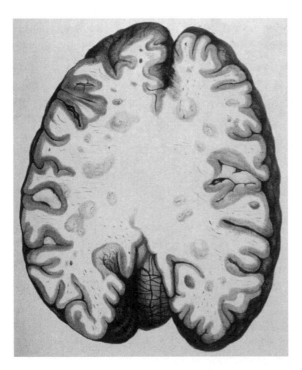

Figure 7.5 William Moxon's illustration of lesions in the white matter of the brain (1875). The appearance of these islets of grey degeneration led Moxon to call the disease insular sclerosis, much favored by Sir William Gowers and Sir William Osler. (Moxon, 1876. Courtesy of the Royal Society of Medicine, London.)

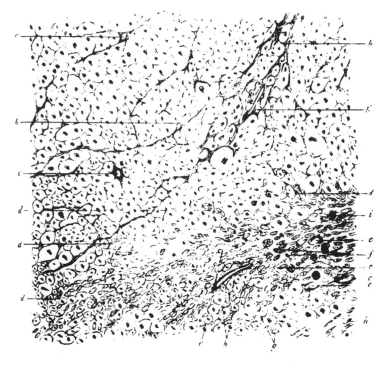

Figure 7.6 Spinal cord section stained with carmine in Moxon's 1875 paper on insular sclerosis. He showed in the lower right areas of sclerosis at various stages with an advancing edge, and areas of axis cylinders with myelin destroyed. (Moxon, 1875. Courtesy of the Royal Society of Medicine, London.)

in hospital, the poor people are found to have grown steadily though slowly worse."

His first case, Emily B., was a 28-year-old woman with progressive weakness. Two years previously, she had a febrile illness that laid her up for several weeks; when she improved, she had weakness and unsteadiness of her left arm and leg. The weakness became progressive and she was bedridden by the time of admission. She told nurses that she believed her illness was the result of the stress of catching her husband in bed with another woman. Referring to himself in the third person, Moxon commented, "On admission her condition corresponded so closely with described cases of *Inselförmige sclerose* that Dr. Moxon concluded that it must be of that nature." She had a dramatic action tremor, with head and limbs quiet at rest but jerky and tremulous with any attempt to move them. Moxon distinguished this tremor from paralysis agitans and chorea. She spilled drinks before they could get to her mouth and could not eat "for fear of her fork." Her speech was staccato, with pauses after each word, and her lips and tongue were tremulous. Sensation seemed normal, but she said she was sometimes numb. She was incontinent of urine. Her disease progressed despite treatment with galvanism, nitrate of silver, tonics, and careful nourishment. Her emotions were unstable and she laughed and cried "far too readily." Her intellect seemed weakened, although her responses were limited by her disabilities.

Postmortem examination showed a shrunken firm brain, with grey patches looking almost like grey matter. (Moxon points out that a case similar to this had been incorrectly reported as *heterotopia cerebri*.) The patches varied in size from a hemp seed to a small nut. The smaller were always spherical, dark grey and soft; the larger irregular, pale, with a white stippling firm enough to resist sectioning. About 40 such patches were seen in each hemisphere, with several patches in the corpus striatum and the thalamus. The grey matter was unaffected. There was a very large lesion around the aqueduct of Sylvius, extending through the pons and medulla. Under the microscope, Moxon saw loss of the medullated fibers, fine connective fibrils, and numerous granular and amyloid corpuscles. He concluded, "In these particulars, the disease corresponds with the cases already recorded by French and German authors." He referred to the cases of Charcot, Frerichs, Valentin, Ordenstein, Bourneville and Guérard, Vulpian, Leube, Bärwinkel, Schüle, Jouffroy, and others.

Moxon's other cases were Matilde, age 23; James P., age 33, a veterinary surgeon; Sarah H., age 37, a servant girl; George N., age 35, clerk; Albert F., age 24, a splint cutter for matches; Harriet B., age 38, a servant; and Edward M., age 32, a footman. All were admitted to Guy's Hospital between 1873 and 1875.

Like Charcot, the great contribution of Moxon was not the issue of being first, but a clarity of presentation that made multiple sclerosis well-known to other clinicians, who could now separate patients with multiple sclerosis from all the other presentations of neurological disease.

*"The recognition of this disease by English physicians will appear sin-
gularly slow at the time (which must soon come) when its characters
are more generally known."*

William Moxon, 1875

OTHER REPORTS

More reports of cases were presented at medical meetings and later published. J. K. Baudry of Missouri published his lecture on multiple cerebrospinal sclerosis in 1874, referring to Charcot, Vulpian, and Clymer.[25]
At the "ordinary meeting" of the Clinical Society of London in 1875, the
presentation by Dr. Thomas Buzzard of a case of multiple sclerosis along-
side a case of paralysis agitans "excited interest."[26] Dr. Buzzard's case of
what he called cerebro-spinal sclerosis was a 33-year-old house painter
who was wheeled into the room in a wheelchair and put beside a patient
with paralysis agitans. Dr. Buzzard began to show how these conditions,
so often confused, could be distinguished. He contrasted the young man's
tremor when attempting to reach for an object with the resting tremor of
the Parkinson patient, which he said resembled the action of rolling a cig-
arette or taking a pinch of snuff.

> *"Asked to rise, the patient with sclerosis made at first several ineffec-
> tual efforts, his whole body being thrown into violent tremors, the feet
> being lifted from the ground when evidently he wished to stand upon
> them; and he attained at last the standing position and made a few
> steps only with the help of an attendant. The patient with paralysis
> agitans rose without increase in tremors, and walked easily, but with
> a hurrying gait, the body bent forward."*

Buzzard pointed out that the conditions could be so well differentiated that there should no longer be any confusion about their diagnosis.
He went on to demonstrate the differences in speech patterns. Once the
patients were dismissed from the room, Buzzard further described the
features of multiple sclerosis. He acknowledged the contributions of
Cruveilhier and Carswell and gave primacy to Charcot for making the
disease known. He said he presented the case not as a clinical curiosity,

but in order to make it known so that others would identify cases earlier in the disease course. He indicated that the patient was being given iodide of potassium and a trial was also being made of the Russian needle-bath, which had benefited another case. It must have been a very effective teaching demonstration.

> "Following the step-wise growth of knowledge concerning a disease entity serves to remind us of the relative transience of our current concepts which, in time, will be replaced or modified by future developments."
>
> J.A. Frith[27]

The first description in Australia was by MacLaurin, who published an elegant clinical description of retrobulbar neuritis in 1873.[28] This was followed in 1875 by a dissertation on MS by Alfred K. Newman,[29] a young physician returning from Aberdeen, and in 1886 a report of MS by Dr. James Jamieson.[30] Frith documented the growing literature on MS in the Australian journals over the century following the description by Charcot.[31] Of interest is the brief note about the work of Dr. N.D. Royle, who found that thoracic sympathetic trunk section "relieved immediately and progressively symptoms of DS (disseminated sclerosis)." He felt that this major surgery should be done as early as possible to improve cerebral circulation and to reduce the venous congestion that preceded the sclerosis.

More cases appeared in the American medical journals. George S. Gerhard of Philadelphia outlined the syndrome and the features as described by Charcot in 1876,[32] and Horatio C. Wood gave a lecture in 1878 on the condition, using Hammond as his source of information.[33] In 1878, Allan McLane Hamilton (1848–1919) of New York City, professor of mental diseases at Cornell University, published a textbook on neurological conditions describing the picture of cerebrospinal sclerosis, referring to other names used for the disorder, *sclérose en plaques disséminées* and insular sclerosis of Moxon.[34] He described three disease stages, much as Charcot. The first stage was a period of episodic symptoms of weakness, poor balance, tremor, and speech disorder. The second was characterized by rigidity of the limbs, contractures, and tremor. In the third stage, the patient had a rapid decline, with bladder and bowel incontinence, bed sores, and dementia. He described a case he had seen only once, discussed one of Bourneville's cases, and the case of Gerhard.

SAMUEL WILKS

Publishing his Guy's Hospital lectures on the nervous system, Samuel Wilks (1824–1911) noted that he had observed the condition characterized by lesions scattered throughout the nervous system, but admitted he did not know what he was seeing until Charcot clarified the disorder.[35] Wilks was said by *The Times of London* to be "the most philosophical of English physicians." His honesty and modesty were characteristic of a

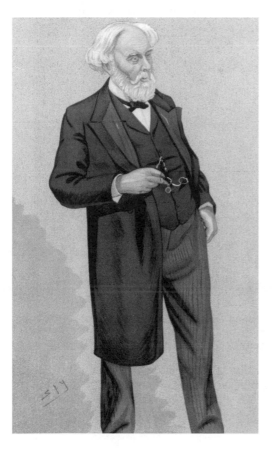

Figure 7.7 Samuel Wilks said he had seen multiple sclerosis but didn't know what he was seeing until he read Charcot's description of the disease. He published two cases, both with pathological examination by Moxon, and one is in Moxon's series (James P., a veterinarian surgeon). Wilks used to accompany Hughlings Jackson on his Sunday rounds and was said by *The Times of London* to be "the most philosophical of English physicians." Notes accompanying his caricature in *Vanity Fair* said that he "has done much to rid ladies of sick headache" and that "he thinks the most wonderful thing in the world is a woman's nervous system." (*Vanity Fair*) (Courtesy of the Wellcome Library, London.)

physician who took pains to give credit to others and was responsible for priority of descriptions being accorded to Bright, Addison, Hodgkin, and Gall. He wrote an early account of lymphadenoma, but gave credit to Hodgkins, wrote the first-known description of myasthenia gravis, and classic work on visceral syphilis, bacterial endocarditis, osteitis deformans, and alcoholic paraplegia.

Wilks described two cases, one of whom was examined by Moxon. The first was a veterinary surgeon, age 33, who had a recurrent neurological disease over two years (James P. in Moxon's series). The second was a woman of 25 who had the onset of neurological symptoms after febrile illnesses and eventually died. The pathological examination of this case, again by Moxon, revealed scattered grey insular patches throughout the cord and brain. Wilks noted that his patients had intellectual impairment but were not depressed, and indeed they often had a happy, emotional temperament and when spoken to were ready to cry, or more likely laugh. He had no comment on cause or treatment.

EDWARD SEGUIN

Edward Constant Seguin (1843–1898), son of Edouard Séguin, pioneer in the care of mental illness, was born in Paris and became a prominent American neurologist who encouraged the use of the thermometer in the United States and wrote widely on neurological conditions. He studied with Charcot, Brown-Séquard, and Louis Ranvier. In 1869, he was appointed to the College of Physicians and Surgeons in New York as the first professor of neurology in the United States. He and his colleagues J.C. Shaw and A. Van DerVeer reported two cases of multiple sclerosis in 1878 with detailed autopsy findings showing the early, intermediate, and late changes in the lesions.[36]

Two years later, Seguin noted the "coincidence of optic neuritis and subacute transverse myelitis." Seguin presented three cases of his own and referred to the two of Erb, making no reference to multiple sclerosis and regarding the coincidence of these features as "accidental." The combination of symptoms was credited to Eugène Devic as Devic's disease in 1894.

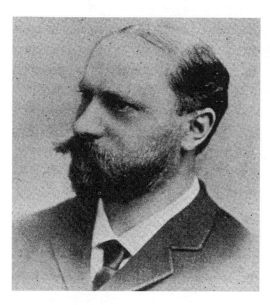

Figure 7.8 Edward Constant Seguin (1843–1898), Paris born and trained, became a prominent neurologist in New York and is often erroneously referred to as the first to describe MS in North America, even though there were earlier reports by Morris and Mitchell, Hammond, Hamilton, and many others. He also described three cases of the coincident occurrence of optic neuritis and transverse myelitis, later to be called Devic's disease, but made no reference to the possible association with MS. (From McHenry, Lawrence C. Garrison's *History of Neurology*, 1969. Courtesy of Charles C Thomas Publisher Ltd. Springfield, Illinois.)

In view of the earlier, clear reports of Morris, Hammond, Hamilton, and other American physicians, it is surprising that credit for the first report on MS in the United States was for many years given to Seguin.[37] This attribution continues to appear in reviews of MS literature.

In the *BMJ* of 1883, Robert Kirkland reported a case he felt was of interest because of its unusual age of onset, as Charcot had indicated that multiple sclerosis was rarely seen after age 30, with age 40 as the outside limit.[38] He described Mrs. G., a lady of 75 who had typical features of MS; the onset of her symptoms came at age 69. She ascribed her progressive problems to the fatigue associated with caring for her ill husband. She had diplopia, failing vision, vertigo, tinnitus, drawling speech, decreased hearing, intention tremor, stumbling gait, wide-based gait, and dragging of her feet. She was no longer able to leave her house. Perhaps the most striking disease feature was her tendency to laugh in a ridiculous manner, but within a few minutes be bathed in tears. Dercum (1894) and Strümpell (1893) published cases with disease onset at ages 57 and 60.

By this time, many European textbooks with descriptions of multiple sclerosis were being translated for American audiences, and American textbooks on diseases of the nervous system all had sections on the disease, most repeating the picture described by Charcot.

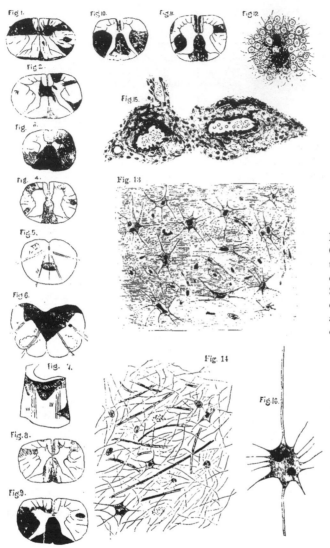

Figure 7.9 Edward Constant Seguin's illustration of the pathology of multiple sclerosis. Seguin described the early, intermediate, and late changes in the disease. (Seguin, 1878.)

References p. 60

WILLIAM OSLER

The earliest Canadian reports were by William Osler (1849–1919), who opened his presentation to the Medico-Chirurgical Society of Montreal in 1879 with the comment:

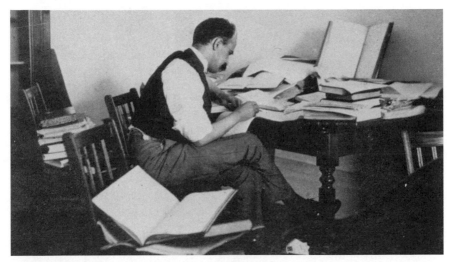

Figure 7.10 William Osler, while at McGill Medical School in Montreal, presented three cases of insular sclerosis to the Medical and Chirurgical Society of Montreal in 1878 and published these cases two years later, the first described in Canada. He had no new ideas about the disease but wanted the condition to be known by his colleagues. (From the collection of Dr. C. Roland.)

"Gentlemen: I wish to bring under your notice this evening a form of Cerebro-Spinal Disease which has not engaged the attention of the Society, and of which, as far as I know, no cases have been reported in this country."

He presented three cases which he felt represented the early, advanced, and final stages of multiple sclerosis.[39]

Osler discussed the case of F. H., age 26, with a marked tremor, slow speech, and normal sensation. "By a happy coincidence, I had Engesser's article in *Ziemssen* on Multiple Sclerosis before me when the patient came in, and the symptoms presented by him corresponded so closely with the description I had just read, that the diagnosis seemed very clear." The diagnosis was later confirmed by the consultants at the National Hospital for Paralyzed and Epileptics in London.

The next patient, James Bennet, age 44, had a wide-based ataxic gait, intention tremor, and could not stand with his eyes shut. He had hyperactive reflexes, slurred speech, and some impairment of intellect. There was a past history of bizarre acts in his social life and at work, and he was in trouble with the law. Osler regarded him as having insular sclerosis, now the term used in the British literature, as there was cerebral involvement. Like many of his era, Osler differentiated this from the paralytic form, for which he used the term multiple sclerosis.

There is minimal history on Osler's third case of multiple sclerosis, S.B., age 46, since he was in a terminal state of paralysis and unable to talk when he was admitted to the hospital. He had ptosis of the right eye, incontinence of urine and feces, and contracture of the left arm. He died five days after admission. Osler also regarded the case as insular sclerosis.

Osler presented careful clinical and pathological observations, but speculated little on the etiology or treatment of such cases, adding nothing new to the growing discussion. He was busy doing pathological correlations during his Montreal years. In a clever approach to epidemiology, Ebers looked at 786 of Osler's autopsies during his eight years at the Montreal General Hospital to determine the number of MS cases. He found one definite case and two possible cases of MS, and concluded that the prevalence of MS in Osler's time might not have been much different from today's.[40]

In his 1892 *Principles and Practice of Medicine*, Osler briefly described multiple sclerosis.[41] Oddly, he said it occurred mostly in middle age, although he noted that Pritchard had described more than 50 cases in children. His description of the signs and the disease course is uninspired and in some aspects peculiar. He repeated the elements of the Charcot triad as the major features.*[42] A few of his comments are surprising: sensation seldom being affected, sphincters affected only late in the disease, and episodic comas being a feature of the disease. He recognized that vertigo, mental change, and spastic legs were common. Osler felt the diagnosis of MS was easy in advanced cases and might only be certain when the disease had progressed to this stage. Earlier, there might be confusion with hysteria and paralysis agitans. He was puzzled by the *pseudo-sclérose en plaques* of Westphal with similar clinical features of tremor, scanning speech, and spasticity, but without nystagmus and postmortem lesions (which we now recognize as Wilson's disease). In keeping with his repu-

---

*In Osler's library was a presentation and autographed copy of Charcot's *Agrégation*.

tation as a therapeutic nihilist, he felt no therapy was of any value, although a prolonged course of nitrate of silver might be tried.

Osler's textbook also had chapters on acute and chronic myelitis and optic nerve disease, but there is little mention in these chapters of the possibility that these conditions might be forms of multiple sclerosis. In his book on cerebral palsy, Osler referred to cases of multiple sclerosis in children which resemble cerebral palsy, but many references to multiple sclerosis in children in the 19th century are undoubtedly to other diseases that resemble MS clinically or have white-matter demyelination.

By 1910, Osler had involved many other authors in the production of later editions of his works. For the sections on the nervous system, he worked with Lewellys Barker (his successor at Johns Hopkins), Edwin Bramwell, Farquhar Buzzard, Harvey Cushing, Gordon Holmes, Smith Ely Jelliffe, Colin Russel, and William Spiller, who will be discussed elsewhere. The chapter on disseminated sclerosis (multiple sclerosis, insular sclerosis, *sclérose en plaques*) was written by Edwin Bramwell, son of Byrom Bramwell. The one and a half pages on this disease had swelled to 18 pages in the 18 years since the first edition.

Bramwell, writing the section on MS in Osler's textbook in later editions, divided cases into various types: classical with the Charcot triad, cerebro-spinal, intermittent or hysterical, spinal, cerebral, and sacral. No one recovers completely or permanently, he said; even those who have long remissions eventually progress, with an average duration of life of ten and a half years, rarely as long as 20 years. No treatment had proved to be helpful, but he used arsenic in small doses as the only medicine. Bramwell had many recommendations for a healthy lifestyle. Marriage should be forbidden. Hot baths are contraindicated. Pregnancy is to be avoided and in what must have been an unusual suggestion in 1910, abortion was justifiable if pregnancy occurs.

By 1910, discussion of diagnosis of MS had advanced due to Uhthoff's observation of optic disc changes, the differentiation from hysteria by Thomas Buzzard, and the discovery of the toe sign of Babinski. In writing the section on MS, Bramwell had the advantage of recent reviews of large series of cases by Sachs, Borst, Hoffman, and Byrom Bramwell, as well as the exhaustive monograph on MS by Müller.[43]

This edition of Osler's noted that MS was among the most common afflictions of the nervous system. It was said to be much less common in the United States than in Scotland and the Continent. This may be due to cases' being overlooked across the Atlantic. Bramwell noted the surprising difference of opinion on the gender ratio in MS. Many (Charcot, Uhthoff, Frankl-Hochwart, Probst, Pierre Marie, Krafft-Ebing, Tredgold) found it more common in males. Others (Byrom Bramwell, Bruns, Berlin) found it more common in females. Still others thought it occurred equally often in the two sexes (Erlangen, Edwin Bramwell, Müller). Bramwell concluded from this confusion that the occurrence of MS was likely equal in the two sexes.

Osler indicated that the onset was usually in the third decade; earlier reports of common childhood cases were undoubtedly in error. Discussing causes, it relegated infection to a process that may aggravate but not cause the disease; the same was true for trauma and environmental toxins. It is interesting to note that Parkinson's disease may still have been confused with MS 50 years after Vulpian and Charcot attempted to clarify the difference. The textbook noted that Embden had seen symptoms similar to MS in manganese workers; manganese causes a form of Parkinson's disease.

SIR BYROM BRAMWELL

In his important 1882 textbook on spinal cord diseases dedicated to Charcot and Erb, Byrom Bramwell wrote that MS was a rare disease, an opinion he would later reverse.[44] He felt that in many cases, there was a history of trauma such as a blow to the head or spine, or exposure to cold and wet. Occasionally MS might occur as a sequel to acute diseases, or pregnancy. In a few cases, there was a distinct hereditary tendency. But he concluded, "In most, the exact conditions which excite the affection are obscure." Although he felt MS was more common in women, he had six cases, five of whom were males. Like Charcot, he divided cases into three stages; the last stage was that of muscle atrophy, the picture of amyotrophy.* Like Osler, he felt that diagnosis was easy in advanced and typical cases, but could be very difficult in early cases. In one of his

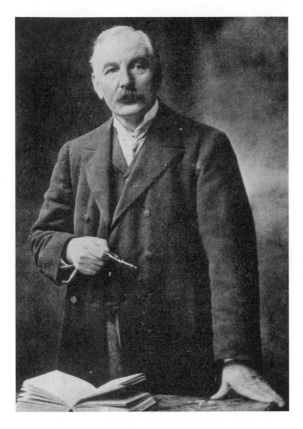

Figure 7.11 Sir Byrom Bramwell (1847–1931), in an age that was still characterized by empirical approach, was a careful observer of diseases such as multiple sclerosis, spinal cord disorders, and brain tumors, measuring and collecting data to assess a theory of observation. It was said of Bramwell, as it was said of Jonathan Hutchinson and William Gowers, if physicians believed they have found something new, they should first consult the writings of Bramwell. McHenry said he touched medicine at all points, and whatever he touched he adorned. (Courtesy of the National Library of Medicine.)

patients, the disease onset was with sudden deafness and "noise in the head" after exposure to hot sun. He outlined how the condition could be differentiated from cerebellar tumor, locomotor ataxia, and Parkinson's disease. His therapy was conventional for the time, consisting of silver, arsenic, hydrotherapy, and galvanic stimulation, but he concluded that the results of these therapies were disappointing.

Bramwell and other authors of this period had a good understanding of the clinical manifestations of multiple sclerosis. Contemporaries were impressed with the neurologist's command of brain diseases as well, and a review on multiple sclerosis in *The Lancet* in 1887 commented:

---

*Because neurologists today seldom see MS patients in the final stages of the disease, the picture of atrophy and widespread amyotrophy is seldom mentioned in current writings. It was often seen when patients lived out the last stages of their illness in hospitals like the Salpêtrière.

"It would seem as if neurologists having wellnigh differentiated all the types of central lesions, were now exploring the peripheral system."

In 1903, Byrom Bramwell was one of the first to note a geographical pattern for MS when he compared the north of Scotland to North America, noting that one in 58 of his patients had MS while a publication from New York indicated that frequency was one in 219 there.[45] He dispensed with the idea of a hereditary predisposition and felt MS occurred in all social classes. He commented that the upper classes get the disease as often as the lower, and indeed, the disease often comes on in "healthy well-marked girls brought up in the country." In concluding the section on causes, he commented that there was such a multiplicity of possible causes put forward that they were all likely to be of secondary importance.

In his detailed description of pathology, Bramwell noted that the white matter is mostly affected, but the grey matter can also be involved; Ribbert's suggestion that the grey matter was a barrier to the degeneration was not his experience. Discussing changes in plaques at different stages and at the center and periphery of the plaque, he said that there is a loss of axons in the center, with preservation elsewhere, though the preserved naked axons did not appear healthy. Although Bramwell noted the earlier observations of Rindfleisch, Ribbert, and others who were impressed with the relationship between plaque and blood vessel, he and certain others were not convinced of this relationship.

Bramwell did not like Charcot's separation of cerebral, spinal, and cerebrospinal MS as the features are often mixed; diagnosing a cerebral form alone was problematic. His description of clinical symptoms and signs of the disease is complete. He said that older writers had felt sensory findings were rare, but this was not the experience of current clinicians. Indeed, Freund found sensory findings in 29 of 33 patients. Although Bramwell fully described the reflex changes in MS, he mentioned a pattern that might puzzle the modern neurologist, but that Thomas Buzzard thought quite characteristic: absent knee jerks with ankle clonus. Again contradicting the earlier Osler description, he noted that bladder symptoms were often present early in the disease, and that

504   DISEASES OF THE SPINAL CORD

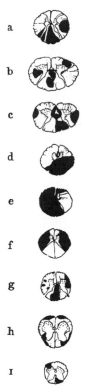

Figure 7.12 Sections through the spinal cord of an MS case of Byrom Bramwell's, which he used to illustrate the widespread lesions in the disease. He noted that lesions were also found elsewhere, and that there was no secondary degeneration seen, indicating to him that the axons were preserved. (Bramwell, 1895.)

FIG. 153.—*Transverse sections through the spinal cord, from a case of cerebro-spinal sclerosis, showing the position and extent of the sclerotic (deeply stained) patches at different heights. About one and a half times the natural size.*

a, upper cervical region; b, cervical enlargement; c, cervical enlargement; d, upper dorsal region; e, mid-dorsal region; f, mid-dorsal region; g, upper lumbar region; h, lower part of lumbar enlargement; i, sacral region.

Sections b, d and h are shown more highly magnified in succeeding figures.

80 percent of Oppenheim's patients had these symptoms. Many patients were constipated, but rectal incontinence only occurred late in the disease. He said memory change was present in 50 percent of patients, emotional alteration in 40 percent, and intellectual impairment in 27 percent.

Bramwell divided cases into various types: classical with the Charcot triad, cerebrospinal, intermittent or hysterical, spinal, cerebral, and sacral. No one recovers completely or permanently; the disease in those who have long remissions eventually progresses. The average duration of life with MS was 10 years, although some patients lived more than 20 years.[46] No treatment had proved helpful and the only medicine he would use on his MS patients was arsenic in small doses. He had many recommendations for a healthy lifestyle.

JAMES STEWART

In 1882, Dr. George Ross presented a case of multiple sclerosis to the same group in Montreal, which heard Osler's presentation of three cases. At the June 27, 1884 meeting of the Medical-Chirurgical Society of Montreal, Dr. James Stewart continued the discussion of this same case, one of multiple cerebral sclerosis with a stroke-like acute onset.[47] The patient was a 47-year-old hotel porter with a three-year history of vertigo, unconsciousness, and on recovery, a persistent speech difficulty. Later he had mental changes, with outbursts of laughing and crying. He had tremor and bilateral optic atrophy with marked visual impairment. He was treated with potassium iodide. The discussion that followed Ross' presentation indicated that the audience regarded such cases as belonging to a category, some due to disseminated sclerosis and others, syphilis. Today we would likely entertain other diagnoses for a single acute event with unconsciousness.

SIR WILLIAM RICHARD GOWERS

It has been said that neurologists in the era of Gowers were like naturalists in a lush tropical jungle, gathering, collecting, classifying, and arranging the neurological specimens around them. Of these neurologists, "none had a sharper eye or a more skillful pen than William Gowers."[48]

In his small 1884 monograph, *Symptoms and Diagnosis of Diseases of the Spinal Cord*, William Gowers (1845–1915) did not discuss MS specifically, but case 3, a man of 28 with a progressive cord lesion, was thought to have slow progression due to a "local sclerosis."[49] He indicated that he did not like the term "sclerosis," which implied connective tissue overgrowth and hardening, while the disease lesions might be softer than normal.* He was unhappy that nonspecific terms such as "chronic myelitis"

---

*Early 19th century English, French, and German literature contain many meanings for sclerosis.

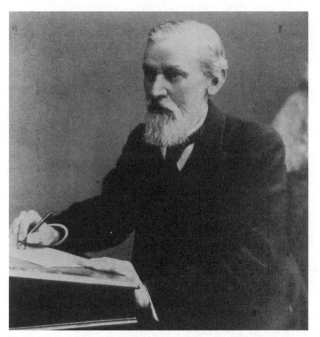

Figure 7.13   Sir William Richard Gowers (1845–1915), one of the greatest clinical neurologists, wrote a perceptive overview of multiple sclerosis in a great textbook of neurology, *A Manual of Diseases of the Nervous System* (see McDonald on Gowers). It has been said that a neurologist who believes he or she has discovered something new should first look it up in Gower's textbook. Foster Kennedy said we would all be better clinicians if we periodically read Gowers. He always took notes in shorthand and felt everyone should do so. He could illustrate his texts well, as his pictures were regularly displayed at the Royal Academy of Arts. (Courtesy of the National Library of Medicine.)

and "degeneration" and "sclerosis" did not differentiate between a pathological process and a disease. When he used the terms, he meant a process; he was resistant to premature classification of diseases when only the process was apparent, although he recognized that clinical history was helpful in formulating the processes into categories.

His classic, *A Manual of Diseases of the Nervous System* (1888), is often referred to as the "bible of neurology," and still available a century later in reprints.[50,51] In it, he discussed current understanding of MS and his personal beliefs about outstanding questions on the disease. He indicated that half the cases of MS had no identifiable cause, and many apparent associations were "influences" rather than causes. Like Pierre Marie, he emphasized that the disease was not related to syphilis. Although a few

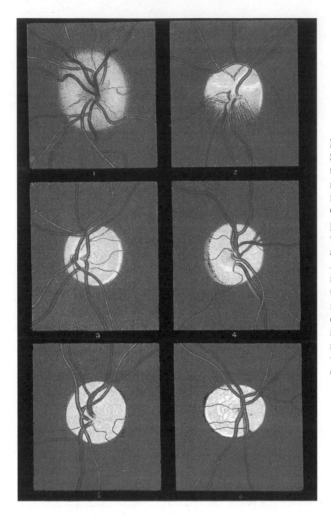

Figure 7.14 Paintings of Sir William Gowers of the appearance of optic neuritis and optic atrophy from various diseases. Gowers was an accomplished artist whose works regularly appeared at the Royal Academy of Arts in London. In these illustrations, Gowers used the term optic neuritis for many acute conditions affecting the nerve head, including meningitis, and tumor as well as multiple sclerosis. (Gowers, 1879.)

cases in siblings had been noted, these were exceptional; he felt there was no evident genetic or familial predisposition. Pathologically, there were scattered patches in the white matter, which appeared shrunken due to the thinning of nerve fibers. The patches were characterized by overgrowth of neuroglia and wasting of the nerve fibers. He emphasized neuroglial overgrowth as the underlying process.

In his 1879 monograph *A Manual and Atlas of Medical Ophthalmoscopy*, with his own paintings of the optic disc and retina, hardly surpassed by later photography, he gave little attention to optic nerve changes in MS. In

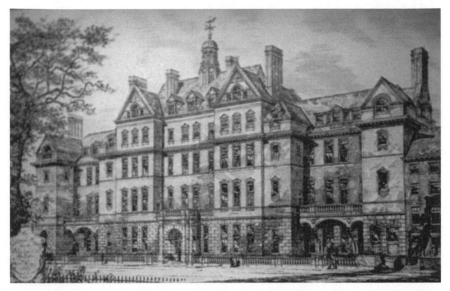

Figure 7.15 The National Hospital for the Paralyzed and Epileptic (1883). The outstanding neurologists at this institution in the late 19th century made important observations of the nature of MS, and their prolific writings made the disease better known to clinicians. It continues today as a center for MS research.

a two-paragraph discussion, he commented that amblyopia occasionally occurs and sometimes without visible optic nerve change, although examination can be difficult due to nystagmus. Charcot had shown that the optic nerve can have the same sclerosis seen elsewhere in the central nervous system, but Gowers said that optic nerve involvement only rarely progressed to complete blindness. Because the axis cylinders are preserved, some function may persist even with loss of the myelin sheath. In the appendix of case histories, Gowers described Maria R. (case 34a), age 20, a general servant with a strong family history of epilepsy, who was "never bright or strong." She developed weakness and tremor with mental change, and after a period of improvement got steadily worse. Her left optic disc showed nasal pallor; it was pale and grey, and she had poor acuity and color perception. Case 34, Thomas A., had optic atrophy bilaterally and intermittent neurological symptoms and signs, which Gowers thought might be lateral sclerosis, but which sound more like MS. Sadly for us, there are no illustrations of the optic atrophy of MS in his own beautiful drawings and paintings, but he illustrated "optic neuritis" from other causes.

Gowers, Clifford Allbutt, and S. Weir Mitchell were responsible for making the 1861 Helmholtz development of the ophthalmoscope a part of the routine physical examination.[52] It was not an easy procedure at first, using a candle or gas lamp to provide the illumination that allowed visualization of the retina by the new instrument. Gowers invented a three-wick candle to help illuminate the retina.*

Gowers was not the philosopher that Hughlings Jackson was, but a thoughtful observer, a "visual" and artist like Charcot, who saw more clearly than others patient problems encountered day to day. Along with Jackson, Russell, Ferrier, and Horsley, he brought fame and glory to British neurology at the end of the 19th century.[53] Foster Kennedy wrote that we would all be better doctors, teachers, and writers if, from time to time, we re-read Gowers' writings.[54] The adage in neurology is still, "If you believe you have discovered something new, first look it up in Gowers."†

Gowers wrote his influential textbook when he was about age 40 and illustrated it himself; his pictures were regularly displayed at the Royal Academy of Arts. He had diverse interests and a lifelong habit of taking notes in shorthand.[55] His hemocytometer was used for half a century. He devised a method of notation for ranges of hearing loss and of musical notation, but these had no more success than his admonition that everyone should learn shorthand.[56] It was said one could always recognize one of Gower's students because they carried an ophthalmoscope and wrote in shorthand.[57,58]

---

*Among his other inventions were the hemocytometer and a hemoglobinometer.

†Others use this quote for Bramwell, or Sir Clifford Allbutt, great physicians who wrote influential textbooks. My admiration for Gowers increased when, after years of reading original texts to try to get the early story of multiple sclerosis correct, I found that Gowers got it mostly right in this very succinct paragraph:

"Our knowledge of the affection is recent. The lesion was, indeed, long since figured by Carswell and Cruveilhier and described thirty years ago by Frerichs, Rindfleisch, etc., but the malady was not generally recognized until re-investigated by Vulpian and Charcot and his pupils and described by Charcot in his widely-circulated 'Lectures.' The apt designation 'insular sclerosis' was proposed by the late Dr. Moxon, who first described the disease in this country."

JOSEPH-FRANÇOIS-FÉLIX BABINSKI

Joseph-François-Félix Babinski (1857–1932) published his thesis on MS in 1885.[59] He worked in a junior hospital position in general medicine (*interne des hôpitaux*) with two physicians, Vulpian in neurological

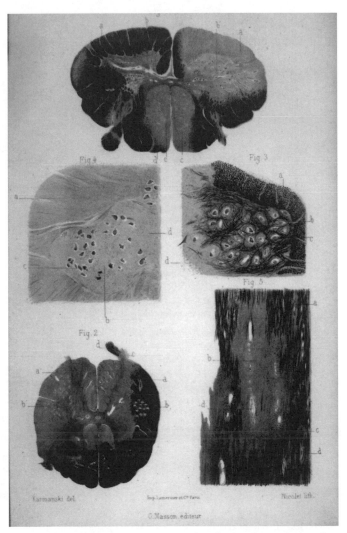

Figure 7.16   Dr. Joseph Babinski's illustrations of multiple sclerosis lesions from his thesis *Etude anatomique et clinique sur la sclérose en plaques*. Paris: G. Masson (editor), Libraire de l'Academie-de-medecine, 1885. Plate 1, facing page 145. (Courtesy of the Wellcome Library, London.)

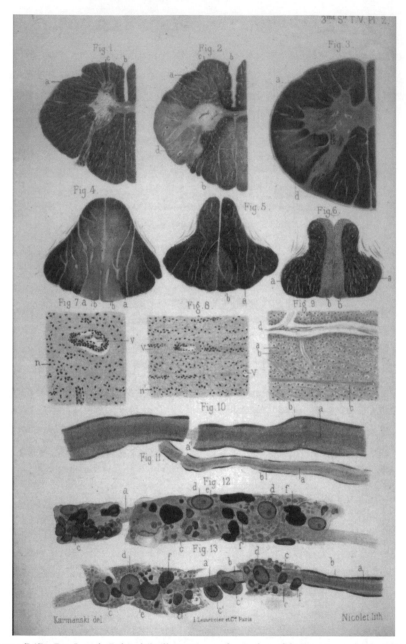

Figure 7.17 Dr. Joseph Babinski's illustrations of spinal cord lesions in multiple sclerosis with microscopic drawings of the inflammatory changes to myelin and axons. *Etude anatomique et clinique sur la sclérose en plaques*. Paris: G. Masson (editor), Libraire de l'Academie-de-medecine, 1885. Plate 2, facing page 147. (Courtesy of the Wellcome Library, London.)

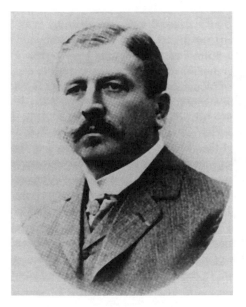

Figure   7.18 Joseph-François-Félix Babinski (1857–1923) is remembered for his description of the "cutaneous plantar reflex" in a 28-line report in 1896. He did one of the early monographs on multiple sclerosis and modern neurologists are returning to his observations as they reflect current findings on myelin and axonal change. (Courtesy of the National Library of Medicine.)

pathology, and Corneil, who was a capable pathological anatomist. Both his chiefs had an interest in MS, and it was natural for him to select this topic for his thesis (*Étude anatomique et clinique sur la sclérose en plaques*).[60] He leaned more toward clinical pathophysiology than to clinico-pathological correlations; this was one of his few studies that relied heavily on microscopic examination.[61] Van Gijn has suggested that this was because Babinski had no talent for drawing what he saw, as Charcot had. In his thesis on MS, the beautiful plates on focal demyelination were drawn by M. Karmomski, a laboratory assistant, and lithography was by M. Nicolet.

Babinski's thesis on MS concentrated on the idea of inflammation and the infiltration of lymphocytes into the plaque, which he felt was important in the pathogenesis of myelin breakdown and formation of plaques.

> *"Destruction of the myelin sheath … results from the nutritive activity of neurolgia and lymphatic cells; as in all inflammation, it is the diapedesis of lymphatic cells and their multiplication in the neurolgia that marks the start on the morbid work."*[62]

Babinski was born in Paris, the son of immigrants who had fled Poland. He completed his medical training in 1884 and became chief physician under Charcot at the Salpêtrière. He was initially less successful and famous than his older brother Henri, who wrote a book on French cooking under the pseudonym Ali-Bab that went into 13 printings. Much to Charcot's disappointment, Babinski was always passed over for an academic position, but his reputation grew. He was an impressive man on the wards—tall, quiet, and thoughtful, questioning every idea and concept. Although he also made original contributions to clinical neurology and the study of hysteria, and, during WWI, to the treatment of war neurosis, he will always be remembered for his paper on the "phénomène des orteils" (the phenomenon of the toes), which became the eponymous Babinski reflex.* Babinski died of Parkinson's disease on October 23, 1932, in Paris.

JULIUS ALTHAUS

Julius Althaus, a prominent neurologist at the Hospital for Epilepsy and Paralysis at Regent's Park, gave two lectures on sclerosis of the spinal cord in 1884,[63] and in the introduction to his book a year later made an important comment: that in many publications, from many countries, the term "sclerosis" had many meanings.

> *"There is no pathological term which is now-a-days so freely and somewhat loosely used in speaking and writing about the diseases of the nervous system as the word sclerosis. We hear and read not only of*

---

*The first mention by Babinski of the reflex that bears his name was a brief note in the Comptes-Rendus of 1896 stating that the normal reflex on stimulation of the plantar surface of the foot was flexion, but in some cases of "paralysis," the response was extension of the toes. A full, two-page account was given in 1898 in *La Semaine Médicale*, a weekly journal, and he called it the phenomenon of the toes (*le phénomène des orteils*). The most effective technique for eliciting the reflex involved having the patient close his eyes, with the leg slightly flexed at the knee, and waiting for the muscles to relax. The lateral side of the plantar sole was stroked without warning the patient of the procedure. He then described seven cases who manifested the phenomenon of the toes. Within months, James Collier in London emphasized the functional importance of this reflex, and over the next few years, Babinski added to the discussion, including the observation of fanning of the toes as part of the reflex.

primary and secondary sclerosis, but also of posterior and lateral scle-
rosis, of descending and ascending, and of insular, disseminated, and
amyotrophic sclerosis."[64]

He noted that sclerosis originally meant certain pathological changes on postmortem examination. It was being widely applied to diagnoses and patients with any obscure and chronic disease of the nervous system, who were than called "sclerotics." He pointed out that the word means "hard" and although many sclerotic patches are indeed hard, others in the fresh state are soft. He defined what sclerosis means in cases of tabes dorsalis, progressive locomotor ataxia, posterior column sclerosis, and Vulpian's posterior leuco-myelitis. Only after discussion of these and other diseases, did he come to the disorder that interests us here, "sclerosis in patches," which he said was also known as multiple, insular, and disseminated sclerosis, the condition described by Charcot.

Althaus wrote a text on the various "scleroses" of the spinal cord; the last section was devoted to MS.[65] He noted that in 1877 he had initiated the name "Charcot's disease" for multiple sclerosis, but Althaus gave up on this term; he did not use it in his chapter or put it in the index.*

Like Osler, Althaus felt sensation was rarely involved in sclerosis, and clinicians of his era overemphasized this feature to separate MS from the tabes dorsalis form of syphilis, even though modern neurologists feel that sensory loss is a common symptom and sign in MS. His description is clear, and he gives a number of sample cases of the early and late stages of the disease. He felt therapy for MS was in its infancy and unsuccessful; it was usually started long after there had been irreparable damage to the nervous system. This comment has a modern ring. However, Althaus advised the use of iodide of potassium, arsenic, and nitrate of silver, as well as electrical therapies.

Modern readers, aware of the nature of acute attacks of MS, will be puzzled by the dramatic onset of MS described by these early writers. Althaus indicated attacks had a sudden onset like an apoplectic attack or

---

*The last record I can find of MS being referred to as Charcot's disease is in a 1910 *Lancet* article by Poorman.

epileptic seizure, which preceded a coma. Sufferers might die, but if they recovered, they regained control over the paralyzed parts and might have complete or partial recovery. Althaus felt some of the dramatic symptoms of MS might be related to an acute infection (a high temperature was often a common symptom). Some cases could be confused with neurosyphilis: patients had headache, dizziness, depression, memory impairment, indifference to daily life, anorexia, and grandiose delirium. Modern physicians feel that many of these symptoms are characteristic of late effects of MS, and not the acute onset of the disease. Like many of the 19th-century authors, Althaus commented on the characteristics of MS in children, saying that the disease could occur at any age. Tremor was such a characteristic of the disease that he specifically mentioned a case reported by Bastian which had no tremor.

J.S. BRISTOWE'S QUESTION

Twenty years after Charcot's lectures on MS, every medical student and registrar was aware of this neurological disease. J.S. Bristowe said in 1887 that he framed a question on multiple sclerosis for the membership exam of the Royal College of Physicians of London, asking about the differential diagnosis of tabes dorsalis and multiple sclerosis.[66] Candidates were competent in their description of these disorders, but only one or two seemed to recognize that the diseases could be confused and could look very much alike. Most of the candidates felt the distinctions so obvious that "no one of experience could confuse them." Bristowe was experienced enough to recognize that the conditions might look very much the same in early stages, and when they were in "partial," rather than in "classical," presentations. He then outlined 10 cases where the diagnosis could be confusing. It is interesting that he commented, as other writers did, on "epileptiform seizures" in multiple sclerosis, which from the description we now recognize as acute weakness and collapse. Bristowe had earlier noted that these are usually brought on by rising temperature.

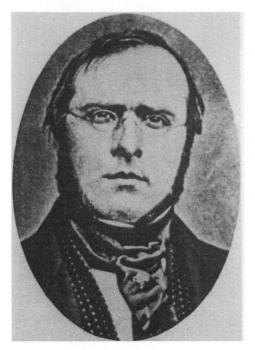

Figure 7.19 Augustus Volney Waller, anatomist and physiologist. He showed the degeneration of the distal nerve fibers following section of the nerve and stimulated interest in how nerve fibers reacted to damage in the peripheral and central nervous system. (From McHenry, Lawrence C. Garrison's *History of Neurology*, 1969. Courtesy of Charles C Thomas Publisher Ltd. Springfield, Illinois.)

OTHER REPORTS

Sir Christopher Nixon reported a case with autopsy findings and a year later Tweedy diagnosed a patient during life and ascribed the cause, as Moxon had, to sexual habits and domestic activities.[67] In 1893, Landon Carter Gray confused the clinical picture by indicating that MS was not uncommon in children with onset ranging from 14 months to 14.5 years, half of the cases coming on after a convulsion.[68] He pointed out that other writers, such as Hodemaker, Unger, Leube, Charcot, and Prichard, had noted childhood cases, and Prichard had collected 50 such cases at the New York Polyclinic.

In 1888, J.A. Ormerod, a Queen Square consultant, published a case in circumstances we might all envy when we are confronted with a challenging diagnostic case in the office.[69] He saw a person with sensory symptoms on the right side, bladder difficulty, and pallor of the right optic disc. Even though Charcot's triad was still in vogue, and diagnosis of MS tended to be made only in the late stages, Ormerod suspected multiple sclerosis. He said, "I had the advantage of the opinion of Dr. Pierre Marie, who was present in the outpatient room" and who was ushered in to assess the case and subsequently agreed with the diagnosis.* If only we all could have an international expert on the condition sitting in the anteroom when we are puzzling over a diagnosis.

In an 1895 textbook on diseases of the nervous system in children, Bernard Sachs devoted 11 pages to multiple sclerosis.[70] He indicated in a footnote that Totzke had recorded two cases evident at birth, others at ages five and 14 months, and 33 cases between ages two and 14 years. Even Sachs doubted those were all MS; the youngest he had seen was age 14 with onset of symptoms after age 10. Pierre Marie had previously reported three cases in infants in 1883, though he later thought he was wrong in the diagnosis.[71]

In discussing the differential diagnosis, Sachs felt that MS could be confused with hereditary tremor in the young, or with the pseudosclerosis of Westphal (later known as Wilson's disease). He felt the latter was "not an important disease (to my knowledge it has not been clearly established in any other instance)." Sachs was concerned that transverse myelitis, which he felt was a separate disease, would be confused with MS, as might hysteria and Parkinson's disease.

PIERRE MARIE

Pierre Marie (1853–1940) was born into a wealthy family; when he decided on medicine as a career, his father objected and insisted he enter law. He passed the bar in law, but then renewed his interest in medicine and entered medical school, to study under Charcot and Bouchard.

He presented 25 cases of MS in his monograph on "insular sclerosis and the infectious diseases"(1884).[72] Marie praised Charcot for giving a masterful description of the clinical and pathological features of the disease. Some of Marie's cases were from a monograph by Kahler and Pick (1879), who noted that onset often followed acute illness.

---

*That patient, who had the onset of multiple sclerosis in 1880, later became a patient of Dr. Ramskill, and MS was confirmed at autopsy in 1887.

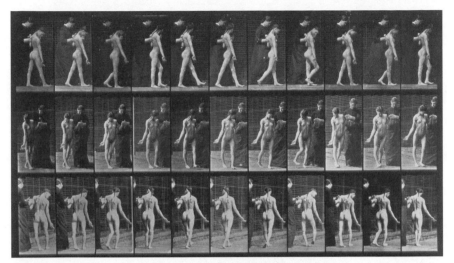

Figure 7.20   A girl with multiple sclerosis walking with her nurse in the Blockley Hospital for the Poor. Photogravure after Eadweard Muybridge, 1887. This was one of the 781 photogravures on animal locomotion by Muybridge carried out at the University of Pennsylvania. (Courtesy of the Wellcome Library, London.)

Marie felt there were three major forms of MS: spastic, purely cerebellar, and cerebello-spastic. He classified the course of the disease into the chronic progressive course: intermittent attacks, chronic remitting course, and patients with increasing improvement or apparent cure. He showed the diagram by Gilles de la Tourette of the foot pattern of a patient with multiple sclerosis trying to walk along a line. The pattern shows the gait (foot pattern) of the patient with spastic *and* cerebellar forms of MS.

Marie said that many of the causes of multiple sclerosis were well-known—overwork, exposure to cold, injury, and excess of every kind. Although these are common precipitants, he said he knew of another cause even more common—infection—"or rather infections." He listed the most common infections he had seen that precipitated MS: typhoid, malaria, smallpox, diphtheria, erysipelas, pneumonia, measles, scarlatina, whooping cough, dysentery, cholera, and other fevers.

Marie confessed that the evidence was not yet conclusive for infection as a cause for MS, and prudent reserve was reasonable from a purely scientific point of view. Although this seems open-minded, in a

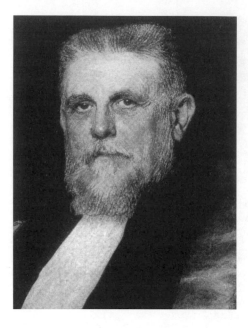

Figure 7.21 Pierre Marie (1853–1940), student of Charcot, was convinced that MS was due to an infection and would soon be swept by the development of a vaccine such as Pasteur had developed for other infections. Although others would criticize his views (Marie did not shrink from controversy) and most would accept only that infections could aggravate the disorder, a century later the idea of a viral cause and a potential vaccine lingers. (Courtesy of the National Library of Medicine.)

footnote, he indicated that most people accepted his theory of infection, and it would be ungracious of him to find fault with those who disagreed, even though some of these disbelievers had been very hostile. He went on to note that some even disagreed with his theory that most epilepsy had an infectious origin, but until that was proven, he would just repeat that he was steadfast in this opinion. He said he had accumulated an even more impressive mound of facts since he first published this theory. He outlined the usual scenario—a person age 20–30 contracts an infectious disease, and during the disease, or in the months that follow, symptoms of multiple sclerosis begin.

Marie confessed embarrassment when the discussion turned to the actual organism involved, for so little was known. He added that some colleagues who had obviously not read his papers had erroneously concluded that he had found *the* organism of MS. He assured them that he had never said such a thing. He felt that many organisms, or more likely combined infections, might initiate MS. He concluded:

"These, gentlemen, are suppositions, and I put them before you without unreasonably insisting upon them. The one point in this discus-

sion which I would fix in your minds is the following fact, a fact
which, thank God, has been well established, viz., that the cause of
insular sclerosis is intimately connected with infectious diseases."

Marie's firm belief in an infective cause for MS would have direct
implications for how therapy was to be directed. He recommended drugs
to deal with the sclerotic and the infective elements of the disease. "It
would follow, then, that iodide of potassium or sodium would be beneficial, as you know how much good may be done ... in vascular sclerosis.
For infection, he recommended mercury, not because it was effective in
syphilis, which Marie knew, no matter how similar the manifestations,
was unrelated to MS, but because mercury could be used for its disinfec-
tive properties.

His lesson ended with an uplifting note, which captured the current
excitement of an age that grasped the germ theory, and the discoveries of
Koch, Pasteur, and Lister:

"I have little doubt in fact, gentlemen, that in the employment of such
a substance as the vaccine of Pasteur or lymph of Koch the evolution
*of insular sclerosis will someday be rendered absolutely impossible."**

In his later writings, Marie mused that he was uncertain about how
common MS was, but noted that Uhthoff had seen 100 cases of ocular
disorder due to MS over six to seven years in the hospitals and poly-
clinics of Berlin, so it was not rare.[73] Hans Uhthoff published an extensive monograph on the eye findings in multiple sclerosis, including
retrobulbar neuritis, the scotomata, and visual field abnormalities.[74]
He felt both sexes were equally affected, and onset was usually
between ages 20 and 30; if a patient presented with a neurological disease after age 40, MS had scarcely to be considered. Although MS was

---

*Pierre Marie was born into a wealthy family, had classical education in private schools, and
initially followed his father's admonition to study law, but after graduation, entered medical
school and later was influenced by his teachers, Charcot and Bouchard. He was said to enjoy
golf, fencing, travel, his own rolled cigarettes, and prune liquor (Swiderski). Like Charcot, he
read and annotated journals on his ride to the hospitals each day. After an active and prestigious career, he suddenly resigned after the deaths of his wife, son, and daughter, but lived
another 17 years.

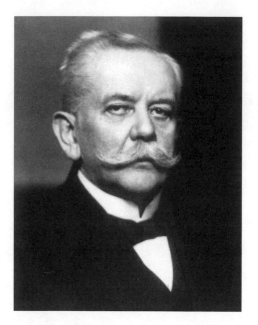

Figure 7.22 Wilhelm Uhthoff collected 100 cases of multiple sclerosis when many felt it was a rare disease. He detailed the ocular and visual changes in the disease. He is remembered for the observation that exercise can cause the vision to transiently decrease. (Courtesy of Hans K. Uhthoff, Ottawa.)

rare in children, he had collected 13 cases from others, but he questioned some of these diagnoses.

HEINRICH OPPENHEIM

As avidly as Marie pushed the infective etiology of MS, in 1887 Heinrich Oppenheim strongly postulated an environmental toxin such as lead, mercury, manganese, copper, zinc, or even carbon monoxide or cyanide as a cause of the disease.[75] There was no specific therapy for MS, Oppenheim said, but things that might be helpful include silver nitrate, potassium iodide, spa baths at Oeynhausen or Nauheim, leeches, and a mild galvanic current applied to the back of the head. This approach to therapy for MS was not much different from that applied by physicians for multiple sclerosis through the 19th century.[76]

CHARLES L. DANA

While European writers were regularly publishing on the features of multiple sclerosis, Americans still believed the disorder was rare, at

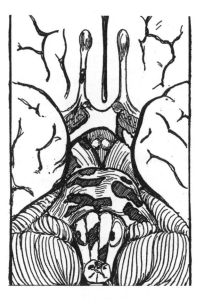

Figure 7.23 Charles Dana's crude illustration of the lesions of MS adapted from an illustration from Charcot. Dana, like many on both sides of the Atlantic, thought the disease was rare in North America. He recognized the diversity of the clinical picture, and also the *formes frustes* such as a progressive spastic paraplegia, which could have other manifestations as well, a purely spinal form, and a purely cerebral form. (Dana, 1894.)

least on that side of the Atlantic. Charles L. Dana wrote in New York in 1894:

> *"In America the disease is, in the writer's experience, rare. The diagnosis, to be sure, is often made, but only two cases verified by postmortems have been reported by American physicians."*

Charles L. Dana, 1894[77]

ARNOLD EDWARDS

Arnold Edwards, a resident medical officer in Manchester, published a small monograph on his review of the literature and his investigation of 33 cases of "undoubted disseminated sclerosis" in 1895. Twenty-three of the cases were male, 10 female. He surveyed 60 published cases and again found males predominated, even though he noted that Charcot's cases were 25 female and nine male, giving the repeated excuse that mostly females made up the population of the Salpêtrière.

Edwards felt MS causes were specific fevers including typhoid, scarlet fever, variola, morbilli, pertussis, diphtheria, typhus, and malaria; other fevers might also precipitate the disease. He believed that microorganisms were not the cause, but the toxins produced by them precipitated the disease in those with a latent tendency to nervous disease. Acute rheumatism, trauma, cold and wet, extreme heat, pellagra, pregnancy, and syphilis were all listed as initiating the onset of multiple sclerosis. Emotional upset such as prolonged grief and fright could also bring on the disease, but this could be quite distant from onset. He mentions a patient who had a severe fright and developed MS six years later. As to the pathogenesis of the plaques, he noted the different opinions of the pathologists. Ziegler (1886) argued that it was primarily a degeneration of the cell elements due to a distance of tissue nutrition, while Rindfleisch, supported by Ribbert and Marie, felt that disturbance of tissues was due to an embolic vascular lesion, which seemed the only explanation for the scattered nature of the plaques, and was supported by the presence of a vessel at the center of each plaque.

Onset was abrupt in only two of the 33 cases, and tremor was said to be the most characteristic of the symptoms. Although many argued that it was a characteristic tremor, Edwards notes that many others found the same tremor in other neurological diseases.

RISIEN RUSSELL

In 1899, Risien Russell wrote an excellent review of the disease, downplaying any role for infection in the cause of MS. He recognized that infections such as influenza could aggravate the condition of a person with MS, if the disease existed in a mild and unrecognized form. In this case, the infection would appear to have caused, rather than brought to light a preexisting condition. He disagreed with Oppenheim, who believed that exposure to environmental toxins such as lead, copper, and zinc was the cause of MS. Russell said that many young ladies whose circumstances would exclude them from "the baneful influences" suggested by Oppenheim still came down with MS, so there must be some more general etiological factor involved. A wise and kindly physician, Russell recognized that pharmacological therapy was unhelpful, but perhaps silver and arsenic were worth a trial for these unfortunate patients. In addition, patients should avoid stress and exposure to cold, physical and mental fatigue, as well as "indulgence in wine and venery." Russell said: "The therapeutic prospects in disseminate sclerosis are gloomy in the extreme."

Although Russell himself had little to suggest for therapy, W. Ian MacDonald noted in an interview with Macdonald Critchley, who was Russell's last house officer, that a few minutes with Russell had a very therapeutic effect on a patient with MS.

THOMAS BUZZARD

One of the cases in the series presented by Moxon in 1875 was a case of Thomas Buzzard. Buzzard presented cases at meetings of the Clinical Society of London and published his views on MS for 30 years.[78–81] Buzzard thought MS relapses were such an "interesting and exceptional feature of the disease" that he published seven cases in what he confessed was "somewhat wearisome detail" in order to make the point about the importance of numerous attacks and remissions as a characteristic of the disorder. He wanted his colleagues to recognize that relapses were an important diagnostic feature and also might hold a clue about the cause of the disease. Like Russell, he rejected the toxic theory and also the suggestion that MS might have a congenital basis. It seemed rare to him in members of a family, and he favored the theory of an inflammatory process in blood vessels caused by an infection.

As to therapy, he said:

"In the present state of our ignorance regarding the etiology of insular sclerosis, there is no advantage in disguising the fact that we are unable to point to any mode of treatment which appears to influence the progress of this disease."

ASHLEY W. MACKINTOSH

Ashley W. Mackintosh of Aberdeen wrote of the difficulty making the diagnosis in the earliest stages of MS. He tabulated all the cases in the files of the great Queen Square neurologist David Ferrier, added some cases of his own, and wrote about the various modes of onset to assist in making early diagnoses. Careful in his analysis of the files, he reduced the number

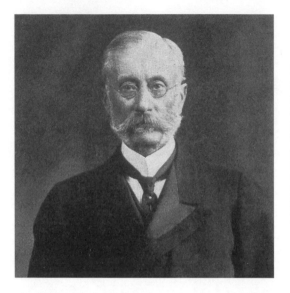

Figure 7.24 David Ferrier (1843–1928) wrote little about MS, although he wrote a great deal on neurological conditions, neurophysiology, and cerebral localization. His careful observation of his patients as a busy consultant was useful when his files on MS cases were reviewed by Ashley W. Mackintosh. (Photographer: Maull & Fox, London, England, 1905.)

to 80 by including only those patients who later developed the cardinal features of MS or who had autopsy confirmation. He said diagnosis was difficult; there were many modes of onset, and it might be many years before the cardinal features appeared, if they ever did. The symptoms at onset might be cerebral, bulbar, or spinal in type. Tremor in the arms was present in 84 percent of patients; nystagmus in 81 percent; optic atrophy in 47.5 percent, and scanning speech in 20 percent. Onset was gradual in 21 of the 80 cases, usually with spasticity in the legs. Gradual sensory and motor symptoms were present in an additional 15 cases. Ataxia and tremor as onset were present in 20 cases, and sensory symptoms alone in 10 cases. Onset was sudden and acute in 10 of 80, with cerebral symptoms in 19 of 80 at onset. Many of the patients had an overlap in their presenting features.

Mackintosh commented on the remarkable variability of features at onset, the frequency of unilateral features, and the frequency of sensory symptoms. Unlike Osler and other early writers, who thought sensory symptoms were uncommon, he insisted that sensory symptoms were in fact highly suggestive of the disorder. He commented:

"The old teaching was that the absence of sensory symptoms was characteristic of disseminated sclerosis; but the writings of Erb, Oppenheim, Freund, etc., have disproved the truth of this."

R.T. WILLIAMSON

By the turn of the century, the clinical and pathological features of multiple sclerosis were well-recognized, as evidenced by the landmark monograph by Eduard Müller (1904)[82] of Breslau, who published an extensive work on the condition, reviewing 1100 references related to MS.

Agreeing with Bramwell, R.T. Williamson in his textbook on *Diseases of the Spinal Cord*, said that MS was not a common disease, even in hospital practice, but was more frequent in England than in America, and judging from the reports from the Continent, common in the country districts of Germany.[83] At the Manchester Royal Infirmary during the 10 years that he was medical registrar, the number of inpatients was 13,864; the number of cases of diseases of the nervous system was 2,294, and of these, 61 were MS, 118 were locomotor ataxia, and six were Parkinson's disease. In addition, there were 10 cases of MS at the Ancoats, Manchester, among 2,870 medical inpatients, of whom only a small proportion had diseases of the nervous system.

Williamson commented that the two sexes were equally affected. Like so many others who noted occasional familial cases, he made little of the association, although he noted that there were several rare reported cases of mother and child having the same disease. One such case was verified pathologically by Eichhorst, and several members of one family with MS were reported by E.S. Reynolds. Death in his cases of MS occurred from emaciation, urinary tract infections, pyemic conditions following paralysis of the bladder, septic absorption from a bedsore, or from some intercurrent disease such as pneumonia or tuberculosis.

Williamson mentioned Buzzard's discussion of an "hysterical form" of MS, meaning that the cases presented with many emotional symptoms, but later on showed typical changes. Progression was often prolonged, and some cases had remissions, and even apparent recovery, as recorded in the cases of Charcot, Oppenheim, Byrom Bramwell, and Maas. He said that there was no cure, and rest, tonic treatment, and good hygiene were of some slight service. He felt that all drugs he had tried had failed, except for quinine.

REFERENCES

1. William Osler. A Clinical Lecture on Erythemia. *Lancet* 1908; 1:143–146.
2. Sherwin AL. Multiple Sclerosis in historical perspective. *McGill Medical Journal.* 1957;26:39-48.
3. Ebers GC. A Historical Overview. In: *Multiple Sclerosis.* Donald W. Paty and George Ebers, eds. Philadelphia: FA Davis; 1998;1-4.
4. Bourneville DM, Guérard I. *De la sclérose en plaques disseminées.* Paris: Delahaye; 1869.
5. Ordenstein M. *Sur la paralysie agitante et la sclerose en plaques generalisee.* Paris: A Delahaye; 1868.
6. Putnam TJ. The Centenary of Multiple Sclerosis. *Arch Neurol Psych.* 1938;40(4):806–813.
7. Ordenstein M. *Sur la paralysie agitante et la sclerose en plaques generalisee.* Paris: A Delahaye; 1868.
8. Ebers GC. A Historical Overview. In: *Multiple Sclerosis.* Paty DW and Ebers G, eds. Philadelphia: FA Davis; 1998;1-4.
9. Bourneville DM, Guérard I. *De la sclérose en plaques disseminées.* Paris: Delahaye; 1869.
10. Echeverria, MG. Sclerosis of both third anterior frontal convolutions without aphasia. *The Medical Record.* 1869;4:1–2.
11. Schüle Hans. Beitrag zur multiplen Sklerose de Ghirns und Ruckenmarks. *Deutsches Archives für Klinische Medicine.* 1870;vii:259.
12. Compston A. The Story of Multiple Sclerosis. Chapter 1 in *McAlpine's Multiple Sclerosis.* London: Churchill Livingstone; 1998:3-42.
13. Hammond WA. A treatise on diseases of the nervous system. Ch. VII: *Multiple Cerebrospinal Sclerosis.* New York: D. Appleton and Co.; 1871;637-653.
14. Compston A. The Story of Multiple Sclerosis. Chapter 1 in *McAlpine's Multiple Sclerosis.* London: Churchill Livingstone; 1998.
15. Ibid.
16. Clymer M. Notes on the Physiology and Pathology of the Nervous System, with Reference to Clinical Medicine. *New York Med J.* 1870;60:225-260; 410-423.
17. Baldwin G. A case of diffused cerebral sclerosis. *Am Insanity.* 1872; xxviii, republished in *J Mental Sci.* 1873; July:304-305.
18. Cook JI. Multiple Cerebro-Spinal Sclerosis. *The Richmond and Louisville Medical Journal.* 1872;14:76-78.
19. Anon. Guy's Hospital. Case of insular sclerosis of the brain and spinal cord (under the care of Dr. Moxon). *Lancet.* 1873;1:236.
20. Anon. Guy's Hospital. Two cases of insular sclerosis of the brain and spinal cord (under the care of Dr. Moxon). *Lancet.* 1875;1:471-473.
21. Anon. Guy's Hospital. Two cases of insular sclerosis of the brain and spinal cord (under the care of Dr. Moxon). *Lancet.* 1875;1:609.
22. Anon. Report on Clinical Society of London. *Lancet.* 1875;1:545.
23. Buzzard T. Case presentation, Clinical Society of London. *Lancet.* 1875;1:545.
24. Moxon W. Eight cases of insular sclerosis of the brain and spinal cord. *Guy Hosp Rep.* 1875; 20:437-478.
25. Baudrey JK in Murray TJ. The history of MS. *Multiple Sclerosis: Diagnosis, Medical Management and Rehabilitation.* Burks J and Johnson K, editors. New York: Demos; 2000:1-20.
26. Buzzard T. Case presentation, Clinical Society of London. *Lancet.* 1875;1:545.
27. Frith JA. History of multiple sclerosis: an Australian perspective. *Clin and Exp Neurol.* 1988; 25:7-16.
28. MacLaurin H. Case of amblyopia from partial neuritis, treated with subcutaneous injection of strychnia. *NSW Med Gazette.* 1873;3:214.
29. Newman AK. On insular sclerosis of the brain and spinal cord. *Aust Med J.* 1875;20:369-374.

30. Jamieson J. Cases of multiple neuritis. *Aust Med J.* 1886;8:295-302.
31. Frith JA. History of multiple sclerosis: an Australian perspective. *Clin and Exp Neurol.* 1988;25:7-16.
32. Gerhard GS. *Cases of Multilocular Cerebro-Spinal Sclerosis.* Philadelphia: Medical Times, 1876;7:50.
33. Wood HC Jr. The Multiple Scleroses. *The Medical Record.* 1878;09/14:224-250.
34. Hamilton AM. *Nervous Diseases: Their Description and Treatment.* London: J&A Churchill; 1878:346-351.
35. Wilks S. *Lectures on Diseases of the Nervous System, Delivered at Guy's Hospital.* London: J&A Churchill; 1878:282-284.
36. Seguin EC, Shaw JC, Van Derveer A. A contribution to the pathological anatomy of disseminated cerebro-spinal sclerosis. *J Nerv Ment Dis.* 1878;5:281-293.
37. Wilson SAK. *Neurology,* ed. AN Bruce. London: Edward Arnold; 1940:148-178.
38. Kirkland R. Disseminated sclerosis at an unusual age. *BMJ.* 1883;1:407.
39. Osler W. Cases of insular sclerosis. *Can Med Surg J.* 1880;1-11.
40. Ebers GC. Osler and Neurology. *Can J Neurol Sci.* 1985b;12:236-242.
41. Osler W. *The Principles and Practice of Medicine.* New York: D. Appleton and Co.; 1892.
42. Osler W. *Bibliotheca Osleriana.* Montreal and London: McGill-Queens Press; 1969:206-207.
43. Müller E. *Die Multiple Sclerose des Gehirns and Rückenmarks. Ihre Pathologie und Behandlung.* Jena: Gustav Fischer; 1904.
44. Bramwell B. *The Diseases of the Spinal Cord.* Edinburgh: MacLachlan and Stewart; 1882.
45. Bramwell B. On the relative frequency of disseminated sclerosis in this country (Scotland and the North of England) and in America. *Review of Neurology and Psychiatry* (Edinburgh); 1903;1:12-17.
46. Bramwell B. The prognosis of disseminated sclerosis. *Edin Med J.* 1917;18:16-19.
47. Stewart J. Multiple Cerebral Sclerosis. *Can Med and Surg J.* 1884; Nov:238-241.
48. Albert DM. Introduction to reprint of *Gower's Manual and Atlas of Medical Ophthalmoscopy* (1879). Classics of Neurology and Neurosurgery Library. New Jersey. 1992.
49. Gowers WR. *The Diagnosis of Diseases of the Spinal Cord.* London: Churchill; 1880.
50. Gowers WR. *A Manual of Diseases of the Nervous System,* 2nd ed. London: J&A Churchill; 1893:vol 2:544, 557-558.
51. Gowers WR. *A Manual of Diseases of the Nervous System.* Vol 2: Diseases of the Brain and Cranial Nerves. 2nd ed. Philadelphia: P Blakiston, Son; 1893.
52. McDonald WI. The mystery of the origin of multiple sclerosis. The Ninth Gowers Memorial Lecture. *J Neurol Neurosurg Psychiatry.* 1986;49:113-123.
53. Albert DM. Introduction to reprint of *Gower's Manual and Atlas of Medical Ophthalmoscopy* (1879). Classics of Neurology and Neurosurgery Library. NJ. 1992.
54. Haymaker, Webb. *The Founders of Neurology.* Springfield, IL: Charles C. Thomas; 1953: p. 292-295.
55. Ibid, p. 292-295.
56. Tyler KL, Roberts D, Tyler HR. The shorthand publications of Sir William Richard Gowers. *Neurology.* 2000; 55:289-293.
57. McDonald WI. The Mystery of the origin of multiple sclerosis. Gowers Lecture. *J Neurol Neurosurg Psychiatry.* 1986;49:113-123.
58. Critchley M. *Sir William Gowers 1845-1915. A Biographical Appreciation.* London: William Heinemann Medical Books; 1949.
59. Babinski J. *Etude anatomique et clinique sur la sclérose en plaques.* Paris: G. Masson; 1885.
60. Ibid.
61. Babinski J. Recherches sur l'anatomie pathologique de la sclérose en plaques et étude comparative des diverses variétés de scléroses de la moelle. *Arch Physiol Norm Pathol.* 1885;5(3):186-207.

62. van Gijn J. *The Babinski Sign—a centenary*. Utrecht: University of Utrecht; 1996.
63. Althaus J. Two lectures on sclerosis of the spinal cord. *BMJ*. 1884;1:893-985.
64. Althaus J. *On Sclerosis of the Spinal Cord*. London: Longmans, 1885.
65. Ibid.
66. Bristowe JS. The early recognition of general paralysis of the insane, and the relations between this disease, tabes dorsalis, and disseminated sclerosis. *Brit Med J*. 1887;1:1-5.
67. Compston A. The Story of Multiple Sclerosis. Chapter 1 in *McAlpine's Multiple Sclerosis*. London: Churchill Livingstone; 1998.
68. Gray LC. *A Treatise on Nervous and Mental Diseases*. London: HK Lewis; 1893:373-378.
69. Ormerod JA. *St. Bartholemews Hospital Reports*. 1988;24:155-161.
70. Sachs B. *A Treatise on the Nervous Diseases of Children*. New York. William Wood; 1895:345-356.
71. Marie, Pierre. La sclerose en plaques et maladies infectieuses. *La Progress Medicale*. 1884;12:287-289.
72. Ibid, p. 287-289.
73. Marie P. *Lectures on Diseases of the Spinal Cord*. Trans. M. Lubbock. London: New Sydenham Society; 1895;153:134-136.
74. Uhthoff W. Untersuchen über die bei multiplen herdsclerose vorkommenden augerstörungen. *Arch Psychiat*. Berlin: 1890; xxi:303-410.
75. Oppenheim H. *Zur Pathologie der disseminierten Sklerose*. Berlin: klin. Wschr. 1887;904-907.
76. Oppenheim H. *Text-book of Nervous Diseases for Physicians and Students*, trans. A Bruce. Edinburgh: Otto Schulze; 1911.
77. Dana CL. *Textbook of Nervous Diseases*. 3rd ed. New York: William Wood; 1894:374-380.
78. Buzzard T. Case presentation, Clinical Society of London. *Lancet*. 1875;1:545.
79. Buzzard T. Disseminated cerebrospinal sclerosis. *Lancet*. 1875;1:304.
80. Buzzard T. Insular sclerosis and hysteria. *Lancet*. 1897;1:1-4.
81. Buzzard T. Brain. *Lancet*. 1904; July:16.
82. Müller E. Die multiple Sclerose des Gehirns and Rückenmarks. *Ihre Pathologie und Behandlung*. Jena: Gustav Fischer, 1904.
83. Williamson RT. *Diseases of the Spinal Cord*. Henry Frowde London: Oxford University Press; 1908.

C h a p t e r

8

Clarifying the Pathology: James Dawson

"Restituto ad integrum."

James Dawson

C harcot's great contribution was the clarification of the concepts of multiple sclerosis (MS). His description of the disease held first place for generations, and we often return to his writings as we change our ideas on the disease. As noted earlier, many knew and described the disorder before he did, and often very well, but it was his clear and confident description of the clinical and pathological features that brought MS to the forefront of medicine. It is a mark of his impact that most of the descriptions over the next five decades were repetitions or small refinements of his clinical and pathological observations. It would be decades into the 20th century before additional important contributions came in pathology, genetics, immunology, and epidemiology. Charcot's pathological descriptions also held, although arguments developed about which tissues or cells were primarily involved in MS. Was it in the glial tissues, as Charcot suggested, or the vessels Rindfleisch suspected? What was the cause of the pathological change? Was it a primary glial hypertrophy, a vascular disease, the result of an environmental toxin, or an infection?

Although it was common for clinicians like Cruveilhier, Rindfleisch, Leyden, Vulpian, Charcot, Mitchell, Moxon, and Osler to follow their patients to autopsy, and to make careful observations of the changes of MS in the nervous system, the first major systematic study of the disease that advanced significantly beyond the observations of Charcot was carried out by James Dawson of Edinburgh.[1,2] His was a remarkable and monumental work on multiple sclerosis published in 1916–1918, heralded as the most important contribution to British neurology in that generation. *The Lancet* said, "It supplied fresh proof of the very high standard of British neurology."

Born in India, James Dawson (1870–1927) struggled against the effects of tuberculosis (TB) much of his life. His initial medical studies at Edinburgh were interrupted by a bout of this illness, and for the next 13 years, he traveled in Canada, the United States, India, and New Zealand where he worked as a lumberjack and as a shepherd. For four years he nursed his brother, who suffered from a form of myelitis.* During this time, Dawson developed bilateral pneumonia, probably as a complication of his TB. Despite these tribulations, Dawson applied to return to the medical studies he had abandoned so many years before and graduated with first-class honors. He took up the study of pathology under J.G. Greenfield, who was then at Edinburgh, and he was awarded a Syme Surgical Fellowship for his thesis on wound healing and inflammation, receiving an MD with a gold medal. His studies then centered on disorders of the nervous system, particularly multiple sclerosis, multiple neuromata, and the spinal cord lymphatic system.[3] Unable to serve in World War I because of his poor health, he became a busy teacher. During that period he published an address on "The Spirit of Leisure and the Spirit of Work," an essay which for many years was presented to each entering Edinburgh medical student.

His research on multiple sclerosis was under Dr. Alexander Bruce, with Dawson as assistant and second author on their first papers. They described the characteristics of the MS lesion, an inflammatory reaction with cells entering from some "central source" and infiltrating the sur-

---

*It would be poetic to suggest it was MS, but it may also have been Pott's disease.

rounding tissues. Bruce was convinced the changes were in relation to the lymphatic system. When Bruce unexpectedly died, Dawson continued to work on his own. His great work on the pathology of multiple sclerosis was published in the *Edinburgh Medical Journal*,[4] and also in versions in the *Review of Neurology and Psychiatry*, and the *Transactions of the Royal Society of Edinburgh*, and finally as a heavily illustrated monograph.

The work was based on the examination of nine cases of MS, one with death relatively early in the course. This acute case gave Dawson the unique opportunity to observe the early changes in the lesions of multiple sclerosis. He started with a long quote from R.T. Williamson (1908) to outline the accepted clinical characteristics of the disease. Then he asked the two central questions. What is the nature of the underlying process? In what structural aspect of the nervous system does it arise?

Dawson had examined nine cases in detail, but his thesis concentrated on a kitchenmaid, L.W., age 28, a patient of Dr. Alexander Bruce, admitted on April 4, 1910 with a two-year history of weakness and tremor, dysarthria, and bladder difficulty. While in the ward, she had an acute brain stem event with right facial weakness, deafness and tinnitus, left arm numbness, right lateral rectus weakness, tongue deviation to the

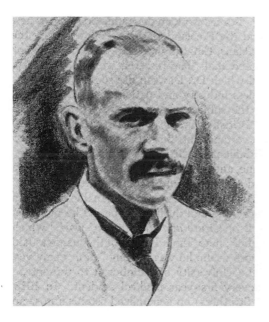

Figure 8.1 James Walker Dawson (1870–1927) made a major contribution to the knowledge of multiple sclerosis by his detailed pathological descriptions, said by *The Lancet* to supply "fresh proof of the very high standard of British neurology." Portrait courtesy of the Armed Forces Institute of Pathology, Washington, DC. (From Portrait in *J Path Bact*, London, 1928; 31:117–121.)

left, dysphagia, followed by blindness, and bulbar failure. She died of an infection on September 5, 1910.

Dawson described the distribution and stages of the lesions. He discussed the lesions noted previously by Marburg (though Marburg was not mentioned), the shadow plaque or *Markschattenherde*. He described cellular changes and then attempted a clinico-pathological correlation of the lesions he noted with her symptoms, signs, and disease course. He said he knew of no other pathological process quite like that of MS—the relative integrity of the specific functioning parenchymatous tissue associated with an enormous increase of the interstitial tissue in definite circumscribed patches.

Dawson reviewed the theories of etiology, quoting Bramwell as saying that the disease could be due to some irritant distributed to the nervous system via the blood vessels, but there might be a congenital vulnerability in the people who develop the disease. These are the exogenous and endogenous theories of the disease. Strümpell and Müller believed it was an inflammatory disease and thus an endogenous disorder, although an external factor could be an *agent provocateur*. Müller thought it was a defect in the glia (as did Charcot) and there could be a

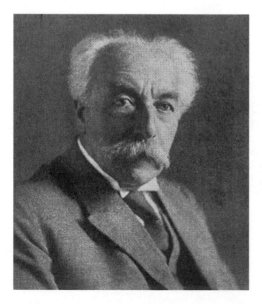

Figure 8.2 Ernest Adolf Gustav Gottfried von Strümpell (1853–1925) wrote a textbook of medicine in 1883, which went through 30 editions and held a place in German medicine that Osler's textbook would soon do in English medicine. He had an interest in neurological disease and wrote of his observations on multiple sclerosis. (Portrait from frontispieces in *Aus dem Leben eines deutschen Klinikers*. Leipzig, Vogel, 1925; by von Strümpell.)

primary form, as well as a secondary form initiated by many external agents. Dawson discussed in detail the theories of an inflammatory process and the underlying defect in the glia. He was initially unimpressed with the toxin theory, feeling that the effects of a toxin would be more diffuse change, but he changes his mind on this later.

Reading Dawson, one is impressed with his clear thinking and his excellent writing. His work bears reading today to see how an investigator struggles with understanding complex theories, and then sets out objectively to unravel the tangled web by observation.

Dawson's Conclusions

The process in MS is a subacute disseminated encephalo-myelitis.

There are no grounds for considering primary and secondary forms of the disease.

Multiple sclerosis is likely due to a specific external agent.

The external agent is likely a soluble toxin.

Somehow the agent enters only certain areas due to some local vascular change.

Some of the recovery is likely due to utilizing other pathways.

Cerebral changes produce the mental changes.

The clinical findings can be explained by the site of the lesions.

Dawson referred to "shadow sclerosis," plaques that have a definite surround. He said that the axon was characteristically preserved and could survive in an area of sclerosis for a long time, but inferred that axons could be lost if they participated in a lot of swelling in acute lesions. He believed, like Charcot, that the nerve impulses could probably be carried by the denuded axons.

Dawson discussed the theories of causation and grouped those which could be assigned to each school. A defect in the neuroglia was postulated by Charcot (1868), Huber (1895), and Redlich (1896), although the latter two thought the ultimate cause was some external toxin or microorganism. Bramwell thought it a developmental disturbance. Rindfleisch had earlier put the primary cause in the vessel, as did Dejerine and Williamson. Marie felt there was a vascular defect, the cause of the vascular change being an infection. Dawson agreed with the vascular theory. He also noted that many investigators were more puzzled and uncertain and did not have a firm belief on the cause of MS.

The paper following Dawson's in the *Edinburgh Medical Journal* was a case report by Byrom Bramwell, with Dawson as the second author, since he had done the pathological examination. This was a case of spastic paraplegia of 15 years' duration in a 45-year-old woman, carefully followed for the last seven years of her life, without any of the other signs of MS. She died of the complications of diabetes. Dawson found characteristic plaques of MS scattered throughout the cord, but not in the brain stem. Unfortunately, the brain was not available for study.

When writing of the life of Dawson in *The Founders of Neurology*, Haymaker commented that little had been added to his 1914–1916 contribution four decades later.[5] Dawson's work was widely quoted for many years, but as usually happens, his hard work and his observations eventually became part of the understood fabric of MS. His name continues to be linked with the appearance of flame-like plaques radiating off the corpus callosum on saggital sections of the brain on MRI, called "Dawson's fingers."*

REFERENCES

1. Dawson JD. The Histology of Disseminated Sclerosis. *Trans Royal Soc Edin*. 1916;50:517-740.
2. Dawson JD. The Histology of Disseminated Sclerosis. *Rev. Neurol Psychiat*. 1917;15:47-166; 369-417; 1918;16:287-307.
3. Haymaker W. *The Founders of Neurology*. Springfield, IL: Charles C. Thomas; Publisher. 1953:174-177.
4. Dawson JD. The histology of disseminated sclerosis. *Edinburgh Med J*. 1924;31:1-21.
5. Haymaker W. *The Founders of Neurology*. Springfield, IL: Charles C. Thomas; Publisher. 1953:174-177.

---

*Dawson's inclusion body encephalitis refers to another Dawson, J.R. Dawson of Tennessee, who described this viral encephalitis in children in 1933 and 1934.

9

The Journal of
a Disappointed Man

W.N.P. BARBELLION

"Never was a half-dead man more alive."
A. J. Cummings, commenting on his brother, 1919

At the beginning of this book, I related the stories of individuals who had features and symptoms of MS before the disease was understood or named. In the 18th and early 19th centuries, a progressive neurological disorder was thought of in general terms, often influenced by external factors, and was treated with common general therapies that fit with these concepts. It is not that there was no theory about progressive neurological diseases; they were understood in the way disease was understood in that era. It is instructive to examine how different it might have been for a patient suffering with MS almost 50 years after Charcot described and named the disorder.

Dealing with a long-standing and disabling medical condition that alters one's feelings and attitudes about life, self, and the future is a struggle known to many MS patients. One who endured the battles, winning some

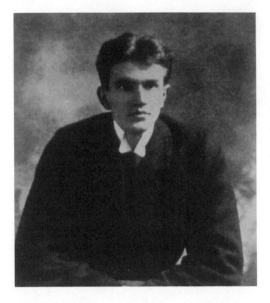

Figure 9.1 Bruce Frederick Cummings took the pen name W(ilhem) N(ero) P(ilate) Barbellion for his chronicle of his life suffering with a progressive neurological disease he would find out after many years was known by his physicians and family to be multiple sclerosis. (From the collection of Arthur Cummings, Esq.)

and losing others to this relentless foe, was Bruce Frederick Cummings (1889–1919). In his diary, he documented a progressive form of MS until his death at age 30, twelve years after the onset of his first symptoms.[1-3]

Cummings wrote under the pseudonym W.N.P. Barbellion, using initials that he felt "concealed the bravado" of Wilhelm Nero Pilate, and added the surname Barbellion, which he took from a confectionery shop sign; it had a sound he thought was "appropriately inflated." By the time he started writing his diary in 1903 at age 13, it was apparent that he had talents for essay writing and mathematics and a love of nature and the outdoors. He dreamed of becoming a naturalist and eventually obtained a position on the staff of the Natural History Museum in London.

By age 18, he was experiencing early progressive neurological symptoms, but was determined to deal with his disease, even though he did not know its name. He said he was going to live his life as planned.

"I am not going to be beaten. If I develop all the disease in the doctors' index, I mean to do what I set out to do if it has to be done in a bath-chair."

He did not know the cause of his illness, but clearly knew it was serious. Over time, he had recurrent numbness and weakness in his limbs, vertigo, depression, decreased sight in one eye, facial numbness, and weakness in his right arm. His blindness increased and he said men looked like trees walking; print was hopelessly blurred. He continued to consult physicians, taking their medicine without any sense of optimism, recognizing that he was worsening. He contemplated suicide and reflected on the fact that his medicines contained arsenic and strychnine.

He thought of attending a Christian Science church, which espoused the belief of Mary Baker Eddy, rejecting medical therapies and substituting spiritual ones. It is not clear whether he ever followed through on this. He consulted a homeopathic therapist in Finsbury Circus, but was disappointed with the results, adding that he had no better luck from the many physicians he consulted.

> *"I could write a book on the doctors I have known and the blunders they have known about me."*

Contributing to Cummings' distress was the realization that he did not understand what was happening to him. He consulted other physicians in hope of an answer. The next physician he saw felt he was quite young to have such a neurological disease (although he did not indicate what the disease was) and suggested Cummings should travel and continue to take arsenic. He was referred to a well-known neurologist, "Dr. H.," undoubtedly Sir Henry Head, who asked him suspiciously if he had ever been with women, and then ordered two months' complete rest in the country. Cummings said:

> *(Dr. H.) "chased me around his consulting room with a drumstick tapping my tendons and cunningly working my reflexes."*

Cummings thought the physicians would advise against his proposed marriage, but when his doctor made light of his paralysis, suggesting that it was related to a recent fall, Cummings felt confident enough to marry Eleanor Benger in September 1915. Perhaps it was not so unusual in that era that his physicians informed his fiancée of the diagnosis of multiple sclerosis, but not Cummings. Although he saw many physicians and neurologists, he still was unaware of his specific diagnosis and only after mar-

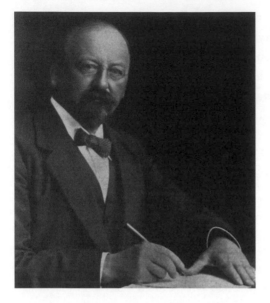

Figure 9.2 Sir Henry Head (1861–1940) was interested in many aspects of neurology, including the effects of visiting Lourdes on multiple sclerosis patients. He made impressive lifelong observations on the sensory system, which included the famous experiment on cutting his own superficial ramus of the radial nerve so that he and Rivers could study the effects. His contributions to spinal reflex physiology and aphasia were also monumental. He was editor of *Brain* and published a volume of poetry, but in the last 20 years of his life had to contend with slowly progressive Parkinson's disease. (Courtesy of the Army Medical Library, Washington, DC.)

riage did he discover the truth; even then he had to resort to subterfuge. He knew he would be rejected for military service, but felt a reason would have to be given. After he was examined, he peeked at the chart to see what diagnosis was used to disqualify him and saw the diagnosis "disseminated sclerosis."

He later looked up Dr. Risien Russell's chapter in Sir Clifford Allbutt's *System of Medicine*. Fortified by knowledge of his condition, Cummings thought he would get on with his zoological projects. He found the chapter in Allbutt helpful, but he said he had to run from the library after reading Dawson's great work on the pathology of the disease. Although he read a lot about the disease after that, he always left a blank in his diary when he came to the diagnosis, as he could not bring himself to use the words. He repeatedly visualized his illness as bacteria gnawing away at his spinal cord, producing a creeping paralysis. He felt he could hear the sound of the gnawing. To drown out the sound, he continually wanted music playing or would lie in bed whistling.

As so often happens, the specter of a serious illness and impending death helped him organize priorities. He became frustrated by the artificial nature of much of life and wanted to strip away the walls and partitions and "walk about with my clothes off, to make a large ventral incision and expose my heart." His diary was originally entitled "A Study in the Nude." He became resigned to his fate, philosophical about his past life and the likelihood of an early demise:

> "I am only twenty eight, but I have telescoped into those few years a tolerable long life: I have loved and married, and I have a family; I have wept and enjoyed, struggled and overcome, and when the hour comes I shall be content to die."

He wrote the hidden dream of most MS patients:

> "It would be nice if a physician from London, one of these days, were to gallop up hotspur, tether his horse to the gait post and dash in waving a reprieve—the discovery of a cure!"

The cure did not arrive and his failing strength caused him to resign his position at the Museum in 1917. At age 28, ten years after the onset of his progressive illness, he made a false diary entry, "Barbellion died on December 32 (1917)," but he did not die for another two years. His journal was published and well-received, and this brought pleasure to his last months.

> "The kindness everyone has shown the journal and the fact that so many have understood its meaning, have entirely changed my outlook. My horizon has cleared, my thoughts are tinged with sweetness, and I am content."

Compston raised the question of whether Cummings/Barbellion may have hastened his own death by taking the doctor's prescription of arsenic and strychnine, but although he did contemplate this at one point, there is little to suggest that he took anything but the prescribed amounts. He died at age 30 on October 22, 1919 in a cottage at Gerrard's Cross.

Barbellion has left us a remarkable record of a young man's struggle with MS at the beginning of the 20th century and the approaches and attitudes of the physicians of the day. His journal, *The Journal of a*

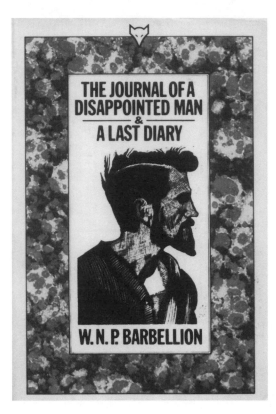

Figure 9.3 Front cover of the recently reprinted Journal and Diary of Bruce Frederick Cummings showing an engraving by John Nash (Hogarth Press, London, 1984) under his pseudonym W.N.P. Barbellion. This edition has an introduction by H.G. Wells and a new introduction by Deborah Singmaster. These poignant and well-written diaries describing his life with MS were erroneously thought by some to have been written by Wells, but he said he wasn't smart enough to write such an account.

Disappointed Man,[4] is still in print. After his death, *A Last Diary* was published. His only other publication was *Enjoying Life*, published in 1919.*

W.N.P. Barbellion, a young man who fought a long and losing battle with multiple sclerosis, is still remembered for his open and honest documentation of his illness. In the words of Peter Clifford, he "embodied that rare fusion of scientific and literary genius which can observe nature and self with equal sensitivity, analyzing with scientific detachment, yet feeling with poetic intensity."

---

*A.F. Pollard, editor of *History*, suggested that H.G. Wells was the real author of this remarkable diary. Wells, who is often said to be critical of Barbellion as an egotist who was seeking immortality, responded that he wasn't clever enough to have written such a book. Others felt the brother, A.J. Cummings, might be the author and pointed to discrepancies in the text. In fact, Barbellion admitted bowdlerizing his journals, so the small discrepancies mean little. He added material later, and rewrote sections, which would explain errors of dates and weather in the diary. A little editing is not an uncommon habit for those who are preparing their diaries for print.

REFERENCES

1. Barbellion WNP. (pseudonym for B.F. Cummings). *The Journal of a Disappointed Man*. London: Chatto and Windus; 1919.
2. Barbellion WNP. *The Journal of a Disappointed Man; and The Last Diary*. Gloucester: Allan Sutton; 1984. Bibliographical notes by Peter Clifford.
3. Murray TJ. The Journal of a Disappointed Man: A Patient's Perspective on Multiple Sclerosis—1909-1919. *Nova Scotia Medical Journal*. 1992;121:59-62.
4. Barbellion WNP. *The Journal of a Disappointed Man and A Last Diary*. London, Hogarth Press, 1984.

10

Experimentation, Meetings, Reviews, and Symposia, 1920–1960

Although there was not a great amount of activity in multiple sclerosis (MS) research between the World Wars, there were two landmark events, one a meeting and one a review. They changed the directions in the study of MS by focusing on the current understanding of the disease. In an age that had many therapeutic approaches, most physicians concluded that none of them was better than using no therapy at all.

Most advances in medicine are recorded by the date of publication of the discovery and remembered in association with the discoverer. We normally do not recognize that a field or discipline can be advanced by a pivotal meeting, by an intelligent review of the state of the art, by the publication of a book, or by the formation of an organization. The understanding of MS was advanced significantly by the 1921 and 1948 meetings of the Association for Research in Nervous and Mental Disease (ARNMD),[1,2] and by reviews by Russell Brain in 1930[3] and Schumacher in 1950,[4] and by the monograph by McAlpine, Compston, and Lumsden in 1955.[5] Another landmark that continues to influence the direction of MS care and research was the formation of the National MS Society by Sylvia Lawry in 1946.

ARNMD held its annual meeting in New York City on December 27–28, 1921 and took as its theme that year the current knowledge and research on multiple sclerosis. The papers from that meeting were published in 1922, with the discussion following each presentation.[6] The papers covered current understanding of pathology, epidemiology, etiology, and clinical features of the disease. This landmark meeting clarified an increasingly confused field; although it produced a few erroneous conclusions, it clarified many more. The meeting's influence was the result of overviews by leaders in the field of MS and was due to the attendance of many leaders in neurology, particularly American neurology, medical professors writing papers and textbooks on neurology, and teaching the next generation of neurologists.

Walter Timme, founder of the ARNMD, began the meeting with a general history of the disease to that date. There was a review of the geographical distribution of MS by Charles Davenport, as well as studies on World War I troops (by Percival Baillie), psychological effects (by Sanger Brown and Thomas Davis), a discussion of the psychopathology by Smith Ely Jelliffe, and a review of the pathology by George Hassin.

The conclusions of the meeting tried to capture a consensus of quite varied opinions and were in keeping with the understanding and state of medical research of the time. In writing the conclusions, the commissioners emphasized that MS was among the most common organic diseases affecting the nervous system. They de-emphasized the importance of the Charcot triad, but continued to emphasize the importance of the abdominal reflexes (lost in 83.7 percent of cases), and the value of temporal pallor of the optic disc as a sign. They concluded that there was no particular psychic disorder characteristic of the disease, that euphoria was not very characteristic, and mental deterioration often absent. They could not support Jelliffe's belief that MS was "schizophrenia of the spinal axis" with plaques induced by repressed tensions.[7] Impressed by the inability to reproduce studies by many investigators that suggested the disease was due to a transmissible virus, spirochete, bacterium, or other agent, they concluded there was no solid evidence for a bacteriological cause, but expected further experiments on this in the future.

Hassin concluded that MS was a degenerative disease due to some unknown toxin, probably an endotoxin. William Spiller disagreed and argued that MS was an inflammatory disease. In answer to the question posed throughout the meeting—whether MS was an inflammatory or a degenerative disease—the commission took the middle road and concluded that it might be initially inflammatory and later degenerative.

Conclusions of the ARNMD Commission, 1921

1. *MS occurs chiefly in the age group 20–40, but can occasionally be seen as early as age 10 and as late as 60.*

2. *Males are attacked more often with a male:female ratio of 3:2.*

3. *MS makes up 1–2 percent of organic diseases of the nervous system, including those due to syphilis.*

4. *The duration may vary from one to 30 years.*

5. *It occurs more in skilled manual workers than in laborers or in brain workers.*

6. *In the United States, it occurs more around the Great Lakes, while in Europe it is more frequent in the Northern parts than in Italy or the Mediterranean area.*

7. *It is not familial or inherited, with rare exceptions, but in the ancestry, there is often evidence of neuropathic stock.*

8. *Acute infections may precede the disease in 10–12 percent of cases, and it occurs no more frequently in those who have or have not had the usual childhood diseases.*

9. *It is not caused by syphilis.*

10. *In a few cases it might be "excited" by trauma, but trauma itself cannot cause it, though it may "awaken" the disease which is already there.*

At this juncture, there was some clarity about the way MS could manifest as signs and symptoms; more uncertain were the male/female ratio, the prognosis of the disease, the role of heredity, and the underlying factors that could explain the cause of the disease.

GENDER

Over the previous 150 years, there had been controversy about whether the occurrence of MS was more common in men, more common in women, or equal in both sexes. Although it seems as though in the first century after Charcot's description it was found more often in men, that Charcot found it two and a half times more often in women was dismissed as a reflection of the predominance of women at the Salpêtrière. Some clinicians recorded MS as more common in women, others more often in men, and still others equally in the sexes. Wechsler told the ARNMD that the ratio was 3 men to 2 women in his survey of 1,970 records. The ARNMD Commission accepted this as the correct figure. Two decades later, Limberg thought it equal in the sexes[8] as did the fledgling NMSS in the late 1940s, and Schumacher found it slightly more in women by 1960.[9] Today investigators seem to agree that it is at least twice as common in women as men. Why the great variation? Partly this was due to the differing patterns of patient referrals to some clinics. There was also a tendency to give men with neurological disease an organic diagnosis, while women were often diagnosed with hysterical or functional labels, like Mrs. Gatty. The situation was also complicated by the fact that many of the multiple sclerosis cases were diagnosed as other conditions, such as neurosyphilis and hysteria; this continued well into the 20th century.

All agreed that the diagnosis was difficult; textbooks and papers emphasized the differential diagnosis and how to separate multiple sclerosis cases from other disease, particularly hysteria (hysterical patients were unlikely to have spasticity with Babinski signs, optic atrophy, nystagmus, and bladder involvement). There are many cases in the early literature of MS in which the case presented was diagnosed in life as "paresis" (syphilis) or hysteria, only to exhibit characteristic changes of MS at autopsy.[10] One sees what one looks for, and often clinicians assessing a patient with complex and multiple neurological symptoms considered neurosyphilis, hysteria, or some other neurological disorder first. In

1948, Foster Kennedy said, "Forty years ago anyone with 'nervous legs' was said to have locomotor ataxia, now he is quickly called multiple sclerosis."*[11,12]

Reports of the Gender Ratio in MS

	Female	Male	Total
Charcot	24	9	34
Ross		More women	
Blumreich and Jacoby	6	23	29
Probst	24	34	58
Marie/Krafft-Ebing/Redlich		More men	
Edwards	10	23	33
Moncovo	12	9	21
Erb	5	4	9
Chovstek	6	10	16
Gowers		Equal	
Spitzka	7	15	22
Wechsler		More men (3/2)	
Kurland (1952)		Equal	

AGE OF ONSET

Charcot said MS usually occurred before age 30 and considered age 40 outside the limit. However, within a few years, cases were being reported with a very late onset. In 1883, Kirkland described a case with age of onset at 69.[13] Strümpell (1893) had a case with onset at age 60, and Dercum (1894) at age 57. H. Charlton Bastian had a case of a man with onset at age 50, which he ascribed to a fall down a flight of stone steps 18 months before. Such late-onset cases occur in the practice of most MS clinicians, although they are infrequent.[14]

---

*I reviewed 50 cases referred to our MS clinic in the early 1980s who, on our assessment, did not have MS; there were none with hysteria, none with neurosyphilis, but many with minor problems such as carpal tunnel syndrome or migraine, which were interpreted as possible MS. Most of these were medical personnel or those caring for MS cases or working for the MS Society. The other large group had a potpourri of other neurological diseases. As one sees what one looks for, many physicians now look for MS, and "see" it when patients with any complex neurological disease appears. It is not uncommon for a patient to be referred with the question, "Could this be MS?"

PROGNOSIS

The conclusions about prognosis varied over the century after Charcot's initial description of MS. Early in the history of the disease, patients were diagnosed at a late stage, and only when they had a typical relapsing and progressive course. Such advanced cases gave clinicians the idea that patients did not live long. Many stated that patients lived only a few years after the diagnosis, but a few felt that patients lived a long time. It is worth noting that Saint Lidwina, Margaret Davies, Augustus d' Esté, Heinrich Heine, and Margaret Gatty all lived for many decades. Only in the 1940s would it be recognized that life expectancy was only slightly less than anticipated.

Duration of MS (Modified from Thygesen, 1953)

Gowers, 1893	3-6 years (quoted by Allison, 1950)
Bramwell, 1917	12 years in 170 fatal and nonfatal cases
Curtius, 1933	10 years in 100 autopsy-proven cases
Gram, 1934	10.3 years in Danish Invalidity Insurance material
Brain, 1936	12.5 years in 11 fatal cases; 13.6 years in those surviving at follow-up
Drobnes, 1937	12.5 years in 46 fatal cases
Sällström, 1942	9.2 years in 285 fatal cases (range 1–41 years)
Carter, Sciarra and Merritt, 1950	13 years in 46 autopsy-proven cases
Lazarte, 1950	13.7 years in 85 fatal cases
Limberg, 1950	27 years from US death certificates. Average age at death: 54
Allison, 1950	19.5 years in 28 fatal cases, 27.8 years in survivors at follow-up
Müller, 1949	16–34 years

There has been confusion about what features indicated a poor prognosis. Birley and Dudgeon (1921)[15] found the most favorable prognosis in those who were having acute attacks, confirmed by Misch-Frankl (1931), Brain (1936), and Miller (1949). MacLean et al. (1950) calculated that those with recurrent attacks became disabled at a rate of four percent per year.[16] Coates (1930) noted that those with a gradual onset were unlikely to have remissions. Thygesen found from his cases that of those with a progressive onset in the first year, 43 percent were dead at 15 years, while of those with relapsing-remitting onset in the first year, only 21 percent were dead at 15 years.[17] It was accepted that those with signs of cerebellar disease had a poor prognosis (Misch-Frankl, 1931; Brown and Putnam, 1939; Thygesen, 1949) and those with a spinal form had a better prognosis (Brain, 1936; Sciarra and Carter, 1950). Thygesen felt that his cases and those of others showed that a late onset had a better prognosis (Brain, 1936; McAlpine 1946; Thygesen, 1949). Others found a better prognosis if the onset was at a younger age (Müller, 1949).[18]

Müller felt that the discrepancies concerning prognosis and other features in the disease were:

"artificial, caused by 'statistics,' and a result of the different prognostic criteria and extremely varying interpretation of 'slowly progressive disease,' 'rapidly progressive course,' 'persistent progression of symptoms,' 'progressive bouts,' etc. The inaccuracy of retrospective evaluation, moreover, contributes to increase the confusion."

R. Müller, 1949[19]

WECHSLER'S TEXTBOOK

Israel S. Wechsler of New York wrote a textbook of neurology in 1927 that went through many printings and had a clear outline of the clinical features of MS, the differential diagnosis, and how to differentiate from other conditions.[20] He concluded with a gloomy look at therapy. He warned that because remissions were a part of the natural history, any therapy would appear to give good results. Because the cause of MS was unknown, there was no specific treatment, and we should not expect a cure. He recommended general tonics such as iron, quinine, arsenic, strychnine, and Salvarsan, although he emphasized that MS is not syphilis. He had seen good results in only two cases (perhaps a result of the spontaneous remissions he mentioned, but he makes no comment on

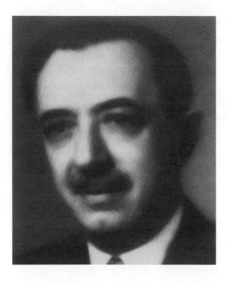

Figure 10.1 Israel Wechsler, born in Rumania, was Chief of Neurology at Mount Sinai Hospital in New York. Although known as a neuropsychiatrist, and a friend of Freud although not a psychoanalyst, his textbook on neurology was very popular and went through nine editions.

this) and admitted that most patients were not helped. Cacodylate of soda by hypodermic injection was often used, he said, but he made no further comment on this therapy for MS. He felt that commonsense measures such as rest and avoidance of exertion were better than medication. Electricity was of no value, but massage could be beneficial, and warm baths could reduce spasticity. Sadly, he concluded that the end result in this disease is incapacity, requiring feeding and nursing care.

THE REVIEW OF RUSSELL BRAIN

Russell Brain's (1895–1966) important review of the state of understanding of the disease in 1930 brought clarity to an increasingly confused field. Brain considered the clinical features and symptoms of MS, the CSF findings, and the treatment of the disease. His paper was a remarkable insight into the understanding of the disease in 1930. It did not represent a consensus; this was the personal conclusion and perception of an outstanding neurologist, assistant physician to the London Hospital and the Hospital for Epilepsy and Paralysis, Maida Vale.*[21]

*Compston assessed the impact of the 1930 review and then followed the changing information and views in the many editions of Brain's textbook *Diseases of the Nervous System* from 1933 to the present. Editions since 1969 have been edited by Lord Walton.

Brain noted there were many reports of greater frequency of MS among those of Scandinavian, Finnish, Scottish, French, Slavic, German, English, and Irish descent compared to those of other populations. He felt the reports of greater rural frequency could not be justified from the inadequate studies. He also could not accept reports that disease incidence was higher in certain occupations: woodworkers, ironworkers, and sailors. Brain reviewed the pathology of the disease and examined the concept that it is primarily a diffuse glial hypertrophy, possibly a reaction to an external agent. He commented that if there were such an agent, it must be able to produce mainly perivascular lesions attended by infiltration of plasma cells and lymphocytes. Such an agent could be a toxin or a virus. Making the same point that Dawson made in 1914, he argued against a toxic cause because toxins are characterized by diffuseness, symmetry in distribution, and timing of their neurological effects, rather than the focal, asymmetrical, and episodic changes as seen in MS. On the other hand, various forms of encephalitis could produce a pathological picture similar to that of MS. Although he respectfully acknowledged the "weighty support" for the toxin theory by Oppenheim, Dawson, and others, Brain thought that infection was a more likely suspect in the cause of MS.

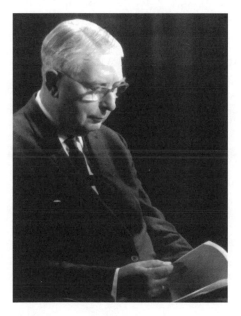

Figure 10.2 Russell Brain (1895–1966), later Lord Brain, contributed substantially to the understanding of MS by his extensive review of the disease in 1930 and his overview of the disease in his textbook editions over the next four decades. He kept careful statistical records on the disease.

Brain looked at the question of which central nervous system tissue is first affected by the disease. Was it the glia, the blood vessels, the nerve, or the myelin? Noting that each had its supporters, he concluded that the myelin seemed to be the constant factor, and the glial reactions were probably a response to the external agent and the breakdown products.

Brain felt Pierre Marie had overemphasized the causal relationship to infection; although he allowed that it could be an aggravating factor (not a cause), a distinct relationship was seen in less than a third of the cases. He gave a list of possible explanations for the apparent relationship of trauma and MS, but felt there was little reason to consider trama a cause of MS. The same applied to cold, heat, and electric shock.

Brain reviewed in detail the numerous reports of transmission and isolation of various infective agents, and the even more numerous reports that failed to reproduce these findings. He concluded that there was no satisfactory evidence that the disease had been transmitted to animals. The recent dramatic story of a virus isolated by Miss Chevassut was still unfolding, and he suggested this work should await confirmation.

He noted that the "classical" picture of MS with the Charcot triad was present in only 10 percent of cases now that milder and partial forms and variations of MS were being recognized. Monosymptomatic, "oligosymptomatic," intermittent, and progressive cases were recognized. He said that verified childhood cases did occur, but were rare; most of the early reports were probably in error, and disease onset was between ages 20 and 40 in 68 percent of cases. The course was variable. Patients might die in months or be working after 26 years.

Brain began his overview of therapy of MS with this perceptive statement:

> *"It is notoriously difficult to assess the value of therapeutic measures in disseminated sclerosis, and most advocates of some particular line of treatment qualify their optimism by alluding to the natural tendency of the disease to spontaneous remissions. That such a qualification is necessary seems to indicate that no mode of treatment is successful enough to achieve, at the most, a greater improvement than might have occurred spontaneously."*

He emphasized good general care and delaying bed confinement as long as possible. The attitude of the physician was important.

"The high susceptibility of the patient to hysterical embroidery of his symptoms demands psychological insight on the part of the physician, whose encouragement and optimism are often of greater value than his pharmaceutical essays."

Brain believed that pyrexial therapy was one of the most important measures, either by malarial treatment, or typhoid vaccine, but probably did no more than retard the progress of the disease. Other methods of inducing pyrexia such as injections of milk, phlogetan, sulfosin, or the spirochete of African relapsing fever, serum from nonprogressive cases, and antipolio serum were tried with more doubtful results.

Arsenic compounds and silver Salvarsan were the most commonly used medications for MS in the 19th century because these were generally used for almost any serious disease. By the turn of the century, these had gained some sense of specificity for neurological diseases since they were useful in syphilis, which affected the nervous system in many ways. Even though these remedies were widely used, Brain concluded there was little evidence that they had any specific therapeutic value in MS. He was also unimpressed with silver Salvarsan, colloidal silver injected intravenously, antimony given intramuscularly or intravenously, sodium salicylate, intramuscular neurotropin, quinine, mercury, vasodilators such as pilocarpine and nitrates, and intramuscular sodium nucleinate. He listed many more drugs used in MS, but concluded they were of no value.

Other approaches to therapy included diathermy with one electrode applied to the vertebral column, particularly advantageous in the spinal form of MS. Deep X-ray irradiation was reported to help half the cases, but Brain thought this was palliative at best and should be used only with caution. Ultraviolet irradiation might give slight improvement. After this very long list of therapies, Brain concluded, "The multiplication of remedies is eloquent of their inefficacy."

Shortly after Brain's review, the transmission experiments of Kathleen Chevassut and Sir James Purves-Stewart were discredited.

Despite Brain's conclusion that therapies had little effect, the array of treatments applied to MS seemed to grow, and Brickner compiled a long list of the most common treatments used in the 1930s,[22] of which Putnam concluded half were probably useful.[23,24]

The discoveries by Glanzmann and Rivers of an experimental model that resembled MS slowly stimulated the growth of research on allergic aspects of MS. Ferraro and others began studies on the immune aspects of the disease.[25,26] Putnam injected oil preparations into the cerebral vessels and produced changes he interpreted as MS-like lesions, fostering the concept that the disease was likely a vascular disorder.[27] By the end of the 1930s, another experienced clinician, S.A. Kinnier Wilson, reviewed the understanding of MS in a textbook of neurology published posthumously.[28]

SAMUEL ALEXANDER KINNIER WILSON (1878–1937)

Some clinicians contributed to the understanding of multiple sclerosis, not by hypothesis or experiment or by discovery, but by carefully assessing their experience with patients and writing this clearly in textbooks and review articles. Hippocrates had warned that experience was fallacious, but experience, especially if critically examined, was an important guiding process in medicine prior to the randomized clinical trial (RCT). This was the case with Hammond, Russell, Gowers, Bramwell, and Brain and in the 1930s with S.A. Kinnier Wilson, who wrote an influential textbook.

The quintessential English clinician and consultant, Wilson was actually born in Cedarville, New Jersey, but his childhood and early education were in Scotland, with medical training in Edinburgh. He was influenced to pursue neurological studies when he was house physician to Sir Byrom Bramwell at the Royal Edinburgh Infirmary. His educational grand tour took him to Leipzig and then to Paris, where he studied with Pierre Marie and Babinski. In 1904, he became registrar and pathologist, later consultant and honorary physician, at the National Hospital, Queen Square. He is remembered primarily for his MD thesis at age 33 on lenticular degeneration, later called Wilson's disease, which won a gold medal from the University of Edinburgh.*[29]

An influential teacher at Queen Square between the wars who helped make this a great teaching center for clinical neurology, he died of cancer before his textbook of neurology went to the publisher. It was completed by A. Ninian Bruce.

His discussion of multiple sclerosis mentioned the early descriptions of Cruveilhier (1841), Abercrombie (1836), and Marshall Hall (1841), but said the first American description was by Seguin (1878), ignoring a number of earlier American reports.

Like Russell Brain, Wilson felt that multiple sclerosis was being more frequently diagnosed because clinicians were getting away from the "rigid schematization of Charcot." He was referring to the fact that previous neurologists hesitated to make the diagnosis if the Charcot triad were not present. He thought MS was quite common, with a frequency approaching that of neurosyphilis, but his experience suggested that there was a slight male preponderance in MS cases. He pointed out that because the clinical picture could be misleading, the diagnosis was only certain when verified by autopsy. Only a minority of patients had some convincing factor as a cause, although he allowed that such factors as stress, infection, overwork, fatigue, and worry could lower the resistance, "vague though that conception might be." He saw a case develop after an *affaire du coeur*, and another in an RAF pilot who had participated in many bombing raids and been shot down three times. Two women developed MS after trauma, one after a mirror fell on her arm, and another when a fan hit her head. He said it was unwise to dismiss such cases as coincidence, and we should keep an open mind on the issue of external stresses and trauma as possible causes of MS.

---

*Webb Haymaker said that when a student referred to this disease as Westphal-Strümpell's pseudosclerosis, Wilson would roll the collars of his white coat together under his chin with his large hands, fold his arms across his chest, fix his audience in a stare, and tell them in his resonant voice the sequence of discovery of the disease, a story in which Westphal and von Strümpell did not fare any better than they would in Wilson's textbook. Denny-Brown told the story of asking Wilson about hepatolenticular degeneration; as Wilson walked away, he turned and asked, "You mean Kinnier Wilson's disease?" Haymaker also reported the story of Foster Kennedy examining a perplexing case of lateral medullary syndrome on Wilson's service for three hours, and being embarrassed when Wilson suddenly asked the patient, "Will you see to it that I get your brain when you die?"

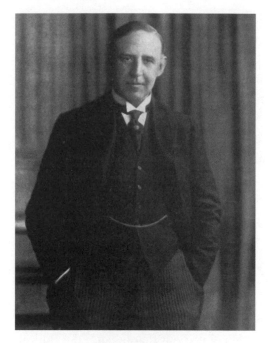

Figure 10.3 Samuel Alexander Kinnier Wilson (1878–1937), the epitome of the English consultant at Queen Square, was born in New Jersey, and educated in Scotland. His great textbook, published after his death, contained a clear presentation of the understanding of the nature and features of multiple sclerosis as understood by an experienced neurologist in the 1930s. (From the collection of Dr. Foster Kennedy.)

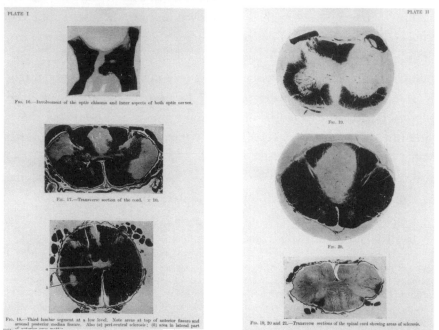

Figure 10.4 I and II S.A. Kinnier Wilson's illustrations of lesions in the spinal cord. (Wilson, 1940)

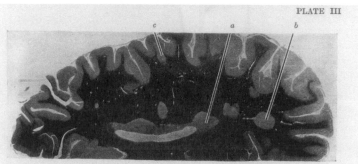

PLATE III

FIG. 22.—Level of the roof of the right lateral ventricle.

(a) Involvement of the outer wall and posterior tip of the ventricle.
(b) Large areas in the adjoining white matter, especially towards the occipital lobe.
(c) Area in the medullary ray of the post-Rolandic gyrus in the precuneus.

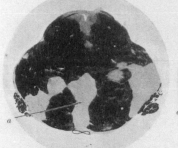

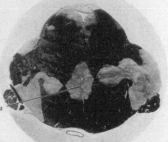

FIG. 23.—Junction of pons and mid-brain.

FIG. 24.—Upper pons.

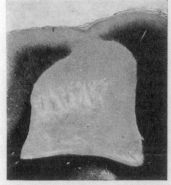

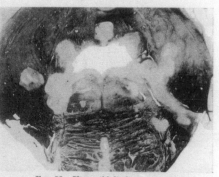

FIG. 25.—Convolution of the para-central lobule.
× 6.

FIG. 26.—Upper third of pons.   × 2½.

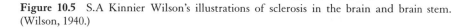

Figure 10.5   S.A Kinnier Wilson's illustrations of sclerosis in the brain and brain stem. (Wilson, 1940.)

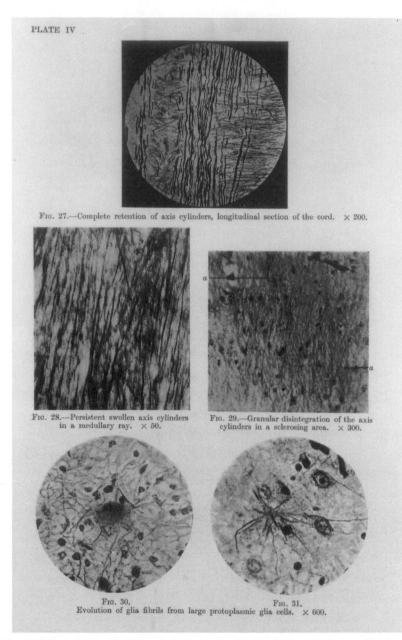

PLATE IV

FIG. 27.—Complete retention of axis cylinders, longitudinal section of the cord. × 200.

FIG. 28.—Persistent swollen axis cylinders in a medullary ray. × 50.

FIG. 29.—Granular disintegration of the axis cylinders in a sclerosing area. × 300.

FIG. 30.   FIG. 31.
Evolution of glia fibrils from large protoplasmic glia cells. × 600.

Figure 10.6 S.A. Kinnier Wilson's illustrations of axis cylinders in plaques showing areas that have complete preservation of axons, others with swollen axons and degeneration. (Wilson, 1940.)

Wilson's description of symptoms and pathology is clear, but conventional. He divided MS into the subjective or predisseminated type, where there were symptoms, but only a few vague neurological signs; the spinal varieties, with features of a myelitis; the cerebral varieties; and the mixed or classical varieties, which may have the "Charcotian triad."

He concluded that transmission studies were unconvincing, and the studies of Miss Chevassut discredited, but the disease might be due to a lipolytic enzyme that disrupts myelin. He was not very positive about the value of therapies for this disease:

"So far as present knowledge goes, the malady is incurable, and statements to the contrary must be received with reserve ... "

"Causal ignorance entails an unfortunate diffusion of therapeutic endeavor and spontaneous remissions make it difficult to assess the value of any particular treatment. The pharmacopoeia has been ransacked for 'nerve tonics,' which flatter only to deceive."[30]

After those comments, it is surprising how many therapies Kinnier Wilson offered his patients. He used arsenic in the form of Fowler's solu-

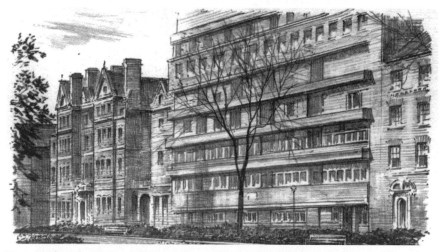

Figure 10.7   The National Hospital, Queen Square, founded by the efforts of the Chandler sisters who were distressed that there was no hospital that would accept patients such as their mother who had a stroke. From the end of the 19th century to the beginning of the 21st century, major advances in MS have come from the consultants and patients in this institution. (Judges Ltd. Hastings England.)

tion, and he was impressed, as were others, by the newer arsenicals. Repeated courses of sodium cacodylate injections were worth trying, and silver preparations and colloidal metals (antimony, selenium, manganese) "did not lack advocates." Intravenous salicylate, quinine tablets, mercury, iodide, lecithin pills, and Löwenthal's lymphoid serum might be tried, he said. There were such glowing reports from abroad of the value of fibrolysin that he tried it on one patient "without any sequel except the final rebellion of the patient." He had good results with pyrexial methods such as TAB vaccine, while others used malaria as a therapy, employing one disease to fight another. He noted that some authors reported remarkable results with whole liver, which at that time was being used for pernicious anemia. Massage and electrical therapy might have "happy if temporary results." No therapeutic nihilist, he. He observed that therapy just mirrored the treatment of syphilis, and although it did little more than slow the disease, such experimentation was important until the cause of MS was found. Finally, he commented on the need for common sense and healthy general measures.*[31]

SETTING THE STAGE 1940–1960

In the 1940s Ferrarro carried out experiments on the immune mechanisms that would stir interest in the immunology of MS.[32] Kabat discovered the increase in gamma globulin in the spinal fluid of MS cases, lending credence to the belief that an allergic reaction may underlie MS.[33] Medawar postulated the concept that the brain was an immunologically privileged site.[34] The development of anticoagulants corresponded with enthusiasm for a vascular cause of the disease, and Putnam influenced many to treat MS patients with the new warfarin.[35–37] Limberg,[38] Bing,[39] and others studied the peculiar distribution of MS geographically. Reese[40] and later Schumacher[41–43] reviewed the changing experience and views on

---

*George Ebers tells the story of a patient, an elderly woman who was diagnosed by Wilson in 1922. She reported he said, "It's DS. Tough luck, old girl. You'll be in a wheelchair in four years. That will be five guineas." In the 1980s, she delighted in pointing out that she had survived Wilson by over 40 years. When she died at age 87, her autopsy revealed three lesions in total. (Personal communication).

the disease, which was helpful to the newly formed National Multiple Sclerosis Society. Cortisone was discovered and caused great excitement in the treatment of rheumatic disease, and it was not long before it was being tried on MS. These will be discussed in more detail in other chapters.

Equally influential in summarizing the state of understanding of MS was the review textbook of the disease, *Multiple Sclerosis* by McAlpine, Compston, and Lumsden published in 1955.[44] Alastair Compston, the son of Nigel Compston, recently wrote that the review was based on 1,072 cases accumulated by McAlpine, and collated painstakingly by Compston, who wrote the first draft. Lumsden wrote the pathology section. Up to the present, with its 1998 third edition, this continues to be a major reference for MS.[45]

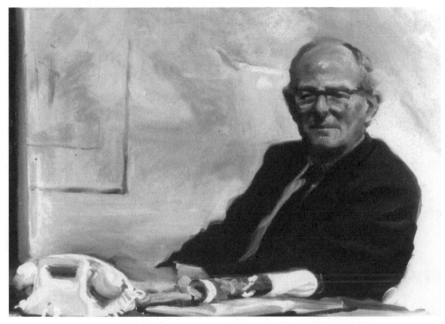

Figure 10.8   Nigel Compston was co-author of the classic McAlpine's *Multiple Sclerosis*, which appeared in 1955, and clarified the clinical, epidemiological, immunological, and pathological aspects of the disease to that date. It was a landmark publication, bringing together the current knowledge at a time when there was great activity in public support for research, interest in epidemiology of the disease, and increasing activity in the new MS societies. Douglas McAlpine accumulated the records of 1,072 cases of MS, and Compston collated most of the material from these records and wrote the initial draft of the book. The third author, Charles Lumsden, wrote the sections on pathology. (Courtesy of his son, Professor Alastair Compston.)

Although terms such as disseminated sclerosis were still in vogue in England up to the 1950s, when this classic work appeared with multiple sclerosis in its title, this became the accepted term in the English-speaking world. McAlpine first used the phrase "disseminated in space and time," for the characteristics of multiple lesions in the nervous system with recurring episodes of symptoms.

During the 1950s, many steps were taken that would influence directions in MS research. Kurtzke developed the Disability Status Scale (DSS), which became the standard for therapeutic trials. Interferons were discovered; these would be studied in MS some two decades later. The HLA system was described. The MS societies of the United States, Canada, and Great Britain began to fund MS research. Swank in Montreal theorized about fat intake as a basis of the disease and developed a diet to treat patients. Waxman showed that the proteolipids of myelin were encephalogenic. Lesions of MS were seen on isotope brain scans.

In 1960, a meeting was held at the Royal Society of Medicine in London to discuss the current understanding of MS.[46] Allison reviewed the epidemiology of the disease, and the strong evidence that there was a geographical north-south distribution of cases. J.H.D. Miller of Dublin showed that although there had been concerns about pregnancy and multiple sclerosis, there were fewer relapses than expected during pregnancy, but more in the postpartum period. Sir Francis Walshe rose in the question period to say this was an important paper, and because there was so much prejudice against married women with MS having babies, the paper should be read before the Royal College of Obstetricians and Gynecologists.

Henry Miller of Newcastle discussed the etiological factors and commented:

> *"If disseminated sclerosis is ultimately shown to have a 'cause' in the conventional sense of the term, this will probably be discovered by a biochemist, an immunologist, a veterinarian, or a geologist. It seems unlikely that it will be revealed to a neurologist, who has studied the disease by his traditional methods for more than a century."*[47]

In assessing possible etiological factors, Miller noted that in the Newcastle experience, one-third of relapses occurred in relation to an infection, but probably any infection, as there was no seasonal pattern noted. If there were an allergic basis for MS, perhaps steroids might be helpful, he speculated, but he noted that sporadic experience with steroids made physicians doubtful of their value. Most results seemed to be similar to those seen in untreated cases, so if there were a benefit, it must be very limited. Miller carried out an 18-month study comparing prednisolone, salicylate, and placebo and found no difference in the rate of progression or disability in any of the groups.[48]

Miller found only six percent of patients had more than one case in their family, and early attempts by David Poskanzer and others did not show any patterns in genetic and blood group studies. The discussion made it apparent that there was still a reluctance to accept a genetic basis for MS. Miller and his group also looked at the possibility that lumbar punctures and surgical operations might have an effect on relapses, but found none. They were surprised to find that the higher Social Class 1 had twice as many cases and the lower Social Class 5 had less than half as many as expected. They had no explanation, but this was also found with polio and coronary heart disease. Kurland, however, commented that in his studies in Winnipeg and Charleston, there was a geographical difference, but no difference with social level, at least in North America, nor was there any relationship to other factors such as water supply, sanitation, or fat intake. At this meeting, there was discussion of the genetic factor in MS, reviewed by Sigvald Refsum of Norway, and the conclusion of the symposium suggested a familial rate of 10 percent.[49]

Even in an age when large case series and statistical methods were being applied, anecdotes still had influence. Dr. Isabel Wilson, noting that one of Charcot's patients fell into a stream, and one of Dawson's cases fell into a swimming pool, raised the question of whether this might indicate a role for wet and dampness and perhaps a spirochete that entered through the skin. Miller spoke of a steeplejack who developed transverse myelitis after working on a steeple in a blizzard, and two miners who developed MS after working waist deep in water in the mines. He thought that strong stimulation of afferent nerves by cold and weather might cause circulation effects on the spinal cord.

Lumsden reviewed the growing interest in immunity, and the nervous system and suggested MS may be the acute event, but confessed he was unsure of the mechanism of the ongoing disease. He discussed the possibility of an antibrain antibody, even though this might not imply cause, and reviewed efforts to demonstrate the basis of experimental autoimmune mechanisms. Vaccines had been used to block experimental allergic encephalomyelitis (EAE), including experiments with BCG. This work might bring future benefits. (It was at this time that Russian workers were attempting an intradermal Margulis-Shubladze vaccine as a "biological test" for MS.)

At the symposium, E.J. Field reviewed EAE and the attempts to modify the disease with therapeutic agents such as X-irradiation, salicylates, ACTH, and 6-mercaptopurine, none of which had much effect. He concluded that EAE was not allergic in origin, another of Field's controversial views about MS. J.P. Finean gave an elegant paper on the new and exciting views of myelin under the electron microscope. Although the layers of myelin had been seen by X-ray diffraction in 1941, and in very early electron microscopic pictures, the beautiful layering of myelin was only seen clearly in 1950 with the newer techniques of thin sectioning and improved electron microscopes. In 1906, Marburg had postulated that a myelinolytic substance might cause the local breakdown in plaques,[50] and at this conference, R.H.S. Thompson put forward evidence for lysolecithin as a lytic substance in the brain.

In the 1950–60s period, therapeutic activism was in the air, and not without justification. The dramatic results with sulfas, penicillin, vaccines, psychoactive drugs, antihypertensives, anticonvulsants, and the developing fields of imaging, angiography, isotope scans, and new surgeries led to the feeling that new and dramatic therapies were around the corner for every illness. Patients expressed amazement, hope, and respect for medical research, and physicians fostered the belief by indicating that if there were just enough funds, people, and resources, who knows what we could accomplish? This placed the practicing neurologist in a quandary as patients asked about new therapies, and there was little to offer. As we saw in the previous century, realizing there was little that helped did not stop physicians from offering something. In clinics there was a second conflict—physicians who were anxious to be able to offer their patients something, anything, were also the ones who were supposed to be the objective, scientifically minded leaders. They were expected to calmly assess the evidence for what would be a better therapy, something that might help more than the many nostrums passed out to calm the anxious and distressed MS patient. But the experts were just as anxious to be able to offer their patients something; when they felt something might help, they had the influence and reputation to make the therapy widely accepted. This can be seen in the wide use of anticoagulants by Putnam, the histamine therapy of Horton at the Mayo Clinic and Hinton Jonez at the Tacoma Clinic, and the blood transfusions and low-fat diet of Swank at the MNI and later Oregon.

One of the most influential neurologists was Tracy Putnam. Tally recorded 126 therapies that he employed in his MS cases.[51] In medicine, the personal experience of the physician has always had great cachet. No matter what the evidence and the experiment showed, the conclusion following the statement by the physician, "In my experience ...," carried greater weight. In the postwar period, great and prominent men, and they were almost always men, held sway by their opinions and their practice.

It was a period when personal experience provided the direction in MS care. However, as physicians judged their clinical experience with long-standing treatments with quinine, arsenic, strychnine, antimony, potassium iodide, and mercury, and found these useless, they also harshly judged newer therapies such as blood transfusion, anticoagulation, antibiotics, and sympathectomies. Just when they hoped to offer their patients something in an age that indicated that new therapies were just around the corner, they saw the therapeutic armamentarium getting dismally short. It was a frustrating time for patients and for neurologists. By the end of the 1970s there was a feeling, also noted in the previous century, that no therapy was of help in the disease, although some medications might modify some of the symptoms. Steroids were being used more, but the growing experience with what we would now judge very low doses was unconvincing, and of minimal benefit at best, with no change in the eventual outcome.

The time was then ripe for the promise of the immunosuppressant, which dominated the MS research field for the next few decades, and the development of the randomized clinical trial to assess more objectively whether a treatment really worked in a disease that was variable and, in the short-term, unpredictable.

REFERENCES

1. Association for Research in Nervous and Mental Disease. *Multiple Sclerosis (Disseminated sclerosis)*. New York: Paul B. Hoeber; 1922.
2. Association for Research in Nervous and Mental Disease. *Multiple Sclerosis and the Demyelinating Diseases*. Baltimore: Williams and Wilkins; 1950.
3. Brain WR. Critical review: disseminated sclerosis. *Quart J Med*. 1930;23:343-391.
4. Schumacher GA. Multiple sclerosis and its treatment. *JAMA*. 1950;143:1059-1065, 1146-1154, 1241-1250.
5. McAlpine D, Compston ND, Lumsden CE. *Multiple Sclerosis*. Edinburgh: E&S Livingston; 1955.
6. Association for Research in Nervous and Mental Disease. *Multiple Sclerosis (Disseminated sclerosis)*. New York: Paul B. Hoeber; 1922.
7. Jelliffe SE. Emotional and psychological factors in multiple sclerosis. In: *Multiple Sclerosis: An investigation by the Association for Research in Nervous and Mental Disease*. New York: PB Hoeber; 1921:82-90.
8. Limburg CC. The geographic distribution of multiple sclerosis and its estimated prevalence in the United States. In: *Multiple Sclerosis and the Demyelinating Diseases*. Proceedings of the Association for Research in Nervous and Mental Disease (Dec. 10–11, 1948). Vol 28. Baltimore: Williams and Wilkins; 1950:15-24.
9. Schumacher GA. Whither research in demyelination disease? In: Research in Demyelinating Diseases. *Annals New York Acad Sci*. 1965;569-570.
10. Sequin EC, Shaw JC, Van Derveer A. A contribution to the pathological anatomy of disseminated cerebro-spinal sclerosis. *J Nerv Ment Dis*. 1878;5:281-293.
11. Association for Research in Nervous and Mental Disease. *Multiple Sclerosis and the Demyelinating Diseases*. Baltimore: Williams and Wilkins; 1950:212.
12. Murray TJ, Murray SJ. Characteristics of patients found not to have multiple sclerosis. *Can Med Assoc J*. 1984;131:336-337.
13. Kirkland R. Disseminated Sclerosis at an unusual age. *BMJ*. 1883;1:407.
14. Noseworthy J, et al. Multiple Sclerosis after age 50. *Neurology*. 1983;33:1544-1545.
15. Birley JL, Didgeon LS. A clinical and experimental contribution to the pathogenesis of disseminated sclerosis. *Brain*. 1921;14:150-212.
16. MacLean AR, Berkson J, Woltman HW, Schionneman L. Multiple sclerosis in a rural community. In: *Multiple Sclerosis and the Demyelinating Diseases*. Proceedings of the Association for Research in Nervous and Mental Disease (Dec. 10–11, 1948). Vol 28. Baltimore: Williams and Wilkins; 1950:25-27.
17. Thygesen P. Prognosis in initial stages of disseminated primary demyelinating disease of central nervous system. *Arch Neurol Psych*. 1949;61:339-357.
18. Müller R. Studies on disseminated sclerosis. *Acta Med Scandinav*. 1949;133(suppl 222):1-214.
19. Müller R. Studies on disseminated sclerosis: p. 214.
20. Wechsler IS. *A Textbook of Clinical Neurology*. Philadelphia: WB Saunders Co., 1928:137-140.
21. Compston A. Reviewing multiple sclerosis. *Postgrad Med J*. 1992;68(801):507-515.

22. Brickner RM. A critique of therapy in multiple sclerosis. *Bull Neurol Inst NY.* 1935-1936;4:665-698.
23. Ibid, p. 665-698.
24. Putnam TJ. Studies in Multiple Sclerosis. *Arch Neurol Psych.* 1936;35:1289-1308.
25. Ferraro A. Primary demyelinating diseases of the nervous system: an attempt at unification and classification. 1937;37:1100-1160.
26. Ferraro A. Pathology of demyelinating diseases as an allergic reaction in the brain. *Arch Neurol Psychiat.* 1944;52:443-483.
27. Putnam TJ. The pathogenesis of multiple sclerosis: a possible vascular factor. *New Engl J Med.* 1933;209:786.
28. Wilson SAK. *Neurology.* Ed. AN Bruce. London: Edward Arnold; 1940:148-178.
29. Ibid, p. 148-178.
30. Ibid, p. 148-178.
31. Haymaker, Webb. *The Founders of Neurology.* Springfield, IL: Charles C Thomas; 1953:409-412.
32. Ferraro A. Primary demyelinating diseases of the nervous system: an attempt at unification and classification. 1937;37:1100-1160.
33. Kabat EA, et al. An electrophoretic study of the protein components in cerebrospinal fluid and their relationship to the serum proteins. *J Clin Invest.* 1942;21:571-577.
34. Medawar P. Personal Papers of Sir Peterrian Medawar FRS, OM (1915-1987, Medical Scientist, Nobel Laureate, Collected by Dr. Robert Reid, Wellcome Archives and MSS, PP/PBM).
35. Putnam TJ. The pathogenesis of multiple sclerosis: a possible vascular factor. *New Engl J Med.* 1933;209:786.
36. Putnam TJ, McKenna JB, Morrison LR. Studies in multiple sclerosis: the histogenesis of experimental sclerotic plaques and their relation to multiple sclerosis. *JAMA.* 1931;97:1591.
37. Putnam TJ, Chiavacci LV, Hoff H, et al. Results of treatment of multiple sclerosis with dicoumarin. *Arch Neurol.* 1947;57:1-13.
38. Limburg CC. The geographic distribution of multiple sclerosis and its estimated prevalence in the United States. In: *Multiple Sclerosis and the Demyelinating Diseases.* Proceedings of the Association for Research in Nervous and Mental Disease (Dec. 10–11, 1948). Vol 28. Baltimore: Williams and Wilkins; 1950:15-24.
39. Bing R, Reese H. Die multiple Sklerose in der Nordwestschweiz. *Schw med. Wchnschr.* 1926;56:30-34.
40. Reese HH. Multiple Sclerosis and the Demyelinating Diseases. Critique of theories concerning multiple sclerosis. *JAMA.* 1950;143:1470-1473.
41. Schumacher GA. Multiple sclerosis and its treatment. *JAMA.* 1950;143:1059-1065, 1146-1154, 1241-1250.
42. Schumacher GA. Whither research in demyelination disease? In: *Research in Demyelinating Diseases.* Annals New York Acad Sci. 1965;569-570.
43. Schumacher GA, Sibley WA, et al. Problems of experimental trials of therapy in multiple sclerosis. *Ann NY Acad Sci.* 1965;122:552-568.
44. McAlpine D, Compston ND, Lumsden CE. *Multiple Sclerosis.* Edinburgh: E&S Livingston; 1955.
45. *McAlpine's Multiple Sclerosis.* Ed. A. Compston. London: Churchill Livingstone; 1998.
46. Multiple Sclerosis: Progress in Research. Report of a Symposium held under the auspices of the Multiple Sclerosis Research Committee, World Federation of Neurology and Medical Research Council Demyelinating Disease Unit, Newcastle upon Tyne. Field EJ, Bell TM, and Cargegie PR, eds. Amsterdam, London: North Holland; 1972.
47. Miller HG, Newell DJ, Ridley A. Treatment of multiple sclerosis with corticotrophin (ACTH). *Lancet.* 1961;2:1361-1362.

48. Miller HG, Newell DJ, Ridley A. Multiple sclerosis. Trials of maintenance treatment with prednisolone and soluble aspirin. *Lancet.* 1961(b);1:127-129.
49. Multiple Sclerosis: Progress in Research, p. 122.
50. Marburg O. Die Sogenannte akute Multiple Sklerose (encephalomyelitis periaxialis scleroticans) *Jahrb Psychiat Neurol.* 1906;27:1.
51. Talley C. *A History of Multiple Sclerosis and Medicine in the United States, 1870–1960.* PhD dissertation. San Francisco: University of California; 1998.

11

Searching for a Cause of MS

And so we must add not wings but weights and leads to the intellect so as to hinder all leaping and flying.

Sir Francis Bacon, 1620[1]

"It is easy to welcome new facts which submit themselves to a favourite hypothesis; but if we resist this first temptation and pursue our own observations with industry and caution, we are presently made aware that the new facts are far more difficult of study than we had supposed. They turn out to be far less simple and uniform than at first they seemed, and they begin to refuse the shelter of the favourite hypothesis which appeared so convenient for them."

Sir T. Clifford Allbutt
(Discussing optic neuritis with spinal myelitis,
later called Devic's disease, 1870)[2]

"... a child one year old who was thrown into a convulsion by having a goose thrown at her, and after the convulsion, the disease (MS) developed."

Landon Carter Gray, 1893[3]

"Spritka saw a case develop from fright in a cigarmaker."

Landon Carter Gray, 1893[4]

"The most difficult things to explain are those which are not true."

A.S. Wiener, 1956[5]

"The amount of time and money which has been expended to determine the causal factors in multiple sclerosis is beyond computing ... the result has been nil."

William Boyd, 1958[6]

"It is possible that the cause of the disease lies buried somewhere in these lengthy protocols waiting to be found by someone ingenious enough to unearth it."

Henry Miller, 1960[7]

"It therefore seems that we should view the aetiology and pathogenesis of multiple sclerosis on a multifactorial basis, like the celebrated 'Chinese Dinner' where a judicious assortment of individual items combine to give a phenomenon whose entirety transends the mere sum of its individual parts."

D.C. Dumonde, 1979[8]

"Lack of understanding about the cause of MS has generated a remarkable variety of hypotheses over the last century. Few mechanisms have not been proposed to explain the bewildering phenomena associated with this disease."

George Ebers, 1998[9]

The *Oxford English Dictionary* defines *etiology* as a medical term meaning the cause or a set of causes of a disease or condition; also the investigation or attribution of the cause or reason for something (Etiology—from the Greek, *aitiologia*—*aitia*—a cause; *logia*—knowledge). Over the last century, Sir William Gowers, Russell Brain, S.A.

Kinnier Wilson, and other clinicians have attributed lack of success in therapy to lack of knowledge of the etiology of the disease.

Etiology is a challenging concept, for suggested solutions often beg other questions. If *this* is the cause of multiple sclerosis (MS), *why* does it happen, and why in *this patient*, at *this time*? That is what Charcot meant when others explained that the glial change, which he thought was the cause, was really due to an abnormality in the blood vessel; he said that just sets the question a little further back. So what is the cause of the blood vessel abnormality?

The philosopher Bertrand Russell said it was characteristic of humans to be able to comfortably keep conflicting views in their minds at the same time. In the past century, we have carried with us different and sometimes conflicting theories of the cause of MS, often developing overarching concepts so that we could retain favored views for which we have some evidence, and still include weaker concepts for which we have less evidence, but not so little that we are comfortable dispensing with them entirely. Thomas Kuhn, the historian of science, said we might hold a number of differing and competing views, but eventually one theory persists, and the one that "wins" does so as much by a band-wagon effect as by reasoned argument, particularly when the evidence is not overwhelming.[10]

In the age of Margaret of Myddle and Augustus d'Esté, illness was felt to be related to external forces, whether the "hand of God," or exposure to cold and dampness, or the stresses of life. D'Esté thought the onset of his visual loss was due to the stress of holding back tears at the funeral of a beloved friend. Heinreich Heine felt his early dalliances had revisited him as a progressive syphilitic illness. Margaret Gatty's physician stated in *The Lancet* that her illness was caused by her tendency to use excessive physical effort in gardening, using heavy tools in the manner of a man.

In the initial medical descriptions of MS by Ollivier, Frerichs, Türck, and others, there was limited speculation as to cause, other than the observation that the disease was sometimes associated with acute fevers or exposure to dampness and cold. Ollivier did not speculate on cause, but noted that the young man he described worsened when in hot spa waters.

Cruveilhier thought the disorder in the cook Darges was due to the same cause as the rheumatic disorders, a general suppression of sweat.

Over the last two centuries, ideas about the cause of MS have changed as new information and observations became available, as experiments were devised to test hypotheses, and as the trends in scientific interest altered and new technologies appeared. It is sobering to recognize that as we enter the 21st century, most of the questions about the cause of MS were formulated by the end of the 19th century. Some environmental ideas, such as dampness and exposure to cold, lasted a century; others, such as trauma and stress, have persisted on mostly anecdotal evidence, but are still in the minds of patients and some physicians today.

New questions have developed in this century about toxins, lipolytic enzymes, geographical factors, diet, genetics, and immune mechanisms. An infective cause was postulated in the late 19th century and, despite a

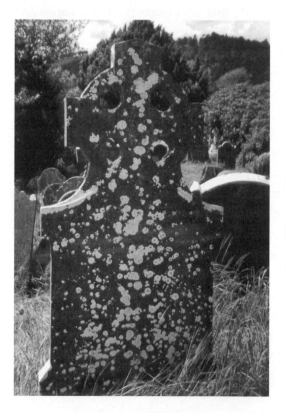

Figure 11.1 Moxon (1875) considered what would cause the patchiness of MS and pondered the similarity to eruptive skin conditions, and also noted the similarity in appearance to the lichen that grew on stones. This gravestone in Glendalough, Ireland, shows the pattern to which he referred. (Photographed by the author.)

lack of substantial evidence, is still a theory because the idea fits the features of the disease so well.

An important question was raised in 1863 by Rindfleisch, who noted in his microscopic examinations that a blood vessel was often prominent in the center of the MS plaque; he postulated that the disorder was due to an abnormality in the vasculature.[11] In 1863, Leyden summarized the state of knowledge of this condition in 34 cases five years before Charcot's lesson on multiple sclerosis. He showed that acute myelitis and the general neurological condition we know as multiple sclerosis are the same.[12] He noted that one of his cases was hereditary, but thought the cause in the others could be exposure to cold and dampness, concussion to the body, and psychic effects such as prolonged worry and sudden fright.

Other questions about which tissue has the primary defect (glia, myelin, blood vessels, or immune cells) continue to occupy investigators. Charcot felt the disorder was one of glial hypertrophy and destruction of nerve tissues, with the "wreck and detritus resulting from disintegration of nerve fibers" being removed by lipid-laden cells.

In 1875, after a very clear outline of the clinical features and pathological findings of MS, Moxon wondered what other conditions might aid in understanding the patchiness of the change in the nervous system.[13] He regarded the pathology as "eruptive" in nature, similar to dermatological diseases, and similar to the process that occurs in smallpox, leprosy, and syphilis. Such patchiness occurs in leprosy of the skin or in the cystoid eruption of bones. Looking for further analogies, he mused that the patchiness called to mind the lichen on a stone wall, or the round puffs of algaceous ferment plant in a changing chemical solution, "pointing clearly to some entirely foreign agency springing into action at the affected spots." He noted that subacute arteritis, of a type occurring in middle age that he called *inflammatory mollities* could affect the vessels to the brain and cause softening and round blotches. However, he confessed that such analogies helped little when there was little knowledge of what caused the vascular change. Moxon concluded that the disease remained of unknown origin.

In 1878, Hamilton said little was known about etiology, but noted that moist cold, emotional excitement, and venereal excesses were suspected by Continental writers.[14] Strümpell and Müller agreed with Charcot that the problem was in the glial tissues, and that glial hypertrophy led to compression of the medullary sheaths. Others considered the defect to be in the myelin itself.[15]

In 1895, Pierre Marie allowing that others felt there was a role for acute illnesses, overwork, cold, injury and excess of every cause, confidently proposed he knew a cause for MS that was even more common— infection, or more correctly, infections.* He listed many infections he had seen associated with the onset or worsening of the disorder (enteric fever, measles, scarlatina, smallpox, diphtheria, whooping cough, erysipelas, dysentery, cholera, and other unnamed infections). Although convinced the cause of MS was an infection, he said he was embarrassed when the discussion turned to which microbe was the culprit. He was upset at the assertion that he had found the microbe, for MS for those who made it quite obviously had not read his papers. He never claimed to have found the microbe and in fact believed that many organisms could be involved in the initiation of MS.[16]

In 1893, Gowers had agreed that infections could be involved, but more as an aggravating factor, and exposure to cold could do the same. He was not sure of the cause of MS and felt that effective treatment would have to await better understanding. Reflecting on the many theories of etiology, he commented: "A minority incriminate factors so diverse as to be destitute of etiological import."[17,18]

His colleague, Risien Russell, agreed in 1899 that infection, like cold and stress, were probably only aggravating factors, but it was wise to avoid physical and mental stress, as well as indulgence in wine and venery.[19] Rejecting Oppenheim's concept of a circulating toxin such as lead, copper, or zinc, Russell said these were highly unlikely causes, as young ladies whose social surroundings would exclude them from such exposure still developed the disease.

---

*In a footnote to his statement, Pierre Marie noted that his theory of an infectious origin was acknowledged by most and it would be ungracious of him to find fault with those who disagreed, even though many of them had been hostile. He added that some had even disagreed with his theory that epilepsy had an infectious cause, but until that case was finally proven, he would just repeat that his opinion on this was unchanged.

Krafft-Ebing said in 1894 that 40 out of 100 cases of MS had a history of heat injury.[20] In 1940, S.A. Kinnier Wilson said heat, like infection, could aggravate MS, but was not a cause; cold might be more important.[21] Landon Carter Gray was sure that when MS occurred in children, it usually came on after a convulsion.[22] Oppenheim believed that all MS begins in infancy and only manifested later in life, probably due to some external toxin.[23]

Charles Beevor felt that certain occupations were vulnerable, a concern often expressed in the German literature.[24] This idea was never emphasized, nor was there much evidence to support it, but the idea would return whenever clusters of MS cases were observed, especially in the workplace. Occupations that were suspected included woodworking, ironworking, farming, working with lead, phosphorus, copper, or aniline dyes; occupations that gave workers constant water exposure; and more recently, working with animals that suffered from swayback disease. Charles Dana believed that MS occurred more often in persons doing skilled manual work than in ordinary laborers or in "brain workers."[25] None of these suggestions about occupational risk have surfaced as relevant in large surveys of MS in recent times.

The idea of a neuropathic constitution coupled with the propensity to many nervous and mental diseases, poverty, and crime was widely discussed early in the 20th century when eugenic theory and practices were in vogue. It persists today under the more respectable mantle of a genetic predisposition to MS. Dana believed many factors could act on a "neuropathic constitution" that existed in some families. These factors included acute infections such as typhoid, diphtheria, smallpox, measles, erysipelas, malaria, myelitis, and encephalitis. MS had been seen in a case of hemoglobinuria, as well as after trauma and concussions.

The idea of causal infection was fading in the 1920s (it was revived in the 1930s), and the concept of some toxin or lytic substance affecting myelin became more prominent, as Marburg suggested in 1906 and 1911. He felt the myelinolytic toxin caused breakdown of the lecithin fraction of myelin.[26] A myelinotoxic substance was also considered by Mott (1913) and Dawson (1916) and was clearly argued by George B. Hassin at the 1921 ARNMD meeting, where he stated that MS was a myelin degener-

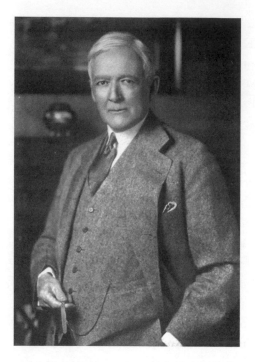

Figure 11.2 Lewellys Barker was a Canadian physician who succeeded Sir William Osler at Johns Hopkins and made many contributions to neurology, discussing the various causes of MS at the 1921 ARNMD meeting in New York. He was said to have produced the first major neuroanatomical text in the United States.

ative disorder, not an infection.[27] What this lytic factor might be was uncertain, but Brickner (1931) announced that he had found a lipolytic enzyme in the plasma of MS patients.[28]

Lewellys F. Barker discussed the exogenous causes of multiple sclerosis at the 1921 ARNMD meeting and indicated it was accepted clinically that infections could produce an exacerbation of MS. A specific infection was unlikely as a cause, but there was also no longer much support for Oppenheim's belief in an environmental toxin.*[29,30] Differentiating a causative agent from an aggravating one, Barker noted that thermic injury occurred in 40 percent of cases, but was likely an aggravating factor, not a cause. He was skeptical about the role of trauma and noted that patients easily incriminate trauma, and "neurologists, who

---

*Barker was a Canadian, who succeeded William Osler when Osler accepted the position of Regius Professor at Oxford. He contributed to the understanding of chronic diseases, geriatrics, liver and kidney physiology, endocarditis, TB, gout, and rheumatic diseases, but his book *The Nervous System and its Constituent Neurons* (1899) was said by Courville to be "the first major anatomic treatment of the nervous system to originate in the United States." His book *Time and the Physician* is an interesting view of medicine in his era.

see many patients suffering from epilepsy, brain tumor, mental deterioration, and other organic processes, are very familiar with the prevalence of this conception." He pointed out that no one has been able to reproduce multiple sclerosis by trauma in animals. Barker concluded that:

> *"If multiple sclerosis is a disease entity due to a single cause that acts in early life, it may be due to some specific infection, but the evidence available is strongly against its being caused by any of our well-known infections, by any ordinary intoxication (organic or inorganic), or by electrical, thermal or traumatic influences."*[31]

Charles Dana believed that MS patients often had skulls of the linear dolichocephalic type.[32] He indicated that people were beginning to agree that there were two types of morphology: either thin patients with high basal metabolism, who were mentally nervous but self-controlled, or the more broadly built, brachycephalic types who tended to be stout, variable in weight, and emotional. He added, "I have never seen multiple sclerosis in a fat man or a woman even when long bedridden."

Dana also believed that MS was more common in males than females (3 to 2)—many others shared this view—and that it was more common

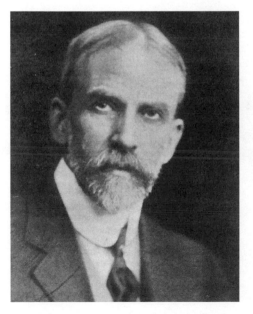

Figure 11.3 Charles Loomis Dana (1852–1935) was a prominent American neurologist who wrote a neurology textbook that went into many editions and printings, but he had some puzzling views on the basis of MS, including a relationship to body type and he said he had never seen a fat person with MS.

in those who came from "neuropathic stock." He felt it was not a familial disease and not inherited, even though there might be rare and doubtful exceptions. He thought the duration of the disease was eight years, but with a range of one to thirty years.

Since Freudian psychoanalysis was a major focus in the early decades of this century, it is not surprising that this should be applied to the understanding of MS. Smith Ely Jelliffe developed an "action pattern theory" of MS using Freudian imagery, suggesting that plaques formed due to repressed emotions, and formed in the area of the brain where the repression was occurring. He referred to MS as a "schizophrenia of the spinal axis."[33] Others shared this view, and Putnam advocated psychotherapy as the most beneficial approach to treatment of MS.[34]

Spiller studied the pathology of MS and wondered whether the primary defect was in the axon, myelin, or glia, concluding it was the glia.[35] Constructing a sequence of events, he thought it was an acute inflammatory disease due to a circulating toxin, focused on the vascular supply to the areas of plaque, affecting the glia. It is interesting that at the 1921 ARNMD meeting, Joshua H. Leiner observed that the axon could be involved, even though not as extensively as the myelin.[36]

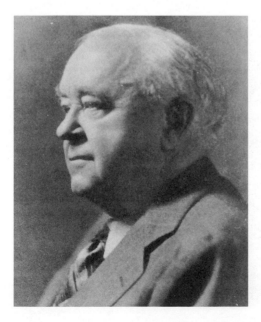

Figure 11.4 Smith Ely Jelliffe (1866–1945) was a prolific author on neurological topics with 1,500 publications and 16 books. He was editor of the *Journal of Nervous and Mental Diseases* for 42 years, remembered as a psychoanalyst, and for introducing Freud and Jung to an American audience. His theories of a psychological cause for MS with stresses causing the lesions in the CNS were rejected by the ARNMD meeting on MS in 1921.

Although writers would always indicate MS was not syphilis, syphilis therapies were used on MS up to the 1940s. The idea of a spirochete as a cause of MS was stimulated by the suggestion of Buzzard in 1913 and encouraged by transmission experiments over the next 50 years. The idea did not take hold: each report of successful transmission or identification was followed by even more negative studies in other laboratories. The Chevassut reports of isolation and transmission of an agent called *Spirula insularis* were soon discredited,[37] as were those of her mentor, James Purves-Stewart,[38] who claimed to have developed a successful vaccine. Dattner's suggestion in 1937 that the cause was a late version of tuberculosis (*metatuberulosis*) found few adherents.

Putnam's thrombosis theory was popular in the era of new anticoagulants, but waned after a few years, even though he continued to treat his patients with these drugs. Putnam postulated that the thrombosis was not due to the vessel walls, but was something in the blood itself, which might be an increase in fibrinogen. His views were controversial, and neuropathologists did not agree with his interpretation of the histology from his thromboembolic experiments.[39]

By 1950, the list of possible etiologic suspects was narrowing. There was no longer a strong belief in stress, cold and dampness, trauma, heavy metal poisoning, or other external toxins as causes of MS. Concepts of allergy and hypersensitivity were being invoked as an understanding of the role of the immune system in MS developed. Schumacher listed a number of factors that might be important in the etiology of multiple sclerosis, including vascular thrombosis, vasoconstriction, allergic hypersensitivity with an antigen-antibody reaction, as well as the pathophysiological mechanisms related to emotions.[40] Lumsden[41] and Reese[42] agreed by the early 1950s that there were two possibilities: a transmissible agent, either a virus or a chemical agent; or a particular nonspecific immune reaction of the nervous system to many causes.

Reese felt the earlier thoughts about a constitutional defect, a relationship to body type, or to an endocrine cause could be rejected. He believed the observations of Curtius[43] and others on heredity were unconvincing and just led to controversy and argument. On the other hand, the menstrual, pregnancy, and postpartum relationships suggested some hormonal basis for faulty fat metabolism. He felt that bacteria were not the cause, but a bacterial toxin had not been ruled out. He believed a viral cause for MS was "extremely unlikely" but could not be excluded, and allergy was an open question. It is interesting that Reese said infection was an unlikely cause since there are no epidemics of MS. (Kurtzke would suggest these in the unusual "outbreaks" in the Faeroe Islands and Iceland a few years later.) Reese was unconvinced by the vascular thrombosis theory, rejecting the wide use of anticoagulants, but was impressed with experiments that suggested a role for vasospasm. He was also impressed with Ferraro's experimental allergic studies, but wondered how much the animal experiments (EAE) related to the human disease.

Major theories of causes of MS listed by McAlpine and his coauthors in 1955 in chronological order were the Strümpell-Müller theory of dysplastic glial development; Marburg's theory of a circulating myelinotoxin; the infection theory; vascular theories of thrombosis or vasospasm; allergic theory; and recent biochemical theories.[44] They postulated that MS was primarily a disease of the oligodendroglia, perhaps induced by hypersensitization or allergy; the cause was not purely genetically determined, but perhaps a genetically determined predisposition coupled with an exogenous factor.

> *"The notion that 'trace elements' play any role specifically in the pathogenesis of multiple sclerosis never really had adherents."*
> Charles E. Lumsden, 1972[45]

The "umbrella concept" that has been prominent in the last three decades has been the possibility of a viral trigger that initiates an immunological reaction that is ongoing in a person who is genetically predisposed.

The idea of an immune mechanism dates back to the work of Glanzmann (1932),[46] and Rivers and Schwentker (1935).[47] Once there was an animal model that seemed to be able to reproduce the scattered plaque of MS, even if it did this only in an acute situation, there was a reasonable model against which theories and potential therapies could be tested. Although initially ignored, the discovery by Kabat[48] on the elevation of gamma globulin in the CSF of MS patients, which would later be shown to be antibody produced in the nervous system, gave further evidence of an immunological process even though it was difficult to show a correlation of the changes with the clinical status of the patient. Interest in the immune mechanisms was spurred on by exciting discoveries about the immune system by McFarlane Burnet and Robert Good and others in the 1960s as well as about ways the body could react to external antigens and learn to react against its own tissues as if they were foreign. MS was an obvious disease to examine as immunological concepts and techniques developed and EAE as the animal model for MS continued to be used, despite concerns about whether the mechanisms were the same.

> *"The premise on which most work on EAE has been based, mainly an understanding of EAE would lead simultaneously to an understanding of MS, has not been proved to date."*
>
> Barry Arnason, 1983[49]

The idea that there may be a genetic factor in MS has a long history—as early as 1863, Leyden noted a familial case of MS among his 34 cases of multiple sclerosis.[50] Other cases were presented by Batten (1908)[51] and most series of investigations at the turn of the 20th century had a few cases in families, though these were often regarded as coincidental, or due to similar environmental influences, "remarkable" but unusual. Davenport made the cogent comment in 1921 that whatever might be found as the exogenous cause of MS, the hereditary factor could not be left out of the explanation.[52] Perhaps MS was similar to many other diseases where the disease only occurs when the constitution or the condition of the person is susceptible, and hereditary factors might be important in determining if, when, and how the disease occurred. Those who wrote the conclusions of the 1921 ARNMD meeting seemed a little unsure that MS "was not a familial disease, and not inherited, with rare and doubtful exceptions." They went on to say, "but in the ancestry there is often evidence of neuropathic stock."[53] This implied, as Davenport suggested, there might be a genetic predisposition upon which other factors could act, a belief that is still current.

Little attention was given to repeated observations of cases of MS in a family, noted by almost all who collected large numbers of patients, until this aspect was systematically studied by Curtius in Germany.[54]

MacKay at McGill collected all the published family cases back to Eichendorst's family in 1896 and graphed the impressive numbers reported in families. He was critical of the Thums twin study that suggested no genetic factor and found a 23 percent concordance rate in identical twins, which is highly suggestive of a genetic factor.[55,56]

Larner at Oxford reviewed viral research in 1986 and said the evidence for a viral cause for MS was less convincing than the epidemiologic data, but all evidence was circumstantial and fragmentary.[57] Despite that, an infectious cause still fit the circumstances best and a century after Pierre Marie, the belief persists. Interest currently focuses on measles, Type C influenza, herpes simplex, parainfluenza 3, mumps, varicella zoster, vaccinia, rubella, adenoviruses, herpes virus 6, Epstein-Barr virus, and others.

We will now discuss current theories of MS causation and the history of these concepts. Karl Popper said in *The Logic of Scientific Discovery* that the most interesting and important aspect of the growth in science is that older and well-established theories are replaced by the new.[58] We have been working for the past century in what Thomas Kuhn would call "normal science," within accepted paradigms that have not changed much, even though the science and technology within the paradigm has advanced impressively.[59] Perhaps in the 21st century the answers to the etiology of MS will come, not from mining the current paradigms further, but from new ideas and new overarching concepts that we have not yet conceived. It is imperative, not just to develop an acceptable concept, because our concepts drive our therapeutic approaches and directly affect how we treat our patients.

THE SEARCH FOR AN INFECTION

"These, gentlemen, are suppositions, and I put them before you without unreasonably insisting upon them. The one point in this discussion which I would fix in your minds is the following fact, a fact which, thank God, has been well established, viz., that the cause of insular sclerosis is intimately connected with infectious diseases."

Pierre Marie, 1985[60]

"It is a tragedy that some problems of multiple sclerosis, not only pathologic and anatomical, but clinical, give rise to so many controversies."

George B. Hassin, 1922[61]

There is no more controversial area in MS than the search for an infection as the cause. Although Charcot postulated MS might be due to exposure to cold and damp, trauma, or emotional stress, developments in bacteriology and the growing acceptance of the germ theory led to consideration in the 1880s that MS might be due to an infection. The strongest proponent was Pierre Marie, Charcot's student and successor to the chair of Neurology at the University of Paris, who argued that not only was MS due to infection (or, as he said, infections) but that the advances of Pasteur and Koch would eventually lead to a vaccine for the disease. It would be a logical step to use their techniques to try and transmit the disease.[62] Despite Marie's strong views, others, including the English neurologists William Gowers and Risien Russell, argued that infection might aggravate the disease but was not the cause. It is sobering to consider that this debate, active at the end of the 19th century, is still alive in the 21st century.

Because there were limited specific medicines or therapies for infection in the 19th century, general approaches to treatment were used, even by those who felt an infection caused MS. When the advances in therapy for syphilis were announced by Erlich, these approaches were applied to MS, not because physicians thought MS was syphilis (they repeatedly pointed out that it was not), but because both diseases affected wide areas of the CNS with devastating and progressive disability. Because both were serious widespread diseases of the nervous system, when advances in understanding cause and development of effective therapies occurred for syphilis, these were applied to MS, where there seemed to be little effective treatment. Antisyphilitic therapies were used for MS up until World War II.[63]

As discoveries were made in other areas of infectious disease around the turn of the century, each was applied to MS. The excitement generated by discoveries in pneumonia, rabies, tuberculosis, cholera, and yellow fever sparked a greater interest in searching for an infective agent in MS, and in using any therapy being developed for an infectious disease on MS patients. There was a possibility, that even if MS were not syphilis, or tuberculosis, or a bacterial infection, it might be an aberrant form of these infections; therefore, there was some logic in the approach. After all, even those who did not believe MS was an infection could not escape the obvious tendency for acute infections to worsen the disease, even if transiently.

EARLY TRANSMISSION EXPERIMENTS

There was great interest in the announcement by Bullock* that he had transmitted MS from man to rabbits.[64,65] A few years before, Farquhar Buzzard had suggested the cause of MS might turn out to be a spirochete.[66] The excitement was increased by the confirming studies of Kuhn and Steiner, who took CSF from MS patients and claimed that they had produced typical MS in guinea pigs and rabbits by an identifiable agent, a spirochete, which they called *Spirocheta myelophthora*.[67,68] This event was confirmed by others, and spirochetes were reported in autopsy material. The situation soon became confusing to clinicians who followed these developments: conflicting reports appeared from other laboratories indicating they could not confirm the transmission experiments. The neurological community, who was watching this closely, were hesitant to make any conclusions. In 1921, Gye (Bullock) again published experiments showing that multiple sclerosis, or a paralytic disease that resembled it, could be transmitted to two out of ten rabbits.[69,70] Gye would later claim transmission to rabbits from blood and CSF of MS patients, but not if the CSF was filtered through a Berkefeld filter, suggesting the causative agent was a filterable agent, probably a virus.

Between 1913 and 1923, many advanced the spirochete theory, notably Kuhn and Steiner, Siemerling, Marinesco, and Petit, but others continued to fail in their attempts to transmit the disease in their experiments. Dr. Oscar Teague of the New York Neurological Institute obtained a grant from the Commonwealth Foundation to review this sit-

---

*There is some confusion in his publications over the next few years; Bullock changed his name to Gye, taking the name of his wife.

uation, and he summarized his work at the 1921 meeting of the ARNMD.[71] He said that five investigators had concluded MS was an infectious transmissible disease, and four disagreed because of their negative results doing the same experiments. Teague did his own experiments and used spinal fluid from acute, chronic progressive, and stable cases of MS. He used a variety of routes of transmission on 220 animals. No fluids showed spirochetes. No animals developed a paralytic disease. In the discussion on Teague's paper, Dr. Tilney indicated that rabbits often developed a paralytic disease and so its presence was not good evidence for the transmission of multiple sclerosis. The controversy did not end, however, and at the same meeting Charles L. Dana stated:

> *"I am assuming that there is an infecting organism at the bottom of the multiple sclerosis lesions. I even assume it is an animal type, i.e. some variant of spirochaetae, hence I place the problem of multiple sclerosis in the domain of animal ecology."*[72]

Despite criticism of the transmission experiments and increasing reports from others who could not reproduce the results, reports of spirochetes continued to appear. Adams, Blacklock, and Dunlop found spirochetes when looking at the CSF from monkeys injected with MS tissue; they said the spirochete looked similar to that reported by Steiner and Kuhn.[73] No one could culture the spirochete, however, and there was growing skepticism in neurological circles, despite the enthusiasm of the proponents of the MS spirochete who continued to report positive spirochete experiments or sightings through the 1920s and 1930s and even in the mid-1950s.

In the meantime, interest in another agent, a virus, became the focus of attention when two articles appeared side by side in *The Lancet*. Kathleen Chevassut, working under the supervision of Sir James Purves-Stewart at the Westminister Hospital, claimed that she could recover a living organism smaller than 0.2 μ, undoubtedly a virus, from 93 percent of MS patients.[74] In a detailed article that fairly reviewed the history and criticism of the spirochete story up to that time, she discussed the isolation of a virus, which bore a resemblance to the agent that caused bovine pleuro-pneumonia. Even more dramatic was the companion *Lancet*

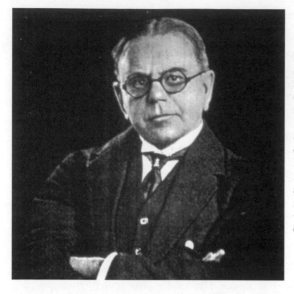

Figure 11.5 James Purves-Stewart was a successful London neurological consultant when he embarked on the experiments to isolate and transmit an agent in MS that he and his research assistant, Kathleen Chevassut, called the *Spherula insularis*. Purves-Stewart published a report of a successful vaccine against this agent, but the research was later pronounced worthless by a Medical Research Council investigation.

paper by her mentor, Sir James Purves-Stewart, a fashionable neurological consultant, who was thanked by Miss Chevassut at the end of her paper for the gifts of a microscope and other apparatus to do her work. In his paper, Purves-Stewart named the virus *Spherula insularis* and announced the production of an autogenous vaccine against the agent, which he had already given to 128 cases of MS, 70 of whom were followed long enough to yield results. Forty of the 70 cases had demonstrated improvement.[75,76] It seemed that Chevassut and Purves-Stewart had not only discovered the cause of MS, but had developed a vaccine that produced clinical improvement.

There was widespread but quiet skepticism from the neurological community to the Chevassut-Purves-Stewart work, but it became more vocal as the duo presented their work to medical meetings. Hans Zinsser said the observations were all artifacts, and even if correct, they would be very surprising on immunological grounds. J.B. Ayer and Tracy Putnam were critical as well and Putnam said that one-half to three-quarters of patients could be expected to improve with any therapeutic intervention.*

---

*Putnam then suggested that the best results were obtained by "conscious directed psychotherapy and re-education," an approach that brought him under criticism some years later, and which he eventually retracted.

Because of growing controversy surrounding the work, Arnold Carmichael at the National Hospital, Queen Square was asked by the Medical Research Council, which had given Miss Chevassut a part-time personal grant for her work, to investigate the research methods and results from the Westminister Hospital where the work was done.[77] Despite lack of cooperation and continual evasiveness by Miss Chevassut, Carmichael was able to present his conclusions at a Royal Society of Medicine meeting in January 1931, indicating that there was nothing of merit in this work.[78] He had attempted their experiment on 19 cases and could not find any evidence of a virus. Miss Chevassut left the conference room in tears. Purves-Stewart returned to his fashionable practice.[79]

In the meantime, French workers were also trying to reproduce the Chevassut results. Pierre Lépine and P. Mollaret reported to the Academy of Medicine that they also could not find evidence of a virus. They felt the spherules and granules Miss Chevassut saw (and cultured) were a contaminant by human serum and of no significance. Despite this, they were also making a vaccine from the material, in the hope that perhaps there was something beneficial in the solution, and were treating patients with it.[80]

It is often said that this ended the work for both Purves-Stewart and Chevassut, but not so. Purves-Stewart would later disassociate himself publicly from Chevassut, but he still believed in the *Spirula insularis*. He continued to take CSF from his patients for isolation of the organism and development of his vaccine, which he continued to use on his MS patients. He retired from his fashionable practice and spent his last days in his lighthouse at Beachy Head, where he wrote an autobiography, *Sands of Time*.[81] In it he talked about his early life and his enjoyable period in training at Queen Square. He dwelled on current world events and was very concerned about the impending shadows of war and the dangers of dictators. Nowhere did he mention the *Spherula insularis* research, nor did he refer to multiple sclerosis or to Miss Chevassut. This clearly was an episode in his life he wanted to forget.

Miss Chevassut did not disappear either. She continued her work, supported by the Halley Stewart Trust, endowed by philanthropist Sir Halley Stewart. The trust provided her personal support and an institute in

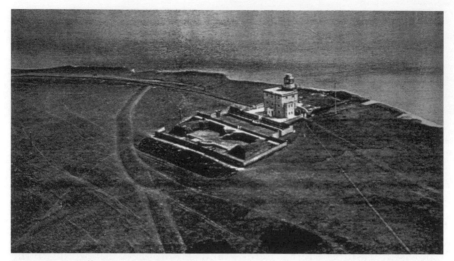

Figure 11.6 Belle Toute Lighthouse, Beachy Head, Sussex, where Purves-Stewart retired to write his fulsome memoirs, in which he made no mention of his then discredited MS work, or the association with the laboratory work of Kathleen Chevassut.

Hampstead with 12 inpatient beds, nursing staff, and a lab assistant. Sir Halley's retired physician son, Dr. B. Halley Stewart, was appointed medical director of the institute, but left after a few weeks because Miss Chevassut resented his presence there. He was back in four months, with the task of establishing a system of controls over her procedures, including lumbar punctures. Miss Chevassut was observed to get around this scrutiny by replacing dummy culture tubes with ones she carried in her lab coat pocket. In the meantime, Dr. S.R. Douglas at the Medical Research Council (MRC) was producing pure cultures of bovine pleuropneumonia virus from the samples Miss Chevassut provided, suggesting these were the virus cultures she was carrying secretly in her lab coat. Braxton Hicks, with Purves-Stewart as coauthor on his paper, injected seven monkeys with Miss Chevassut's vaccine; one developed a form of paralysis. Dr. Norman Howard-Jones, house officer at the Metropolitan Hospital, Kingsland Road in 1933, remembers Miss Chevassut in her white coat, "brewing her autogenous vaccines" and providing them to neurologist C. Worster-Drought, who used the vaccine to treat his MS patients. Miss Chevassut became increasingly discredited and drifted from sight. However by 1935, 550 patients had been treated with the Purves-Stewart vaccine.

The search for a specific organism in MS did not end there, even though Tracy Putnam stood up at the 1930 meeting, during the criticism of Purves-Stewart's virus work, and said the interest in a spirochete was lessening as fewer and fewer spirochetes were being reported each year, "and Professor Steiner who had been particularly interested in the etiology of disseminated sclerosis had substantially retracted the conclusions that he and Kuhn reached 12 years before ..." Steiner and Kuhn continued to report finding spirochetes in the brains and spinal cords of people who died with MS, and would do so for the next 22 years. Their last report appeared in 1952 when most others had lost interest.[82–86] By 1952, Innis and Kurland[87] summarized all attempts to transmit the disease and concluded that all were negative or inconclusive; in 1955, Lumsden found that there was little to suggest a viral infection because injecting material from acute plaques into cultures of human nerve cells had no effect on cell growth.[88]

Interest was briefly sparked again when Rose Ichelson of Philadelphia reported in 1957 that six years earlier she had devised a culture medium that grew a few spirochetes from MS CSF, but modification of the culture resulted in a heavy growth of spirochetes in a few days.[89] She reported that 59 of her 76 cases (78 percent) had positive cultures, whereas all the normal controls were negative. The organism was a spiral with a loop at one end, resembling a tennis racquet. She called it similar in appearance to that of the *Spirocheta myelophthora* of Steiner. In a subsequent paper, she reported that there were positive skin reactions in 62 of 72 MS patients injected with a polyvalent ultrafiltrate of the organism. Soon after, there were a few reports confirming the presence of a living organism in some MS cases, but the same year, a flurry of groups attempted the experiments and showed no evidence of a spirochete or any other living organisms. Careful study of the experiments by a group under John Kurtzke showed the Ichelson work to be invalid. The group did find an organism that resembled the Ichelson spirochete in one instance, but it was from a patient with a past history of meningoencephalitis who did not have MS.[90]

In the second edition of McAlpine's *Multiple Sclerosis*, Lumsden reviewed the Ichelson spirochete observation and the five studies that seemed to confirm it (Simons 1957 from CSF; Simons 1958 from autopsy

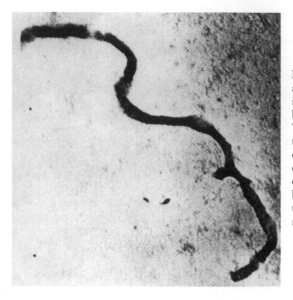

Figure 11.7 John Kurtzke attempted to reproduce the finding of spirochetes in MS as noted by Ichelson, but failed to do so. There were some cases of contamination in all groups (MS, other neurological disease, schizophrenia, and normals), but only one had an organism that resembled Ichelson's organism, and this was from a patient who did not have MS.

tissue; Ahrens and Muschner 1958 from autopsy tissue; Myerson, Wolfson, and Sall 1958 from CSF) and the seven studies that could not confirm it (Harding et al. 1959; Hoffmann and Schaltenbrand 1959; Mavor, Gallagher, and Schumacher 1960; Kurtzke et al. 1962; Scherrer, Mattmann, and Wüthrich 1962; Vinnik and Grann 1962).[91] He noted that the interest and publications disappeared after the 1962 nonconfirmatory studies. He observed that experienced pathologists know that spirochetes are often contaminants in the animal sera media of the type used by Ichelson (here he noted that not all the spirochetes the confirming groups noted were "scratches on the glass" as suggested, perhaps facetiously, by Hoffmann and Schaltenbrand.) Also he said that saprophytic spirochetes were present in the bedsores of virtually all patients, as he had confirmed in a previous study; he felt this was the basis of the observation by Ichelson and others. Lumsden had the opportunity to examine some of Steiner's slides, which had earlier shown spirochetes, and he noted that there were very few spirochetes. They were not related to the plaques and were related to the walls of vessels. They were undoubtedly a postmortem contaminant or a terminal sapremia.

Le Gac hypothesized that the organism responsible for MS was a Rickettsia based on positive serology in 38 of 52 patients.[92,93] Ross could not confirm this, and although it was not accepted as a concept by the neurological community, it led to a well-publicized Le Gac therapy based on the treatment of a Rickettsial infection.

David Sackett referred to ideas such as the spirochete cause of MS as "zombies"—just when you think the ideas are dead, they arise from the grave. In 1987, Gay and Dick reviewed the evidence for a spirochete relationship, and while dismissing the attention to EAE as a model and a virus as a cause, they suggested the spirochete *Treponema denticola* as a cause of MS.[94] They were able to detect IgG and IgM antibody to this spirochete in the CSF of 16 cases of MS. The spirochete story did not end here. There were newspaper reports of a spirochete found in MS patients in a European clinic in the 1990s, but this has not yet appeared in the medical literature.

The neurological community was disturbed to read in 1994 that a prominent and internationally known German neurologist had carried

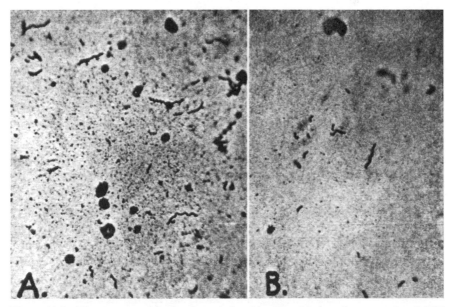

Figure 11.8   The controversial spirochetes isolated by Rose Ichelson from a smear of CSF culture from a patient with MS. She said it was identical to the organism seen by Steiner, which he called *Spirocheta myelophthora*. Some would suggest the appearance of the long strands of silver staining material represented an artifact of silver aggregation, but others felt they were probably saprophytic spirochete contamination from pressure sores (decubiti). (Ichelson, 1957.)

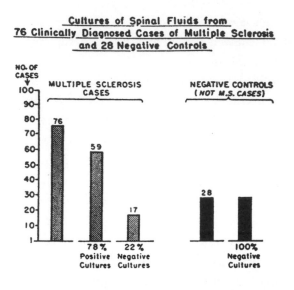

Cultures of Spinal Fluids from 76 Clinically Diagnosed Cases of Multiple Sclerosis and 28 Negative Controls

Figure 11.9 The impressive rate of positive cultivation of spirochetes from MS spinal fluid (CSF) by Rose Ichelson (78%) with none found in control CSFs. However, there were periodic reports of spirochetes being isolated from tissue CSF and transmission to animals between 1919 and 1957, but with even more studies that could not corroborate these findings. Some authors would argue that the structure seen was an artifact or contamination by a saprophytic spirochete. (Ichelson, 1957.)

out unethical experiments involving the transmission of MS materials to humans during World War II (the "Schaltenbrand experiment").[95] In 1940, Georg Schaltenbrand attempted to establish a viral etiology for MS. He thought he had induced an MS-like illness in monkeys by injecting them cisternally with CSF from MS patients. His next step was to see if CSF from the monkeys would induce MS in humans. He felt the experiment was justified in *verblödete Menschen* (demented individuals), and four demented individuals were injected intracisternally with CSF from monkeys who had a spontaneous encephalomyelitis; six people were injected with CSF from monkeys who had been injected with CSF from MS patients. Although MS was never induced, because of a finding of a pleocytosis (not a surprising result) the experiments were continued; eventually 45 people were injected. In his 1943 book on the work, Schaltenbrand indicated that the experiments should be done on a larger scale, but this was unlikely because of the ongoing war. His work was exposed first in 1950 and defended by Pearce Bailey (Schaltenbrand had trained with Harvey Cushing and Bailey in the United States before establishing the University Clinic at Wurzburg), but exposed again by Shevell and Bradley in 1994. Although much of the documentation has mysteriously disappeared, the unethical nature of these experiments was recently reviewed by Shevell, who also documented the active participation of another prominent neurologist, Julius Hallervorden, in euthanasia programs in Nazi Germany during World War II.[96]

In 1962, Adams and Imagawa noted higher levels of measles-neutralizing antibodies and complement-fixing antibodies in the sera and CSF of MS patients, although the increase was modest, about twice that of controls. It was not increased in most cases and was also found in other conditions.[97] John M. Adams, professor of pediatrics at UCLA, wrote a small monograph suggesting that MS was a childhood-acquired disease.[98] Coincidentally, the measles vaccine became available the next year and was widely used, leading to speculation that if we looked 20 to 30 years in the future, we should see a reduction in the incidence of MS.* Murray[99] and Poskanzer[100] noted that measles may occur later in the MS patient group, and it is interesting to note that Augustus d'Esté had measles at age 14, in 1808, 14 years before the onset of his first symptoms of multiple sclerosis. Perhaps this is just an epiphenomenon in MS as similar increased titers were reported to a long list of viruses. Sibley and Foley[101] and others noted that the antibodies were slightly higher in MS patients to a variety of viruses, not only measles, and the list has grown to include type C influenza, herpes simplex, paromyxovirus, parainfluenza 3, mumps, varicella zoster, vaccinia, rubella, Epstein-Barr virus, and adenovirus.[102] Unconvincing and unconfirmed reports have even suggested that rabies, herpes simplex, and parainfluenza type 1 viruses could be isolated from MS tissue. Others have visualized viral-like products under the electron microscope, but many other techniques to confirm the presence of an active virus have led to the conclusion that a virus is not present. But absence of evidence is not evidence of absence, and the search continues.

At an important meeting in Newcastle upon Tyne in June 1971, advances in virological and immunological aspects of MS were discussed. The major topic centered around the research on a measles link,[103] stimulated by the observation that subacute sclerosing panencephalitis (SSPE) was due to measles. However, even though there was an increase in antibodies to measles in MS populations, it was minor compared to the

---

*At the time of writing, 37 years after the introduction of measles vaccine, there is no evidence or suggestion that MS is decreasing, and there are suggestions it may be slightly increasing.

marked levels in SSPE, and not all patients had the increase. In the midst of all the discussion about measles as a causative factor, an exasperated Geoffrey Dean addressed the audience:

> *"Will anyone please tell me as a physician, why we have this contin-ued talk of measles, measles, measles? Is it that measles is simply a nice model to play with, or have we any other real reason for giving this tremendous emphasis on measles?"[104]*

Dean felt that MS was clearly a disease of the environment and point-ed out that not a single African in South Africa was found with the dis-ease, and measles was rampant there.

Walton summarized the discussion succinctly,[105] acknowledging that he was "outside the field" and said it would seem that measles as a possi-ble cause was related to the identification of SSPE as a measles disease of the nervous system, the developments in slow virus disease in kuru and Creutzfeldt-Jacob disease, and the identification of some increase in the measles antibodies in many MS patients. The ideas, exciting as they might be, continued to carry the Scottish verdict: "not proven."

Larner posited that there were epidemiologic clues suggesting a viral cause.[106] Epidemiology can only point toward possible causes, and although evidence does point toward an environmental factor in MS, it does not show that the factor is viral. The search for a viral cause gained some support from migration studies and family studies that suggested as cause an environmental agent in early adolescence. It seemed a logical explanation for the appearance of 24 cases of MS in the Faeroe Islands between 1943 and 1960; this had the appearance of a "point source epi-demic."[107–111] It appeared that some factor or agent initiated the disease before 1943, when MS appeared—by 1960 it had disappeared. The only major event on the islands during that time was the arrival of British troops (1940–1945). A possible lead came from the work of Cook and Dowling,[112] who noted that exposure to small house pets was more com-mon in patients with MS. Canine distemper was unknown on the Faeroes before 1939; after that date, military officers brought dogs to the island. Could canine distemper be the cause of MS on the Faeroes, and perhaps be responsible for the high rates of MS on the Shetland and Orkney

Islands of Scotland, where canine distemper was endemic? Kurtzke also reported a wartime "epidemic" of MS in Iceland that occurred just after an epidemic of canine distemper.[113] Tantalizing as this association was, MS also had a high prevalence in regions of Iceland where no distemper had occurred for 70 years,[114] and the elimination of dogs from Reykjavik failed to prevent a high prevalence there. Further questionnaire studies could not confirm the association of MS with small pets.*[115]

In the 1960s, great anticipation surrounded the new concept of a slow virus infection, first demonstrated by the Icelandic veterinarian Sigurdsson in sheep with visna and scrapie. Gajdusek[116] and others formulated the concept of a slow virus in neurological disease, one that could infect cells and, after a very long incubation period, cause disease. Following the dramatic demonstration of transmission experiments in kuru and Creutzfeldt-Jacob disease, Gajdusek listed in *Nature* (Oct. 17, 1964) the diseases he felt were prime candidates for the inoculation protocols; first on the list was MS. Sibley and others attempted to transmit MS to monkeys and other animals over the next decade, but were unsuccessful. Sibley injected 50 animals and after six years of work, concluded that MS was not a transmissible disease.[117–121] All other transmission experiments failed as well. Currently, many believe, as did Gowers a century earlier, that the virus, if present, is probably a triggering agent rather than the cause.

In 1963, Poskanzer, Shapiro, and Miller advanced the concept that the virus that causes MS was likely more common where the disease was rare, figuring that exposure early in life was protective, as was true with polio. Only if exposed to the virus after puberty would one likely develop the disease at a later time. Moving from a low- to a high-incidence area would not increase the likelihood of the disease as the person was already immune. Presumably moving from a high-incidence area to a low-incidence area would increase the risk.

Poskanzer et al. noted the similarity between MS and polio and suggested this supported the possibility of infection as a cause of MS.[122] In a

---

*During the much-publicized discussions of a possible risk of MS from small lap dogs, many pets were given away or met an early end.

study of a cluster of 11 cases in a population of 150 in a rural Nova Scotia community, Murray[123] found that all cases were living in the community during only one year, 1951, and the last major polio epidemic in Nova Scotia occurred in this region in that year. The average age of measles onset (12–14) was unusually late in this group. Murray concluded, however that a genetic link between the cases, with all fitting into two family lines, was more likely. Compston and colleagues showed that age of viral infection in children was an independent risk factor for MS.[124]

There were a few unconfirmed reports of the identification of a viral cause for MS in the 1940s, but the possibility of an underlying viral infection or viral trigger gained momentum during the late 1960s and early 1970s and in 1972, the National Institutes of Health (NIH) and the National Multiple Sclerosis Society jointly funded a $10 million program aimed at elucidating the cause of MS at the University of Pennsylvania School of Medicine under Donald Silberberg and at the Wistar Institute under Hiliary Koprowski, who would direct the virology studies. Gilden et al. relate the three-decade search for a viral cause for MS and the system organized to acquire fresh autopsy material when word arrived of the death of a person with MS.[125] Researchers were not able to grow virus from MS brain tissue and had negative results from transmission experiments to chimpanzees, various rodents, and chicken embryos.

In 1976, Richard Carp reported that tissue culture cells were inhibited in growth when exposed to brain and spleen tissues from MS patients.[126] The experiments were hailed by *The Lancet* as a milestone in MS research. The study was first on 10 patients, then expanded to 71 MS patients and 45 non-MS patients. The "Carp agent" was said to be small and similar to the scrapie agent in size, and both could cause similar cell inhibition. There was a difference, however, as the "Carp agent" could be neutralized by sera from MS patients, while the scrapie agent effect could not. The Carp agent eventually disappeared from the scene when the observations could not be confirmed.

Lumsden said that eliminating infection from the possible causes of MS was a heavy responsibility, but after over a century of unsuccessfully searching for a specific bacteria, spirochete, or virus as the cause of MS, most scientists no longer believed that such a specific infective agent

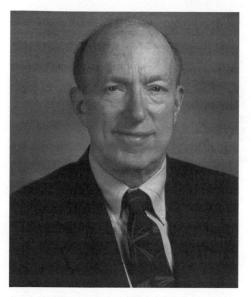

Figure 11.10   Dr. Donald Silberberg led a major project assessing the role of viruses in MS. (Courtesy of Dr. Silberberg.)

would be found in MS tissue. Viruses that have been suspected of causing or triggering MS include measles, Epstein-Barr virus (EBV), rubella, mumps, HSV, HZV, HHV-6, canine distemper virus, Marek's virus SV5, JC, animal retroviruses, human retroviruses, HTLV-1, and new retroviruses. But because the idea of an infectious trigger fits the scenario so well, the theory of some involvement of infection continues to be popular. Recently, interest in a number of organisms such as EBV, Clostridium pneumonia, human herpes virus type 6 (HHV-6), and Chlamydia pneumoniae[127] was sparked by new experiments.[128] It is known that HHV-6 can cause a latent CNS infection, and protein and DNA from HHV-6 have been identified in inactive MS plaques. The finding of increased HHV-6 IgM titers and HHV-6 DNA in the serum of MS patients suggests a recent active viral infection with this agent.[129,130] Although suspicious, this is not proof of cause, but it is just as possible that the HHV-6 products are unrelated, as they can be found in many cells. However, another recent study by Ross in Winnipeg found 17 percent of MS patients had a history suggestive of herpes zoster compared to 5.4 percent in a general group and 6.8 percent in a group of patients with other neurological diseases.[131] Again, this is suggestive but still circumstantial evidence. Studies of HTLV-1 were pursued as a possible link as the myelitis form of that disease can look similar to MS.

A recent study of antecedent infections in patients enrolled in the General Practice Research Database (225 patients who developed probable or definite MS and 900 controls) showed an increase in respiratory infections prior to the development of MS and a five-fold increase over controls in the occurrence of infectious mononucleosis, suggesting respiratory disease can trigger the onset of the disease.[132] EB virus has been suspected as a causative agent since the report of Bray et al. in 1983 and supported by the later observations.[133–136] Whether the role is causative or indirect is uncertain, and EB virus could be just one of the many agents that can trigger the disease.*

Recent studies by Kurtzke et al. of 7,500 French responders to a nationwide survey of MS revealed 260 born in North Africa, most of whom were from Algeria and emigrated to France at the end of the Algerian war of independence in 1962. The researchers presumed that those who developed MS after one year of immigration "acquired" the MS in France. This group had a prevalence rate 1.54 times that of France, and a mean interval of 13 years after immigration. The researchers felt that analysis of this population suggested MS was primarily an environmental disease acquired after childhood, requiring a prolonged exposure, then followed by a long incubation period, probably due to a widespread but as-yet-unknown persistent infection, which caused MS in only a small number of those infected.[137]

Another theory of a viral relationship is the idea of molecular mimicry, in which the viral antigens resemble antigens in normal tissues (in this case myelin). If immunologically active T cells are exposed to the viral antigen, they might cross the blood–brain barrier of someone who is genetically predisposed, and the T cells would misidentify the myelin antigen for the viral antigen and cause the inflammatory response, damaging the myelin.[138]

---

*EBV, a member of the herpes virus family, was first noted in the electron microscopy of cells from Burkitt's lymphoma (1964) by Epstein, Achong, and Barr, and four years later was noted to be the cause of infectious mononucleosis. It is one of the most successful viruses, infecting 90 percent of humans and persisting for the lifetime of the person; it probably evolved from a nonhuman primate virus.

New variations in the approach to infectious diseases continue to appear; the most recent is the advent of prion diseases. A prion is a *pro*teinaceous *in*fectious particle that lacks nucleic acid, which distinguishes it from viroids and viruses. Nobel Prize winner Stanley Prusiner put forward the idea of a new category of disease that could be inherited, infectious, or sporadic, and due to a proteinaceous infectious particle called a prion. Prions may be involved in various dementias, Creutzfeldt-Jacob disease, fatal familial insomnia, Gerstmann-Sträussler disease, and kuru, as well as a number of animal diseases, including scrapie and bovine spongiform encephalopathy. As in the earlier concept of slow viruses, the possibility of MS as a model for such a prion disease seems logical, but remains to be demonstrated. Although there has not been a demonstration of the actual existence of prions, the data accumulating show what Prusiner called a "convincing edifice" for their existence and role in neurological disease, and he postulates there could be effective therapies developed for prion disease. But Prusiner does not yet list MS in his personal list of possible disorders as prion disease.

> *"Some of the postulated links between infection and chronic illness may quickly be proved wrong and rapidly fade from consideration, but others may reveal new worlds for disease treatment and prevention."*
> Bennett Lorber, 1999[140]

There have been two parallel hypotheses for the cause of MS—an infection initiating the onset and the relapses, or an immune injury, probably autoimmune, that causes onset and relapses. A third hypothesis, now more prominent, is that an infection precipitates an immune response, which then results in the relapsing and progressive course of the disease.

EPIDEMIOLOGY: RACE OR PLACE?[141]

In 1886, Hirsh described the new epidemiology, which he first called "geographic pathology," as the medical history of mankind. Since the premise of epidemiology is that disease does not occur randomly, but in patterns that reflect the operation of the underlying cause,[142] the remarkable patterns of

MS distribution in the world lead one to believe that an understanding of these observations could tell us about the nature of the cause. Similarly, understanding the cause should explain the geographical patterns.

Although the concept of a definite geography for MS was slow to develop, there were early indications that there were differences in the distribution of the disease in different regions and different groups. The concept of a medical geography of a disease was common in the late 18th and early 19th centuries.[143] That disease could be distributed differently in different regions, and in different countries, in rural versus urban areas, near the seaside or in the mountains, in different ethnic groups and social levels was a common way to understand disease. The early suggestions that MS was different in certain social groups, in different workers, in Scotland versus America, and in rural versus urban areas, was a common comment in the writings about MS at the end of the 19th century. We have since become familiar with the world map of MS, but similar maps of disease were commonly drawn for malaria, dysentery, hepatitis, tuberculosis, yellow fever, and cholera, especially by the French, who used the maps for strategic purposes in military campaigns. Even the general public accepted the idea that the local environment could be related to the cause or improvement in a disease. This had therapeutic implications because it was healthier to move yourself to another climate for certain conditions.

Charcot himself thought that MS was prevalent in France, not well-recognized in Germany, and uncommon in England. Bramwell later noted that it was more common in neurological practice in Scotland than in America. It may have been thought an unusual neurological disease initially, but by the end of the 19th century, it was recognized as one of the more common neurologic diseases in the hospitals and clinics of Germany, France, Austria, and the United States. For instance, over seven years, Uhthoff collected about 100 cases of MS in the hospitals and clinics of Berlin.[144] Because the frequency of multiple sclerosis was often debated, there were attempts to better measure how common the disease was, in comparison to other well-known neurological diseases, and also, how frequent the disease was in the population (prevalence) and how many new cases appeared each year (incidence). Although Charcot and others felt MS to be a rare neurological curiosity, others found many cases in their clinics and wards, and Charcot recognized that MS would be recognized more often when the features of milder cases and the *forme frustes* of the condition were better known.

Early in the 20th century, there were reports of a low rate of MS in Boston with one case per thousand "nervous cases." It was more common in New York City with a rate of two to seven per thousand "nervous cases," but there was a higher rate of 18 per thousand among the Jewish patients at Montefiore Home.[145] In 1905, Van Wart had found a rate of 44 per thousand among 500 cases of neurological disease and concluded that in Louisiana and surrounding states the disease was frequent. Bramwell found a rate of 20 and later 32 per thousand neurological cases in Scotland.[146,147] Rates varied from 27 per thousand patients in Manchester to 60 per thousand in a more rigidly selected group of neurological patients at the National Hospital for Paralyzed and Epileptics in London.[148] Many scientists observed that MS was much less frequent in the United States than in Europe, and in 1892, Charles Dana said that in his experience, it was rare in America.[149]

In 1922, Charles B. Davenport systematically studied the frequency of MS among army draftees in World War I.[150] He showed higher MS rates in the urban areas, and the highest rates among people living near the Great Lakes and in Washington, Maine, Pennsylvania, Kansas, and Mississippi. He wondered if increased incidence could be related to other diseases that had a similar distribution such as goiter, or to a particular group of people, such as Swedes and Finns, many of whom live in that part of the country. He found higher MS rates in urban communities, in those with higher white-to-black population ratios, and in people who lived near the sea.

In 1926, postal surveys of physicians in Switzerland by Bing and Reese[151] and a subsequent survey by Ackermann suggested that MS was more common in the predominantly Germanic, northern Swiss cantons than in the French and Italian cantons.

Allison did the first systematic study of MS morbidity in a population in northern Wales in 1928, using a defined population, diagnostic criteria, and examination of all cases.[152] By 1930, in his review of MS, Russell Brain said that there was an incidence of 20 per million, with more in urban areas and more in men (3 to 2).[153] In 1938, Steiner noted that MS was common in New York, but in six months, he had not seen a single case in New Orleans.[154] After 1950, major systematic studies were done to map the geographic frequency of MS.

There has been confusing information about gender distribution of MS. Some researchers reported many more men, other equal numbers in the sexes, and others more women. It is puzzling that a 1922 review of 26 studies of MS showed a consistent predominance of 58 percent male to 42 percent female.[155] Only six of the studies showed a slight female predominance. Although there had been suggestions that MS occurred more in certain occupations, Morawitz disagreed, indicating that every occupation and social class was involved.[156]

Putnam noted that at the Boston City Hospital in 1931–1935, there were 50 cases of subacute bacterial endocarditis, 101 new cases of polio but 203 cases of MS.[157] Despite this, he said that polio was much better known to the laity, who donated large amounts of money to this cause, while the more common MS received little attention and was regarded as a rare disease.

Kinnier Wilson summarized the epidemiological data in his posthumously published 1940 text.[158] The disease was a common neurological disorder close to syphilis or brain tumor, he said, with 1,398 cases seen at The National Hospital, Queen Square out of 15,923 admissions (8.7 percent of admissions) between 1908 and 1925. Russell Brain found 8.1 percent of admissions for MS, but a slightly higher rate for neurosyphilis (10.1 percent). Bailey reported MS was 7.4 percent of the nervous and mental defects found in World War I recruits. MS was said to be "widespread" on the Continent, especially in Switzerland from the studies by Bing. It was less common in Italy, Japan, and the United States. It was more common in those of Finnish and Scandinavian extraction, and less so in the French, Slavs, Germans, Scots, English, Irish, Italians, and blacks in diminishing order. MS seemed to be more common further away from the equator. The north-south pattern was also found in the British Isles. Dean found low prevalence in South Africa. MS incidence is absent in the native Bantu, and low in Hungarian Gypsies, the Inuit, North American Indians, and Japanese.[159]

Objecting to the conclusions of previous writers, Putnam declared in 1943 that MS was certainly not a rare disease in the United States,[160] by

TABLE 1

Crude death rates for multiple sclerosis for selected countries and specified years

Country or city	Approximate annual mean temperature		Year	Multiple sclerosis deaths per 100,000 population
Canada......................	Montreal................	42	1944	2.3
Scotland......................	Glasgow.................	47	1945	3.7
England and Wales............	London.................	50	1945	2.3
Holland.......................	Amsterdam.............	50	1940	2.0
United States.................	New York City.........	52	1945	1.1
New Zealand..................	Christ Church..........	53	1942	1.5
Australia.....................	Melbourne.............	58	1945	1.2
Italy.........................	Rome..................	60	1942	0.5
Venezuela.....................	Caracas................	67	1945	0.1
Egypt........................	Alexandria.............	70	1940	0.1
Hong Kong...................	Hong Kong.............	72	1936	0.0
Tanganyika	Dar-Es-Salaam..........	79	1936	0.0
Nigeria.......................	Lagas..................	80	1938	0.0
Straits Settlements............	Singapore..............	81	1935	0.2

Figure 11.11 Crude death rates for MS from selected countries presented by Charles Limberg at the ARNMD meeting in New York, 1948. His work on epidemiology convinced the neurological community that the reports of geographical variations in MS were genuine. (Limberg, 1948.)

1950 it was evident that MS was among the most common neurological diseases and the most common serious neurological disease in young adults. Merritt, who was then an advisor to the new National Multiple Sclerosis Society, estimated in 1948 that there were 50, 000 to 90,000 cases of MS in the United States, but that same year, Limberg gave his estimate as 150,000[161] and a decade later Schumacher increased the estimate to 250,000.[162] (The NMSS now gives that estimate as 500,000.)

Part of the changing picture of MS incidence related to the decrease in the diagnosis of neurosyphilis and hysteria, while neurologists were increasingly able to make a confident diagnosis of MS. Clinicians had often been reluctant to make the diagnosis of multiple sclerosis, for there were no reliable tests. Such a diagnosis meant labeling the person as having a serious progressive disease believed to have a grave prognosis, which could not be altered by any treatment. Physicians who did not have available consultation with a neurologist

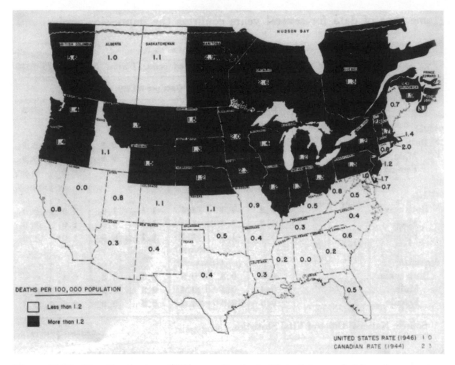

Figure 11.12 The distribution of MS mortality in the United States, dividing the states into those with rates above (black) and below (white) 1.2 per 100,000 per year. The north–south gradient was clear. (Limberg, 1950.)

were also reluctant to make the MS diagnosis. Even in large cities, consultation was available only to those who could afford the fees. Talley documented the paucity of neurological consultations available for people with MS in most areas of the United States, as well as in urban areas where the mobile and immigrant populations could not afford the fees.[163]

By 1948, Charles Limberg provided data at the ARNMD meeting that deaths per 100,000 population were certainly lower in New York (1.1) compared to Glasgow (3.7), London (2.3), and Montreal (2.3), similar to reports from Australia (1.2), and higher than in Rome (0.5) or Hong Kong (0.0).[163] Limberg demonstrated the picture of the north–south gradient in death rates from MS in the United States and Italy. He paid particular attention to the unusually high and rising death rates from British Columbia: 1940 (0.9); 1941 (4.0); 1942 (4.8); 1943 (5.9); 1944 (5.6). Kurland would later show

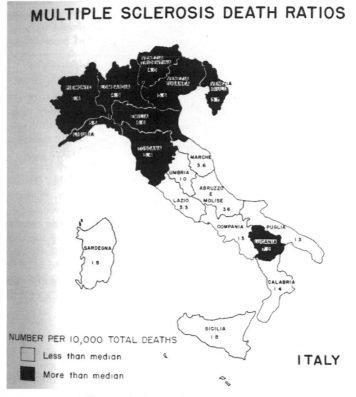

MULTIPLE SCLEROSIS DEATH RATIOS

NUMBER PER 10,000 TOTAL DEATHS

☐ Less than median

■ More than median

ITALY

Figure 11.13 Using a different calculation, showing those areas above (black) and below (white) the median death rate for MS in Italy, Charles Limberg again showed the north–south pattern of MS. (Limberg, 1950.)

that such figures were due to other neurological conditions, such as cerebral atherosclerosis, being added to the totals.[164] Other figures given by Limberg suggested different criteria and collection of data: the duration of the disease was 20 years in Holland and 40 years in Canada.

Limberg calculated a prevalence rate of 35 per 100,000 population in the United States and estimated there were 50,000 American cases. At the same meeting, Alexander MacLean and his colleagues presented the estimate of 64 per 100,000 population in Olmstead County served by the Mayo Clinic.[165] They noted that their figure was higher than that of Kolb in Baltimore (17.8), which demonstrated the north–south gradient, and their figures were also higher than those of Bing and Reese in Switzerland (36.4).

Leonard Kurland, just beginning his postgraduate training in neurology and epidemiology, was impressed by the papers presented by Limberg and MacLean at the 1948 meeting and made a decision to direct his work toward MS. He was recommended for further training at Columbia by Pearce Bailey, but wanted an opportunity to work with the plethora of data available at the Mayo Clinic. He went there instead and remained there through his long career, making important contributions to the epidemiology of MS as well as amyotrophic lateral sclerosis, Parkinson's disease, and many other conditions.

"I did a study comparing Winnipeg and New Orleans, working closely with the neurologists and others at those sites. The neurologist in Winnipeg was the Dean at the time and made it easy to get medical students to go over the charts one by one. But when we had the cases, I asked each to assess them, the New Orleans people looking at the

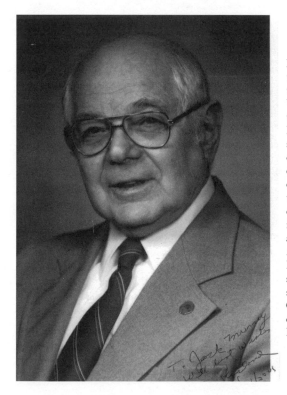

Figure 11.14 Leonard Kurland was a public health physician in the 1940s as a TB control officer. When it was suggested he get further training, he decided he had little interest in pursuing TB, as streptomycin had just been introduced, and he was interested in epidemiology. He decided to work on MS, as he was impressed by the work of Charles Limberg on epidemiology of the disease and was influenced by the paper presented at the 1948 ARNMD meeting by Alexander MacLean from the Mayo Clinic. When Pearce Bailey suggested he go to Columbia, he said he wanted to go to the Mayo Clinic where they had an extensive database. (Courtesy of Dr. Leonard Kurland.)

Winnipeg cases and vice versa. They disagreed on a quarter of the cases. I realized then that I needed training in neurology so that I could evaluate the cases myself.

When I saw the work of Limberg on MS in the United States and the great study of a rural community by MacLean and Berkson and others, I determined that this is what I wanted to study. Pearce Bailey was the new head at NINDB, and he wanted me to go and train with his close friend Houston Merritt at Columbia. But I wanted to be able to work with the data at the Mayo Clinic demonstrated by MacLean in his paper on MS in a rural community, and so I did. I was a physician in the Public Health Service then and all the years at the Mayo, and I couldn't have been able to do the studies I did without that support for my salary, some for assistants and for travel. Over the years we published over 1,200 papers using the Mayo data, not all of them neurological."

Leonard Kurland, 2001
(Personal Communication)

In looking for an etiological factor or factors, Kurland warned that diagnosis could be uncertain, and the disorder might be a syndrome rather than a disease. The difficulty was illustrated by a study in 15 New York and New Jersey hospitals in 1930–1939, which found 33 cases of MS in 25,000 deaths, but at autopsy, one-third were found to have other conditions. There were 11 other hospital cases of MS found at autopsy that were not diagnosed clinically before death. Surveying the data to 1950, Kurland found no convincing evidence that the disease was increasing.[166–168] Early reports of many cases in children, some as young as 18 months, undoubtedly were other neurological diseases that shared some of the clinical and perhaps pathological features of adult multiple sclerosis. Kurland noted the confusion of the 19th century over epidemiology of MS, but acknowledged that the important recent work of Allison in Belfast, Bing and Reese in Switzerland, Müller in Sweden, Schaltenbrand in Germany, and the "remarkable report" of MacLean to the ARNMD in 1947 giving the Rochester incidence, prevalence, and survival rates established important information on the disease.

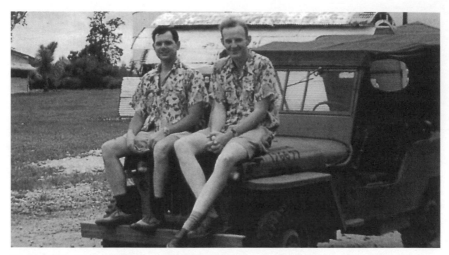

Figure 11.15 Leonard Kurland and Donald Mulder on a neurological epidemiological study in Guam, 1955. In their studies there, they found only one case of MS and it was in a man who had spent six years in the northern United States. (Courtesy of Dr. Leonard Kurland.)

Prevalence was double that reported elsewhere, and median survival was 35 years, compared to earlier reports of eight, 10, and 12 years in studies in hospitals. Limberg in 1950, and Goldberg and Kurland in 1962, reviewing the prevalence of MS in 33 countries around the world, confirmed a striking geographical pattern for MS.

Kurland believed that up to 1948 there had not yet been valid evidence of a variation in the geographic distribution of the disease. In that year, Limberg found that deaths from MS were more common farther away from the equator. The growing evidence from North America was particularly convincing; it covered such a huge geographical area, and the language, medical practice, medical certification at the time of death, and the coding of death were similar throughout. Death rates from MS were higher in Canada and in the northern United States than in the southern United States in the initial studies by Kurland, who looked at New Orleans, Boston, and Winnipeg.

Registries began to be developed in the 1950s because of the growing interest in determining the prevalence and distribution of MS. Most floundered because of inadequate methodology, but for the next few decades, and even now, areas studied will claim they have more MS than other areas because their study shows more than the outdated and incom-

plete figures from other areas. It is particularly common for cluster observations to be generalized to the community at large by the public and
even the medical community. Some clarity was brought to the field by the
review by Donald Acheson, later the Chief Medical Officer of Great
Britain, writing in McAlpine's textbook of MS.[169]

Clear data are often difficult and the confusion may be fostered by
selecting data by diagnostic terms. In an era when the disease was called
by so many names, by different physicians, other conditions were often
included in the survey sweep. Kurland noted that the apparent increase
in incidence in British Columbia was due to the inclusion of cerebral atherosclerosis in the figures for multiple sclerosis. The public continues to
confuse amyotrophic lateral sclerosis with multiple sclerosis, and the conditions are often thought to be similar processes by many physicians inex-
perienced with neurology since both conditions are neurological,
progressive, and called sclerosis.

The most extensive study on MS incidence was done with the
remarkable data at the Mayo Clinic for Olmstead County, covering the 80
years from January 1, 1905 to January 1, 1985, identifying 208 incident
cases (57 males and 151 females), fulfilling modern criteria for MS. The
data suggested a trend toward an increasing risk for development of MS,
but improved case ascertainment, diagnostic techniques, and increasing
knowledge of MS still leave this an open question.

Much of the published information is problematic. As Kurland
pointed out, case or anecdotal reports and case series have no denomina-
tors and thus no rates. If they note some tantalizing association, there is
nothing to use for comparison.[170] Retrospective case control studies suffer from selection bias and also recall bias by the patients. Cohort studies
are difficult and expensive, and we are fortunate to have the resource of
the Mayo Clinic data on Rochester, Minnesota, and Olmstead County.

Migration studies are more interesting, but more problematic. Even
patients will immediately ask when they hear there are high and low risk
areas, "what happens if people move?" The question is difficult to answer
with confidence because the numbers are so small, and the confounding
factors in population studies make them difficult to interpret and tempting to overinterpret.

Nothing changes if the person who has MS migrates elsewhere, of course, but what of the risk to those who do not yet have MS? Moving from an area of high risk to an area of low risk, such as moving from northern Europe to South Africa[171,172] or from the northern to southern United States[173] is associated with a reduction in risk if the move occurs in childhood. This has given rise to the concept of a risk age earlier than 15 for an environmental factor.

Acheson et al. commented on the difficulty of accumulating meaningful data on the influence of environment on MS. Data often relate to where the patient currently lives, or died, but the important time might be where the patient was born, or where he or she was at age 12.[174] Some studies are hard to interpret because they have been attempted in communities with populations that are very mobile, such as Denver and San Francisco. Acheson's studies recorded birthplace because it was accurate information that was easy to retrieve. He found a correlation with the total hours of sunshine and with the average December solar radiation. This does not indicate cause, but these results might be expected from the north–south distribution.

Poser said that the earliest reports of epidemiology of MS commented on the increased prevalence in persons of Scandinavian decent.[175] Percival Bailey noted this in his survey of U.S. troops after World War I.[176] Davenport, Brain, and McAlpine also commented on the higher incidence in northern European countries.[177–179] This was also noted in northern U.S. studies by Steiner, Ulett, Limburg, and Bulman and Ebers.[180–183]

Since the 1950s it had been accepted that MS had an unusual distribution in the world.[184] MS increased in frequency with geographical latitude both in the northern[185] and southern hemispheres.[186] Alter noted that the geographic distribution above and below the equator had a parabolic gradient that increased sharply with latitude, and although the curve dramatically increased at increasing latitudes, it appeared to be lower or absent in very far north and south latitudes.[187] In Europe, MS incidence was highest in central Europe and less north and south of that area. In the United Kingdom, the prevalence varied from 309/100,000 in the Orkney and Shetland Islands, to 178/100,000 in northern Scotland, and 100/100,000 in the south of England.[188] A survey in 2000 of 100,230 patients registered in 13 general practices in England and Wales gave a lifetime prevalence rate of 1 in 500 for MS.[189]

Groups that seem to be relatively resistant, even when living within high-incidence areas, include the Hutterites in western Canada, blacks, Hispanics, and Asians in the United States, and the Maoris in New Zealand. Kurland and Kwang-Ming Chen studied MS in a population of 100,000–140,000 on Guam and found only one definite case. That young man had spent six years in Detroit before the onset of MS. There had been two probable cases and some cases of retrobulbar neuritis.[190]

Milton Alter's career in studying the epidemiology of MS began as a senior medical student in 1955. The Dean of the University of Buffalo required a doctoral thesis before graduation, and Alter selected the relationship of dietary fat and MS. Adler was drafted into the military while a resident with A.B. Baker in Minnesota, and Baker steered him toward Len Kurland at the NIH where military service could be fulfilled. Kurland was studying the epidemiology of MS so it was a happy fit. Kurland had done a comparative study of Winnipeg and New Orleans, and Alter was to continue this work by studying Halifax, Nova Scotia, and Charleston, South Carolina, supervised by Dr. Sydney Allison of Belfast who had the experience of a study of Northern Ireland. The results showed that Halifax had three times the rate of MS of Charleston.

Kurland next selected Israel as a place where a consistent evaluation by the same physician could assess people who came from very different areas. After further training with H. Houston Merritt, Alter began the study in Israel in the neurology department headed by Professor Lippman Halpern. It was an excellent experiment, for the patients with MS or suspected MS who could be assessed came from many different regions and countries. Alter and Uri Leibowitz examined each case, making over 1,000 assessments by standardized criteria. They found that Jewish immigrants from Europe had higher MS rates than those from African-Asian countries, and Jewish immigrants from the United States and Canada had high rates similar to those of northern European Jewish immigrants. Native-born Israelis had rates similar to those of European immigrants. These initial studies were followed by two decades of further work, which included migration studies. They showed that migration to Israel from a low-risk area (e.g., North Africa) was associated with a higher risk of MS if migration occurred before adolescence. Further, the offspring of low-risk area immigrants had a higher risk, similar to that of European and American immigrants, strongly implicating an environmental factor. Alter and his colleagues are now studying the MS risks in Israeli Jews and Israeli-born Jews.[191]

Bulman and Ebers[192] felt that the higher MS prevalence rate in the northern United States and in Canada was related to individuals of Scandinavian descent, and that might also explain the high incidence in Olmsted County, Minnesota, where 25.7 percent of the population are of Scandinavian descent, in contrast to 4.7 percent for the United States in general.[193,194] Poser speculated that the distribution of MS incidence might be traced back to the Vikings over 1,000 years ago.[195] They invaded most European countries, settled in Normandy and Sicily, and engaged in trade with widespread lands. They migrated to the east and established the Russian state, and under the name Varangians, became part of the Byzantine army that saw action over the whole Byzantine Empire. They participated in the Crusades. The habit of capturing, keeping, or selling women and children was widespread in the Middle Ages and, along with the slave trade in men, could be important factors in genetic dissemination. It is an appealing theory that would fit with the geographical distribution of MS and suggest that geographical-environmental distribution may represent instead where people of Viking ancestry migrated.

Sutherland[196] in Scotland confirmed Davenport's observation[197] that there was a higher risk of MS in those of Nordic descendants than in Celts. Skegg in New Zealand used the novel technique of assessing the number of Mc/Macs in the telephone book to show that MS risk was higher in communities that had a higher number of residents with Scottish ancestry.[198] Compston pointed out, however, that Mc and Mac do not differentiate between those of Nordic and Celtic ancestry, as one could see if the phone directories of Glasgow and Belfast were consulted.[199] Ebers confirmed the Scandinavian influence in Canada and the importance of a genetic factor by powerful data from concordant twin studies.[200] Studies in the United Kingdom showed a correlation between

HLA-DR2 and other markers of genetic susceptibility in northern Europeans and regional variations in MS.[201]

Dean found 10 cases of MS in South Africa in 1958, but 42 cases over the period 1959–1968 and posited an increase in frequency.[202] He felt that most factors stayed the same, and this suggested an infective agent introduced from high-risk European countries by immigrants and by South Africans who use air travel to go abroad. By 1985, Rosman and colleagues were suggesting there was an MS epidemic: they had found five new cases in Pretoria and Wonderboom (pop. 319,868), an eightfold increase since Dean did his study, but these numbers were small and might just represent better case finding.[203] Dean also looked at the risk of MS in nurses and physicians and found no increased risk when death rates were calculated from U.K. statistics and from information in the British Doctors' Smoking Study. Dean also found that the prevalence of MS in U.K.-born children of West Indian, African, and Asian immigrants was similar to that in indigenous people, a strong argument for the environmental influence.[204] This may be related in part to uncertainty about prevalence figures from the country of origin compared to the U.K. Compston recorded the various controversies these figures might precipitate.[205]

The north–south gradient in incidence and prevalence of MS is seen on a wide map, but some locations do not follow the expected rate of nearby areas. Sardinia has a much higher rate than Italy, and studies from 1955 to the present suggest Sardinia's incidence is high and increasing.[206]

The highest MS rates have been recorded in the Shetland and Orkney Islands off the coast of Scotland. In all the studies, there was surprising uniformity in the clinical features of MS, regardless of the geography or the incidence rate of the area. Some variations were noticed, with a higher incidence of Devic's disease in India and Japan and higher rates of transverse myelopathy and optic neuropathy in Asians. Factors to explain the geographic difference included factors later felt to be important: amounts of solar radiation, annual temperature, and the number of neurologists in these regions.[207] That the geographic distribution was not an artifact, however, was convincingly demonstrated by the Israeli study by Alter et al., which showed a difference in the prevalence depending on the region of origin of the immigrants to Israel.[208] Alter reviewed the possibilities that might explain the geographic and migration study differences, looking at solar radiation, temperature, toxins and deficiencies, sanitation, and diet. He noted that many factors did not seem to apply, but that it was interesting that the distribution of animal fat in the diet followed the same parabolic curve north and south of the equator that MS followed.[209]

Kuroiwa defined the study of MS in Japan in three periods: 1) the period of neglect (1910–1950), in which it was thought that MS was non-existent (the view of Professor Miura who was a pupil of Charcot); 2) the period of recognition (1950–1970) in which cases of MS were increasingly recognized; and 3) the period of development (1972–1975 and beyond), when the incidence, epidemiology, and characteristics of MS were better defined. The prevalence rate was initially calculated as two to four per 100,000 population, lower than in most Western countries, but there was no north–south gradient in Japan.[210]

Cluster studies are often reported to MS clinicians, but how to investigate such events—three students in the same class who later develop MS; four people living on the same street, etc.—is challenging. Presumably, if there were some external factor, it would have been many years before. A "fishing expedition" often leads to some potential and intriguing observation, some common factor in the cases, but often not translatable to other situations or MS in general, and therefore, likely to be coincidental.

Whenever there are groups or clusters of MS cases, it is tempting to look for an association that might explain the occurrence. In 1947, Campbell et al. reported that four people doing work on sheep swayback developed an MS-like disease, and this sparked great interest, as swayback is an animal demyelinating disease related to copper deficiency.[211] It was soon recognized that swayback did not occur in some areas with high incidence of MS, and copper studies in MS patients were negative. Lead was suspected in the six cases living close together in Berkshire County, England in 1950, but again there was no evidence of increased MS in lead workers or in high-lead areas.[212] Other heavy metals were suspected, including mercury, zinc, and magnesium, but these were all found not to be causative factors. Such ideas recur, however, and in recent years, concerns about mercury from dental fillings led to many patients having costly and painful dental work based on no evidence of cause or benefit. Seven out of 307 nurses working in Key

West, Florida were found to have MS, but Dean could not show an increased incidence in medical personnel in the U.K., suggesting there was no increased risk from contact with patients.[213]

Campbell studied lead in relation to MS in a number of English counties and found six cases within 500 yards of each other in a small village in Berkshire. There were three cases in another village and two in the county, and he attributed this unusual prevalence to high lead content in the soil and water. Sutherland mentioned the occurrence of three girlfriends, three neighbors in the same street, and two gamekeepers who lived in succession in the same house.[214] Every MS neurologist can cite similar reports from their patients. Coincidence? Probably.

In the eight cases in Duxbury, Massachusetts, there were intriguing possibilities, but it transpired that seven of the eight had their onset elsewhere, and moved to Duxbury, a nice place to retire.[215,216]

Eastman et al. reported a cluster of 14 cases in the community of Mansfield, Massachusetts (population 10,000), and noted that between 1932 and 1936, all lived in Mansfield and most within the same block, during a period when there was water contamination.[217] Koch et al. reported six cases in the 450 people in Mossyrock, Washington, but all the cases were related in two families.[218]

Murray examined a rural Nova Scotia community of 150 people where there were said to be 14 cases of MS.[219] Examination of the cases demonstrated a problem seen in many suggested clusters—two of the patients were brothers with muscular dystrophy, and one patient had ALS. Another, related to the MS cases, had untreated myasthenia gravis for 20 years with marked atrophy, but as many of her family were thought to have MS, it was assumed that her episodic weakness was also MS. That left 10 cases of verified MS. A two-year study showed many potential relationships, such as a Scottish background, all were teetotalers, all drank unpasteurized milk in their childhood on farms, ate a high-animal fat diet, and were well-educated. These were not unusual features in the other members of the community. The MS cases had measles relatively late (average age 11.8). It was interesting that all lived in the same area in 1952 when the last large polio epidemic in Nova Scotia occurred in their community, a relationship that was commented on by

Poskanzer et al.[220] Murray also noted that six of the ten cases were related in two families, suggesting a possible genetic factor as well. The studies of Poskanzer in the United States, Murray in Nova Scotia, and Compston in Wales gave rise to another possible association noted in many individual reports—late onset of childhood infections.

The Faeroes are a small number of Danish islands between Iceland and Norway, settled by the Norse Vikings over a millennium ago. Intensive search for all MS cases on the Faeroe Islands in the 1970s revealed 25 cases among native-born residents up to 1977.[221–225] All had onset between 1943 and 1960 except for one case that had onset in 1970. Researchers excluded four cases in Faeroes who had prolonged residence in foreign countries and five among Danish-born Faeroes. The 24 cases met the criteria for a point-source epidemic. The median year of onset was 1949, and the cumulative risk of MS for Faeroes in 1940 was 87 per 100,000. Researchers noted that British troops occupied the Faeroe Islands in large numbers beginning in April 1940 and continuing throughout World War II. During the war, all but three patients resided in locations where troops were stationed, and those three were also in direct contact with the British. In 1979, Kurtzke suggested that this constituted an "epidemic" related to the introduction of British troops (or their baggage). He speculated that if this were so, MS was a transmissible disease, probably infectious, with only 1 in 500 of the exposed individuals being affected.[226] In 1980, Kurtzke described another "epidemic" of MS in Iceland in the postwar period without the rapid appearance and disappearance seen in the Faeroes.[227] Those studying infections in relation to MS discussed a "window of vulnerability" in adolescence, and in his studies of the "outbreak" in the Faeroe Islands, Kurtzke suggested there was a latency period of six years. Canine distemper was suspected as a potential factor in the Faeroes, an idea supported by the work of Cook that small animals might be linked to the disease.[228] In dogs, there is a canine encephalitis that resembles the pathologic appearance of multiple sclerosis that was called "akute multiple Sklerose des Hundes" by Scherer.

Shatin postulated that gluten intolerance might explain the world distribution of MS, since MS was more common in northern wheat-eating areas such as Winnipeg, but less common in the more southern corn-eating areas, such as New Orleans.[229] This idea was incorporated into some of the diets advocated for the treatment of MS, such as the MacDougall diet, which advocated among other things, gluten-free food choices. In 1997, Carlyle hypothesized on epidemiologic grounds that there was a "vitamin MS" deficiency in those who get MS and felt this as-yet-unknown "vitamin MS" was due to inadequate vegetables, fish, and game meats in the diet.[230] Others are interested in the possibility that there may be a vitamin D deficiency in areas with less solar radiation, which would fit with the general distribution of MS in the world. Because pretreatment with 1.25 dihydroxy vitamin D can prevent EAE, or reduce it if given later, this will be further studied in MS patients.

At the same time as epidemiologic studies from South Africa, Switzerland, England, Finland, the clusters in Iceland, the Faeroe Islands and Norway, the parallel growth in genetic information on MS gave rise to the obvious conclusion that this disease had a complex polygenic origin.

THE GENETICS OF MS

"Every man is endowed at birth by his parents and ancestors with a type of constitution built of anatomical, physiological, immunological and psychological material which will help determine his course through life and his reactions to environmental stress and injury."

J.A. Ryle, 1931[231]

"The plethora of studies and facts is not easy to synthesize and interpret."

N.C. Myrianthopoulos, 1970[232]

"The only feature within a given community that is known to be associated with an increased risk of the disease is the occurrence of the disease in a relative."

John Prineas, 1970[233]

Although the acceptance of a genetic factor in MS is relatively recent, the question of a genetic or familial relationship has long existed. Virtually all the early authors on MS, including Leyden, Charcot, Erb, Oppenheim, Duchenne, Marie, Gowers, and Russell noted familial cases in their series, but thought MS was rare, and each downplayed the importance of these occasional cases. Charcot himself wondered about the possibility when he was told of a familial case by Duchenne.[234] Gowers said MS was seen in some siblings, but its occurrence was "quite exceptional."[235] It was hard to ignore the nine cases in one generation reported by Hervouet in Toulouse in 1893[236] or the case of a mother and son with the disease reported by Eichhorst.[237]

Charles L. Dana felt heredity was a predisposing cause of MS in a small proportion of cases, but this was because of the inheritance of a "neuropathetic constitution." His belief was common in the late 19th century and persisted for the first half of the 20th century.[238] Some families were thought to have a "taint" that made them prone to many neurological disorders as well as behavioral and mental abnormalities; they were also thought to be susceptible to enviromental factors such as cold, habits, lifestyle influences, and unacceptable attitudes. Being of "neuropathic stock" meant they and their families were particularly susceptible to diseases of the nervous system, such as hysteria, epilepsy, neurosyphilis, dementias, and specific debilitating and chronic neurological diseases, such as multiple sclerosis. Some groups were singled out as being more likely to be neuropathic stock. If this were the basis of multiple sclerosis, then little could be done to alter the situation therapeutically, as the person was destined to succumb to illness due to a weakened constitution. This widespread belief was one of the reasons people often denied any evidence of neurological disease in the family.

Although early writers dismissed the idea of genetics to explain more than one case in a family, they acknowledged that such families often had members with many neuropathic disorders. James Jackson Putnam and Charles Dana were among the prominent neurologists who believed that many MS patients were from families with an inherited neuropathic constitution. After the turn of the 20th century, these ideas began to blend with the rhetoric of those with racial and eugenic agendas. Certain immigrant populations were felt to have a tendency toward neuropathic constitutions, but some of the prejudices were hard to maintain when the populations with the higher incidence of multiple sclerosis tended to be the white, blonde, blue-eyed Scandinavians, and the Scots, British, and Germans, rather than the Italians and other Mediterranean groups, the Jews, and the Afro-Americans.

If predisposing risk for MS was instead an external factor, such as stress, trauma, diet, infection, toxic elements in the environment, overexertion, or exposure, then potential prevention or therapy was a distinct possibility. Even if the agent were seen to be internally mediated, such as hormonal imbalance, menses, or pregnancy, or a disorder of the digestive system, therapy would then be a possibility.

There were five major theories about the cause of MS in the last decades of the 19th century: a derangement of glia, a vascular disease, an infection, an internal metabolic disorder, or a toxin. None was totally discredited, although each had its prominent supporters, and they continue in some form even today.[239] The 20th century would add the possibility of a genetic basis, an immunological mechanism, and the most widely discussed, a combination of many of these possibilities.

In the *Louisville Medical News* in 1882, J.W. Holland published the story of a family with three cases of MS.[240] Dr. E.S. Reynolds reported two families in *Brain* in 1904 and commented that although William Gowers and Risien Russell said such observations were "exceptional," it was likely that more would be found when more was known about the disease and its variant forms.[241] He also observed the association of mental illness and thyroid diseases with these cases.

Curshmann in Germany reported familial multiple sclerosis in 1920,[242] and Davenport in 1922[243] was convinced about the role of a familial factor and the link with Scandinavian ancestry in the United States. He emphasized heredity, internal factors, and constitution as predisposing conditions. Although most patients have no family history of MS, a significant number do have this history. After presenting accounts of hereditary MS, including MS in three siblings, Davenport made the following insightful comment:

"In conclusion, may I be permitted the suggestion that, whatever may be eventually proven to be the endogenous cause of multiple sclerosis,

the factor of heredity cannot be left out of account? Just as tumors inoculated into a mouse will, or will not, grow, according to the racial constitution of the mouse, and just as the bacillus tuberculosis that inhabits the body of all of us does or does not flourish there depending upon the constitution and condition of the individual, so there are probably internal conditions that inhibit, and others that facilitate the development of this disease or the endogenous factors upon which it depends."

Charles Davenport, 1922

Not all researchers were convinced. Even the clear-thinking Russell Brain would admit in 1930 only that familial cases were rare, and if not due to chance, were likely due to exposure to a common environment or to similar infections.[244] Convincing evidence of a genetic factor had been noted by Curtius in Germany in 1933, showing that 10 percent of MS cases had a positive family history, or 42 times the expected rate of the general population as calculated by various studies at the time.[245] He noted 84 other reports in the literature and did a systematic study of 3,129 relatives of 106 subjects living in Bonn and Heidelberg. Ten additional cases of MS turned up, giving a relative risk of 1 in 40. No cases occurred in a control population. The report was criticized because the diagnosis of MS was not always certain in the relatives. Curtius believed that any nervous disease in the family indicated a constitutional predisposition, and he noted greater numbers of people with neurologic, psychiatric disease, and developmental defects than in a comparison group with fractures, giving weight to the idea that MS patients come from "neuropathic" family stock predisposed to neurological disorders. His studies were downplayed. They came at a time when information about genetic impurity was a sensitive issue in Germany. The risk in relatives was confirmed again in 1938[246] when Curtius and Spur reported on 444 relatives of MS cases and found four cases of MS.

In his 1936 study of twins, Thums came to a conclusion completely opposed to that of Curtius, since none of his monozygotic twins was concordant at the time of study.[247] In contrast, McAlpine studied 142 cases and found eight examples of familial incidence in two parent-child groups and six sibling pairs.[248] McAlpine also saw four cases of conjugal MS and knew of four others.

Although there were occasional references to Curtius' work over the next decade, attention to a genetic factor did not occur until Russell Brain referred to Curtius in 1940 and Roland MacKay in Montreal reviewed the familial cases in all reports from 1896 to 1948, demonstrating that this was not an occasional or unimportant factor.[249] He documented all familial cases from Eichdorst's early report in 1896 to publications in 1948. He showed a concordance rate of 23 percent in monozygotic twins, clearly indicating a genetic factor, later confirmed by Canadian and British studies.[250] MacKay's study was a model for data collection, accepting only cases in the literature with good descriptions and diagnostic standards. He collected 79 cases of familial MS, in 188 individuals with 26 autopsies, including five instances from his own practice.*[251] MacKay noted various problems of clarity concerned with the issue of MS diagnosis and the role of heredity and said some of the reported cases were other familial neurological diseases—this is the error of the *inexpert*. However, many neurologists who believe there is no hereditary factor in MS excluded the diagnosis when there is more than one case in the family—this was the error of the *expert*!

Other familial cases were added by the survey of Pratt, Compston, and McAlpine,[252,253] who found a positive family history in 6.5 percent of 1,003 relatives of 310 cases, and by Moya (1962)[254] with a collection of 4,500 cases from the literature, which showed a familial rate of 1.8 percent. Myrianthopoulos reviewed the literature up to 1970 of the various twin studies, including a very large one of 60 twin pairs he had done with MacKay. Using rigid diagnostic standards, after a further five-year follow-up, these cases showed a concordance rate of 15.4 percent in monozygotic twins and 10.3 percent in dizygotic twins. With more liberal diagnostic standards, the rates were 23.1 percent and 20.7 percent, hard-

---

*Roland Parks MacKay (1900–1968) was described by Robert Aird as one of America's great neurologists. He graduated second in his class at the University of Toronto (Charles Best of insulin fame was first), and trained with Henry Woltman in neurology at the Mayo Clinic. He was professor of neurology in Chicago on various faculties and served as president of the National MS Society.

ly the difference to be expected if the disorder were primarily genetic.[255] Perhaps the most unexpected finding was the high rate in both groups.

The annual report of the British MS Society in 1966 declared confidently, "MS is not hereditary, it is not infectious or contagious, and it is not a mental disease." Perhaps this statement was based on the feeling that this would be reassuring to patients and their families, even though the evidence for a genetic factor was mounting.

Accepting that there is a genetic factor involved in MS and that it may have originated in the Nordic countries has given rise to the view that the distribution of MS in the world relates to where these people migrated rather than to any local environmental factor, but this remains speculation. Researchers have pointed to areas of local "epidemics" such as the Faeroe Islands and risk altered by immigration to suggest there is an environmental factor. The environmental risk is thought to be a viral infection, since the risk of certain infections may vary according to geography. During the last two decades, it has become clear that there is a genetic factor in MS, suggestive but not yet conclusive evidence of a viral "trigger," and the geographical explanation is still uncertain and much debated.

The human leucocyte antigen (HLA) system was described as a leucocyte blood group system by Dausset in 1958;[256] soon after, researchers recognized that this system determined the fate of the transplanted organs, as the major histocompatability complex (MHC). These systems controlled the individual response to foreign antigens. Following weak but tantalizing indications that MS might be associated with blood group O, in 1972 researchers found a relationship with HLA-A3.[257,258] Soon after, 2,500 patients were HLA typed, and an association was noted with the HLA class II antigen D/DR2, which suggested a genetic link for MS. There was an association with antigen Ld-7a (later called Dw2) in 70 percent of Danish patients. Reports over the next few years on families, populations, and different races became a confusing situation. By 1976, Compston showed a relationship of MS with HLA-DR2, which was a stronger link.*[259] Looking for a genetic factor, Compston found 19 per-

---

*A full review of the HLA system was provided by Jan Klein and Akie Sato.

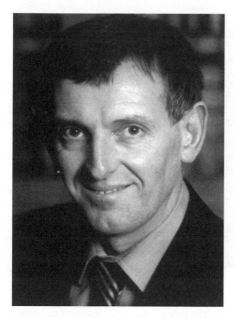

Figure 11.16 Professor Alistair Compston of Cambridge is the current editor and lead author of McAlpine's *Multiple Sclerosis*, a landmark publication in MS, which was initially drafted by his father (1955) Nigel Compston. Over the last 25 years, he has contributed to the epidemiology, genetics, immuno-pathology, treatment, and the history of MS. He was Chairman of the MRC Cambridge Centre for Brain Repair 1992-2000. (Courtesy of Dr. Alistair Compston.)

cent of the population was DR2 positive in assessment of HLA types, but in MS patients the percentage was 55. The complicated story was reviewed by McDonald in his Gowers lecture.[260]

Although MS appears to be a sporadic disease, another family member with the disease can be found in 10–20 percent of some series. More suggestive of a genetic disorder is the finding that MS occurs in 2–5 percent of siblings and nonidentical twins, but in 23–33 percent of identical twins.[261] This latter observation is of great importance, because although it shows that there is a genetic factor, the disease is not present all the time in the second identical twin, so some other factor(s) must operate to determine if the disease appears in the genetically predisposed person. Also, half-siblings have a reduced risk of MS, even if raised in the same environment as the MS patient. If a person with MS had been adopted in childhood or infancy, there was no increased incidence in the adopting family, suggesting that there is no environmental risk factor. Further, first cousins raised in different environments from the MS patient have the same lifetime risk of MS as those raised in the same environment, suggesting no risk factor in the environment. Perhaps the external triggering factor is not in the local environment, but in the individual. In

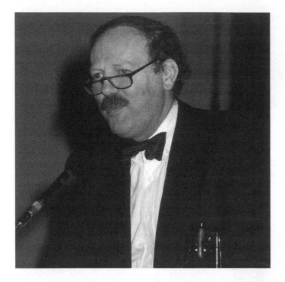

Figure 11.17 George Ebers carried out the largest genetic study to date, utilizing the Canadian Network of MS Centers. His studies also include monozygotic and dizygotic twin studies, studies of adopted MS patients and their families, and many epidemiological studies and clinical trials. Ebers also published on Sir William Osler's contributions to neurology, and like Osler, Ebers is a Canadian who was appointed a professor at Oxford University. (Courtesy of Dr. George Ebers.)

other words, it could be a common infection to which all are subject that acts as a trigger in the predisposed individual.

Since the observations by Jersid, Fog et al. in 1973, and Compston et al. in 1976,[262] it has been recognized that the presence of the HLA-DR2 allele substantially increases the risk of MS. The only population without this association is that of Sardinia. The Scots have the highest frequency of this allele in the general population. Although HLA-DR and D polymorphisms are associated with a risk for MS, they do not correlate with the type or rate of progression in the disease, although recent work suggests some other receptors and genes may be related to the course of the disease.[263]

Unsuccessful efforts to identify the specific genes that determine disease susceptibility have been made, and it would seem that genetic predisposition must be much more complex than a simple gene disorder. Major histocompatability complex (MHC) genes seem to be important, though less than in diseases such as narcolepsy, rheumatoid arthritis, and diabetes. There is evidence of gene coding for human leukocyte antigen (HLA) DR antigens in many, but not all, MS patients, so the HLA DR haplotypes are not sufficient, or perhaps even necessary, to produce the disease.[264] A systematic screen of the human genome was completed in

1996, which provided evidence for linkage of MS to HLA, and identified six new chromosomal regions, which may contain susceptibility genes for multiple sclerosis.

A major genetic study of MS patients has been undertaken in Canada by Dessa Sadovnick, George Ebers, and The Canadian Genetic Collaborative Group surveying 20,000 Canadians coast to coast, and now entering its fourth phase. This is the largest genetic study on MS and has already provided important information on the risk in relatives of MS cases, in identical and nonidentical twins, and in the families of MS patients who were adopted.[265]

THE VASCULAR THEORY

For a number of reasons, a vascular basis for MS has been considered from the earliest days, when the pathology was being examined under the microscope. In the early 19th century, lenses for microscopes were of poor quality, one of the reasons many French clinicians paid little attention to microscopy. But even with a crude microscope, Eduard Rindfleisch (1836–1908) noted in 1863 the consistent location of a blood vessel in the center of MS plaques.[266] He saw that there were changes in blood vessels and nerve elements secondary to inflammation combined with hyperemia in the plaque. In addition, he recognized perivascular cell infiltrations and fatty changes in the neuroglia. He suggested that the search for a primary cause of MS should address alteration of individual blood vessels and their ramifications.

> *"If one looks carefully at freshly altered parts of the white matter ... one perceives already with the naked eye a red point or line in the middle of each individual focus ... the lumen of a small vessel engorged with blood. ... All this leads us to search for the primary cause of the disease in an alteration of individual vessels and their ramifications; all vessels running inside the foci, but also those which transverse the immediately surrounding but still intact parenchyma are in a state characteristic of chronic inflammation."*
>
> Eduard Rindfleisch, 1863

In 1882, Ribbert suggested that the vascular lesion in the MS plaque was a thrombosis of the vessel secondary to infection of the bloodstream, and that was the cause of the disease.[267] This theory was pursued by Pierre Marie, who was convinced of the underlying role of infection, but he also agreed that infection might then produce a vascular change that produced the plaques of MS.[268] Others, like Dana, felt the pathology was primary in the vessel and related to local thrombotic or vasospastic change.[269] The vascular theory was favored by many and persisted even when other theories arose over the next century. It was considered seriously again when experiments performed in the 1930s suggested that it might be possible to produce experimental MS by altering the blood supply to the brain.[270,271] The vascular association is being re-examined today.

Tracy Putnam did experiments in 1931, injecting cod liver oil into the carotids of cats and dogs which seemed, to Putnam at least, to produce patches of demyelination resembling the lesions of MS.* He did some further experiments blocking the carotids with various oils to produce these lesions, but his work, presented to many meetings, was received with skepticism. Even Putnam would admit that it would be fair to say pathologists were particularly unimpressed; they did not think the lesions looked at all like those of MS. Despite the criticism, the idea caught the attention of others, and Hurst and Cook did their own experiments in 1943 by injecting olive oil and egg yolk (a "mayonnaise") into one carotid of animals. This produced some demyelination, but even they did not claim it resembled MS. They suggested the changes looked more like Binswanger's disease, a dementing disease with a pattern of widespread white matter change related to hypertension and ischemia in most cases.[272]

---

*Tracy Putnam (1894–1975) studied with Stanley Cobb in 1929–1932 while waiting for a neurosurgic post. He took a research position to study MS and read over 1,000 books and papers on the subject. Over the next few years, he published many papers on what would become a lifelong interest in and focus on multiple sclerosis. His idea that the phenyl portion of the barbiturates accounted for the anticonvulsant properties of barbiturates, although incorrect, led to his discovery with Houston Merritt of the value of diphenylhydantoin (Dilantin). After a successful period in Boston, he accepted the directorship of the Neurological Institute of New York, which "proved a grave mistake," and he later moved to Los Angeles.

It was hard to ignore the perivascular location of the inflammation and the plaques, so it was logical to treat MS patients with anticoagulants when they were discovered. Putnam used various anticoagulants after 1939 to address what he felt was the basic problem of MS, a vascular disorder due to abnormal clotting.[273] He reported on 74 cases of MS treated with the new anticoagulant, dicoumerol. Thirty-one patients dropped out of the study, but he concluded that patients with the more acute relapses benefited while the patients with progressive MS did not. His results were published in 1947 and discussed at the ARNMD conference in 1948.[274] There were confusing studies of coagulation in MS patients in the 1940s with reports of low or high prothrombin times in MS. The observation that retinal periphlebitis occurred in some patients with MS seemed to confirm the suspicion that there was an underlying vascular disorder, but McAlpine thought this was an incidental finding.[275]

Putnam never wavered in his belief in anticoagulation as a therapy of MS up to the time of his death in 1975 at age 81.[276] Many neurologists tried this new therapy and some claimed improvement in certain patients, as one might expect from the variable course of the disease. Brickner used vasodilators to treat MS during the 1940s,[277] but by this time, enthusiasm for therapies based on a vascular thrombosis or vasospasm was fading.

Speculation about a vascular cause for MS surfaced again when Swank and others developed a theory and approach stating there was a dietary factor in MS related to the effect of high fat intake on vascular flow.[278–280] The logical treatment approach would then be a low animal fat diet (Swank Diet), and Swank continues to treat patients with this approach a half-century after he originally proposed it. Swank approached the vascular concept from a different direction, altering blood lipids and coagulation through diet. He published his work in a series of articles and a book between 1953 and 1956, and his dietary approach has had widespread appeal in the MS community.[281]

In 1966, Cyril B. Courville published a monograph arguing the case for a vascular embolic cause of MS,[282] building on the historical arguments of Rindfleisch (1863), Dawson (1916), Siemerling and Raecke (1911, 1914),

Putnam (1935–1947), Marburg (1942), and others who saw a relationship of the plaque to a blood vessel. Courville discussed a case from the English pathologist William McMenemey of Maida Vale Hospital, London, who provided him some blocks of wet pathological material. The patient was a woman with multiple sclerosis and in the small areas of early demyelination, there were vessels whose lumens contained small fat globules. Courville thought the fat globules in this one case resembled those seen in traumatic fat embolism, and although he admitted one swallow did not make a summer (and he did not find such fat globules in the several other cases he had studied), he was impressed enough to build a case for a vascular fat embolic cause for MS on the basis of this patient. His many earlier publications focused on the vascular relationship, but he was now writing when the interest and belief in a vascular cause had waned, as attention had shifted to the burgeoning sciences related to immunology, epidemiology, and viral diseases as a way to explain MS.

THE IMMUNOLOGICAL THEORY

"Certainly one of the most lengthy and unfinished chapters in the history of MS research has been the search for the postulated 'immune defect' believed to cause MS."

George C. Ebers, 1998[283]

The theories of etiology of MS that arose in the 19th century posited a degenerative, vascular, infective, environmental, or toxic cause. Early in the 20th century, the genetic concept slowly grew, and only in the last half of this century was there a strong sense that an immunological mechanism might underlie the basis of the disease, though the seeds of this idea had been laid much earlier. Waksman said that the paradigm shifts from vascular to infection and later to immune mechanisms occurred slowly, as the understanding of what was occurring in the MS plaque developed, with studies by Adam and Kubik in the 1950s and by McDonald and Prineas in the 1970s.*[284–289]

---

*Reviews of the pathology of the plaque can be found in Dawson 1916 and 1917–1918; Lumsden 1970; Prineas 1985; Raine 1993, and Prineas and McDonald 1997.

There were early observations on animal models of immune reactions (EAE), on postinfectious encephalopathies, and later on experimental allergic neuritis (EAN), but serious consideration of immune mechanisms in MS grew in the 1960s, became a focus of research activity in the 1970s, was a predominant concept in the 1980s, and has been a basis of therapeutic attempts since then.*[290-293]

In his 1986 Gowers lecture, McDonald outlined the four main lines of evidence for an immunological abnormality in MS: an elevation of CSF antibodies to various viruses; elevated CSF gamma globulin; the presence of immunologically competent cells in the plaques; and the number of helper and suppressor cells in the peripheral blood, which change with changing activity of the disease.

Outbreaks of encephalomyelitis in the late 1920s led many researchers to speculate on the relationship of acute postinfective encephalopathies and MS. The idea that MS could be related to a hypersensitivity reaction dates back to the observation of Glanzmann (1932), a Swiss physician, who noted postinfectious CNS involvement in chickenpox, smallpox, and vaccinations.[294] Ludwig Van Bogaert had put forward the idea at the International Congress of Neurology at Bern the year before that a phasic hypersensitivity allergic reaction might explain MS.[295] The creation of a model of experimental allergic encephalomyelitis in 1933 by Rivers, Sprunt, and Berry[296] and Rivers and Schwentker in 1935[297] and experimental demyelination supported an allergic concept of demyelination.[298] Ferraro and Jervis showed that they could produce paralysis in monkeys by repeated injections of brain substance over nine months, which resulted in a disseminated inflammation of the CNS with foci of demyelination. In 1951, Lumsden[299] seemed to strongly support the possibility that a similar process could be operating in MS; up to the present day, variations on the EAE model are used to assess possible changes and effects in MS and the likelihood that drugs might be effective against the disease. EAE was later produced by Freund's complete adjuvant, produced in 1942 by Freund and McDermott. For years there were concerns that EAE was not MS, but it

---

*The history of the neuroimmunology of MS has been detailed by Byron Waksman.

has been an important and lasting model for study of processes that probably go on in the human disease as well.

Ferraro summarized the immunological theory in 1944 and attempted to classify and unify the demyelinating diseases as expressions of an allergic reaction in the nervous system; this work was influential in turning interest to the immune phenomena in MS.[300] In 1948, Peter Medawar suggested the brain was an "immunologically privileged site" because it did not show the usual rejection of skin allografts when they were placed within the nervous system.[301] As early as 1885, Paul Ehrlich had noted that aniline dyes injected into the circulation did not stain the central nervous system, suggesting that there was some protective barrier present. The later presumption was that the vasculature was different or that it was due to the absence of a lymphatic system.

McAlpine suggested that MS was an immune reaction following an infection, setting up a process that might be recurrent.[302,303] Writing in a later edition of McAlpine's book, Lumsden commented that evidence to support this theory was mounting but still indirect.[304]

Damashek and others postulated a concept of autoimmunity as a cause of certain diseases, but only when immune thyroditis and other conditions became evident was there some consideration that this might explain diseases like MS. In the 1960s there was increasing excitement about the concepts developing around graft–host rejection and its variants. Models in the nervous system, such as experimental allergic neuritis, were examined by Waksman and others. These were thought to be delayed hypersensitivity-type reactions. Waksman says there was a lull in EAE research during the 1960s and early 1970s, but as immune mechanisms were being elucidated and new genetic models became available, the studies continued and became important in attempts to predict what agents might be therapeutically useful in MS. If an agent prevented EAE or reduced its effects, it was considered for trial in MS.

Byron Waksman described his first research job in 1949, when he was hired by L. Raymond Marison of the Massachusetts General Hospital to work on EAE in rabbits, a model Marison had described two years before. Waksman had just finished his immunology training and said there were only a handful of immunologists interested in EAE,

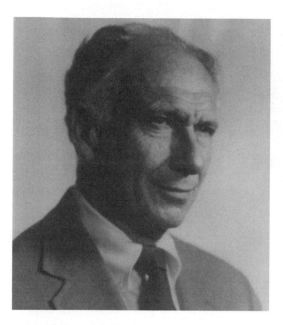

Figure 11.18 Dr. Byron H. Waksman began his half-century of work on the cellular immunology of MS with studies of EAE at the Massachusetts General Hospital in 1949. His studies of the autoimmune process and the role of immunoregulatory lymphocytes and of cytokines in MS and other neurological diseases were important contributions. In 1979, he became the Research Director of the National MS Society and encouraged researchers in MS and the collaboration and interaction between MS investigators. He suggested a study of interferons in the treatment of MS. (Courtesy of Dr. Byron H. Waksman.)

notably Ferraro, Alvord, Kabat, and Freund.[305] He described the state of knowledge, the limited experimental tools available in the immediate post-World War II years, and the lack of people to talk with about immunity and the nervous system. In 1951 he published a paper on EAE and hypothesized that it was a new kind of delayed or tuberculin-type reaction occurring in the nervous system.[306]

By 1950, neuropathologists believed that central and peripheral demyelinating diseases were toxic, degenerative, or perhaps infective processes with macrophages (gitter cells) arising locally by activation of local microglia as an injury response. These processes acted as scavengers to clear up the products of myelin/tissue breakdown, as Charcot believed. Autoimmunity was not accepted as an important pathogenic mechanism despite the work on EAE in the nervous system, phakogenic neuritis in the eye, and Dameshek's work on autoimmune hemolytic anemias.[307]

Waksman next showed that proteolipids of myelin were encephalitogenic a few years after Kies, Robz, and Alford had discovered myelin basic protein as an encephalitogen. He vividly described the early work on immune mechanisms through studies of EAE and EAN (experimental allergic neuritis) in the 1950s and 1960s. That was part of the para-

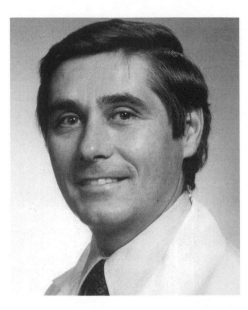

Figure 11.19 While pursuing a career dedicated to MS research, Dr. Barry Arnason also mentored a new generation of MS clinical investigators. (Courtesy of Dr. Barry Arnason.)

digm shift that recognized autoimmunity as a common underlying neuroimmunologic mechanism in many diseases and acknowledged the central role played by lymphocytes and macrophages in the production of destructive lesions in the nervous system.*

Witebsky suggested criteria for defining the presence of an autoimmune disease: specific autoantibodies, a corresponding antigen, and the induction of an analogous immune response in an experimental animal. As Ebers points out, it could be argued that these criteria are justified, but further knowledge of immunology has shown they are not adequate to prove the case.[308]

An intriguing observation that might help us understand the puzzling clues to immunity and infection and the distribution of MS in the world was the suggestion that local factors can play a role in the expression of a disorder when there is a genetic predisposition. The nonobese

---

*Waksman said he worked to encourage young investigators, and the results were evident in my interviews with leaders in MS research, who often pointed to Waksman's influence. Jack Antel of Montreal gave an example by showing the intergenerational influence in the MS community. Waksman influenced Barry Arnason, who was the mentor for Jack Antel, who was the mentor for Joon Whan, who received the Founders' Award of the American Academy of Neurology for his MS research.

diabetic mice (NOD) developed by Makano in Japan did not develop diabetes when they were shipped to New Zealand, but did when they were shipped to Edmonton, Canada.[309] The explanation seemed to relate to the diet and cleanliness of condition early in life and to viral infections. If the mice were reared germ-free in early life, they developed diabetes. Could this relate to the situation of MS? As early as the 1960s, Poskanzer suggested there might be a relationship between MS and sanitary surroundings in early life; perhaps in warmer tropical areas, infections occurred earlier. The same distribution in the world is true for polio and may relate to age of exposure.[310,311]

In the 1970s, Albert Aguayo in Montreal carried out transplantation experiments in the peripheral nervous system. These techniques would later be applied to the central nervous system, and efforts continue today to develop methods to increase myelination and stimulate remyelination. In the 1980s, interest in the cytokine system showed it was central to the destruction occurring in the plaques, and an excess of cytokines could be the basis of the fatigue in MS. In 1988, Lisak suggested that various aspects of this immunologically mediated disorder might be amenable to therapeutic intervention: the inflammation; the destruction of myelin; the astrocytic proliferation and scarring; and the decreased conduction.[312] To these aspects we can now add the axonal damage that may be the result

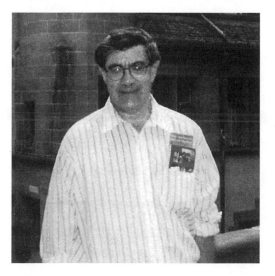

Figure 11.20 After a distinguished career in MS research, Dr. John L. Trotter (1943–2001) died as this book was in its final stages. (Courtesy of Lippincott, Williams, and Wilkins.)

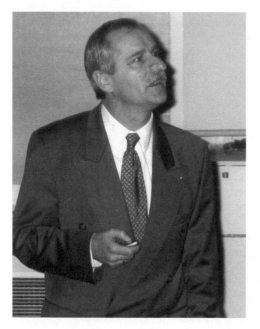

Figure 11.21 Professor Hans Lassmann of the Brain Research Institute in Vienna, founded by Heinrich Obersteiner. Lassmann began his research on MS under Henry Wisniewski in New York, studying EAE. His laboratory has explored two parallel lines—understanding the mechanisms of immune surveillance and brain inflammation, and the immunopathology of MS. Exploring the heterogeneity of the MS lesions, Lassmann's group has collaborated with Wolfgang Bruck in Berlin and Claudia Lucchinetti and Moses Rodriguez at the Mayo Clinic. (Courtesy of Dr. Hans Lassmann.)

of these other four processes and which may govern the extent and rate of progression of MS.[313–315] It has recently been recognized that the underlying process is more extensive than previously realized, more ongoing and more advanced, when we formerly thought symptoms indicated an intermittent and transient process in small isolated patches. There may also be common genetic susceptibility factors for autoimmunity coexisting with other genetic disease-specific or environmental factors that make up the individual's personal risk for a disease like MS.[316]

Research on the immunology of MS has been extensive in recent years, and Ebers reported a comment of Helmut Bauer that over 7,000 papers have been written on this topic. Ebers recently reviewed the background and theory of immunology in MS.[317] Much of current therapy is based on the concept of modifying the immune system.[318]

Despite 50 years devoted to the exploration of immunity as a primary basis for the pathophysiological changes in MS, the evidence still remains mostly circumstantial. That there is an immunological process present is evident. Whether it is the cause or the mechanism by which the cause acts is still unclear.

TRAUMA, STRESS, AND
ENVIRONMENTAL FACTORS

Since MS was recognized, external factors have been considered as a cause or at least a precipitant of attacks of MS. Although such ideas began in the 1830s, by 1970, an anonymous neurologist writing in a British MS Society pamphlet indicated that MS could be precipitated by infection, emotional strain, physical injury, pregnancy, fatigue, and overexertion.[319]

Trauma

It is natural for patients who are experiencing the onset or an exacerbation of MS to wonder if the event is related to something that happened in their lives, a stressful event, an episode of physical exertion, an injury, or a fall. It is likely that none of these is anything more than coincidental, but an association has been discussed in the medical literature for many years and is worth reviewing, especially since this continues to be an issue in the courts. Cases in the courts are often won on the basis that trauma seemed closely related; even if it did not cause the disease, it might have aggravated it.

In 1863, Eduard Rindfleisch felt MS could be caused by damp and cold, injury, emotional stress, prolonged worry, or by an acute illness.[320] Leyden agreed with these factors and included concussions to the body as a possible cause.[321] Although Vulpian seemed to believe in the role of trauma and related a case of MS following an ankle sprain, Charcot made only passing mention of trauma and was more impressed with the effects of emotional factors as a cause. Hammond in the United States believed that blows to the spine from railroad accidents could be a factor.[322] Almost all authors in the late 19th century listed infections, trauma, exposure to cold and damp, emotional factors, and acute infections as factors in the development of MS.

H. Charlton Bastian at University College Hospital, London, reported a patient with a later onset than usual, one far beyond the outer limit of 40 suggested by Charcot and related to trauma. His patient developed MS after age 50, which Bastian related to a fall down a flight of stone steps a year before. Eighteen months later, the patient began to drag his leg. His symptoms improved, but returned four and a half years later, and his disease then had a progressive course. Autopsy showed characteristic scattered grey patches throughout the nervous system.[323]

In 1889, S.V. Clevenger indicated in his book on spinal concussion that multiple sclerosis could be caused by a blow to the head or spine, but he was equally convinced that such a blow could cause syphilis (tabes dorsalis).[324]

In 1897, Mendel reported four cases with onset of MS within a year of skull or spinal trauma.[325] Church and Peterson felt factors like overwork, trauma, and cold exposure might be important, but they also felt there was likely a familial neuropathic tendency in these patients,[326] as evidenced by the familial cases reported by Erb, Oppenheim, and Duchenne.

At the turn of the previous century, Klausner found prior trauma in 19 percent of the MS cases he studied.[327] Hoffman found it in 8 percent.[328] The conclusion of the meeting on MS in 1921 was that MS "appears to be excited by trauma, but trauma cannot itself cause the disease."[329] Despite this conclusion from the experts of the day, there have been reports of the association of MS with trauma for the subsequent 75 years.

Russell Brain, in his landmark review of the status of MS from the viewpoint of a perceptive physician analyzing the literature to 1930, seemed to cover all bases and gave a list of reasons why a factor may appear to be associated with MS—1) coincidence; 2) trauma of the nervous system may be confused with MS; 3) trauma may induce changes in pre-existing but latent plaques; 4) bedrest from trauma may make an MS patient less able to compensate for current MS problems such as incoordination; 5) the trauma may be due to the disabilities fostered by MS; and 6) the trauma might damage the nervous tissue and make it susceptible to the virus of MS.[330]

S.A. Kinnier Wilson said trauma as a cause was "a *questio vexta* to which no ready answer can be returned."[331] He described a young woman who dropped a heavy mirror on her right forearm, later developed weakness and pain in the limb, and then developed neurological signs that progressed to the picture of MS. A third case was a woman who developed MS after a fan fell on her head. He acknowledged that a mirror falling on the arm and causing MS was an untenable proposition, but the disease might be "lit up" by the injury. He noted worsening of MS in another man who was caught in a snowstorm. Wilson cautioned that it would be unwise to disavow such external influences and we should keep an open mind, judging every case on its merits (a difficult challenge in an era of evidence-based medicine).

In 1933, Harris noted the association of spinal or head injury in 6.3 percent of his MS cases,[332] and the next year Von Hoesslin found 11.2 percent of 516 MS cases had suffered trauma in the previous two months.[333] Taking a more selective view, including only severe injury, Keschner in 1950 found an association of trauma with MS in only 1.7 percent of cases, but still concluded that trauma could aggravate the disease.[334] Until this date, the reviews had been uncontrolled so it was not evident how much trauma would be found in the normal population or in a comparison disease.

Richard Brickner and Donald Simons studied 50 MS cases randomly selected from a large group, although they did not indicate how they made the selection; they looked at the relationship of emotions and stress to their MS patients.[335] They detailed the cases of patients who suffered marital strife, job anxiety, motor vehicle accidents, recalcitrant children, worry about spousal health, examination anxiety, family deaths, burglary, or fright by a mouse. One case outlined in detail was a woman with MS who left her lover, who then threatened suicide with a gun. In the meantime, she had taken up with another man and taken a job to repay a debt so that she did not have time to prepare meals properly. She then developed her second attack of MS. Bricker and Simons reasoned that MS could relapse under stress, although they allowed this was "not scientifically final." Stress was a possible cause of aggravation of MS, but they did not suggest it was the cause of the disease.

The first controlled study on the relationship of trauma and the onset of MS was by McAlpine and Compston in 1952, following a preliminary study by McAlpine in 1946.[336] The study found trauma in the three months prior to MS onset in 36 of 250 patients (14.4 percent) compared to 13 (5.2 percent) of 250 controls, which was suggestive of a relationship.[337]

However, two years later, a Canadian study by Kurland and Westlund showed no difference in trauma experience in 112 MS patients and 123 controls.[338] Study of other "trauma" found that deterioration in symptoms occurred in 8 of 57 surgical operations (14 percent),[339] and in 1985, Kelly found that all 14 MS patients who had thalamotomies experienced severe disease exacerbations within three weeks.[340] In 1968, Alter and Speer matched 36 MS patients with two controls each and found no association between head trauma or surgery and MS.[341]

Sibley (personal communication) said that in 1975, Dr. Harry Weaver, the new director of research for the NMSS, said there was a discouraging history of research using EAE as the tool; he suggested to Sibley that they study the patients themselves for clues as to cause. Sibley then began a systematic study of environmental causes for MS including infections, stressful life events, and trauma, and over an eight-year period concluded that common viral infections were the main environmental risk factor, especially viral upper respiratory infections, and that stress and trauma were not important. In 1991, Sibley et al. reported on 170 patients who were followed monthly for a mean of 5.2 years and 134 age- and sex-matched controls.[342] The study did not support an association for trauma, closed head injury, or major surgical procedures.[343–347] In 1993, Siva et al. at the Mayo Clinic[348] and Gusev et al.[349] in 1996 found no association of head trauma and MS onset or exacerbation; the latter study had more head injuries in the control group.

Because this issue was unsettled in the literature and in the courts, in 1999 the Therapeutics and Technology Assessment Subcommittee of the American Academy of Neurology (AAN) reviewed the history and evidence for the association of physical trauma and of stress in MS onset and aggravation of disease. Their review was by very rigid standards of evidence, classifying the published data into categories of strength of evidence.[350] As the AAN committee pointed out, the reports are difficult to assess as many are small, uncontrolled, and mostly of lower-order Class 3 evidence. The committee also recognized that memory bias is an issue when people with an acute illness are asked for associated phenomena, and that trauma is very common, occurring in one-third of the population in any year. However, they added that the issue is important because if trauma and stress are linked to MS, this would have implications for advice to MS patients about how they live their lives and could have important legal implications.

The review found no Class 1 evidence, and only Class 2 and 3 studies were available to make conclusions. Such a review must decide how close in time the trauma must be to be relevant, and what kind of trauma is relevant. The American Academy of Neurology review is a good example of how current evidence is assessed in an attempt to find factors associated with MS.

Stress

Most patients will relate that stress has a definite role in the worsening of their disease. Over the last 150 years, medical writers have noted that stress is an aggravating factor. But is this really true?

Anecdotes that stress precipitated worsening of the disease abound in literature. In 1822, Augustus d'Esté was grief-stricken while attending the funeral of a beloved relative, and on the first page of his diary, he indicated that when leaving the funeral, he noted that his vision had deteriorated, and he had to have his letters read to him.[351,352] It still is not clear what influence stress has on MS, if any. There are groups who feel very strongly that stress is an important influence in aggravating symptoms and bringing on attacks of MS, and there are also those who believe this is an illusion, if an understandable one. It is understandable, they say, because at the onset of MS, or when a new attack of symptoms occurs, the patient will look to see what might have caused it, and stressful events are easy to recognize in normal life. But is there actually a relationship that suggests stress worsens, let alone causes, MS?

Charcot mentioned trauma and other factors, but confessed he did not know the cause of MS, though he was impressed with the role of issues related to the "moral order," such as grief, anger, illicit pregnancy, and the stresses of a false social position. For some reason, he particularly pointed to female teachers in this latter category. In males, stress might have related to loss of caste. Having been "thrown out of the general current," men were too impressionable and ill-provided with the means of maintaining what, in Darwin's theory, is called the "struggle for life."[353]

Moxon felt two of his eight patients had their disease precipitated by stressful events—one from the death of her sister's child, and the other from finding her husband in bed with another woman.[354] Russell,[355] Bramwell,[356] McAlpine,[357] and Adams[358] also felt their experience with MS patients confirmed an important role for stress.

S.A. Kinnier Wilson admitted that only a minority of MS patients have some convincing factor as a cause, although he allowed that such factors as stress, infection, overwork, fatigue, and worry could lower the resistance, "vague though that concept might be." He noted that one case developed after an *affaire du coeur*. He related the story of a Royal Air Force pilot who crossed the English channel on missions 200 times and was later shot down three times in air fights with minor injuries. Four months after the last of these incidents, he developed diplopia and tremor and a few years later had the clear signs of MS.[359]

There was a great deal of interest in stress as a factor in physical as well as emotional illness in the 1950s with the publications of Selye on stress and the general adaptation syndrome and the discoveries surrounding cortisone and ACTH.[360] The general belief was that stress could adversely affect the brain and other organs, and that a natural defense mechanism was by corticotropin production so ACTH and cortisone administration would imitate a natural protective physiological mechanism. At this time, patients were being given ACTH by Houston Merritt and his colleagues.[361]

Patients comment frequently that they can associate some stressful event with exacerbations of their disease. Brickner and Simons found this in only 14 percent of their cases,[362] and Pratt found this in 58 of 229 cases.[363] Philippopoulos et al. found that 35 of 40 patients had a stressful episode just before the onset of their disease.[364] Retrospective questionnaires are fraught with methodological problems, and most case-control studies have not confirmed the association of stress and MS. Pratt could not support this association,[365] and Baldwin found as many traumatic events in the lives of controls as in MS patients, but the MS patients had less stability in their lives.[366] Malmgren asked patients on each visit about seven types of stress and could not confirm a relationship of stress to disease exacerbations.[367]

The recent studies of Rabins[368] and Franklin et al.[369] provide marginal, if any, evidence for any association of stress and MS. Grant,[370] however, found severe threatening events in 62 percent of his MS patients, but only in 15 percent of controls. In 1991, Warren noted that 56.8 percent of patients with an exacerbation of MS had had an intense emotional event in the six months prior to the event, compared to 28.4 percent of patients in remission.[371,372]

One of the more interesting studies is that of Nisipeanu and Korczyn, who reported in 1993 on the experience of attacks of MS in relation to the Persian Gulf War.[373] There appeared to be a lower rate of attacks immediately after the war than before, suggesting that acute severe stress might actually reduce attacks of MS. However, the results of the study are not strong evidence as the numbers are small and the period of study is short, and because it is well-documented that attacks decrease over time.

In 1997, Sibley reported the final results of the study mentioned above under the discussion of trauma,[374] concluding there was no association of MS with stress, but the AAN committee noted marginal evidence for an association of MS with job and marital stress.[375] The AAN committee concluded that there was Class 2 evidence both for and against an association of stress and MS, but there were reasons to regard the possible association as weak. There is a recent observation that new lesions on MRI may be more frequent two months after major stress, but this is again circumstantial, weak evidence.[376]

What is the conclusion of all the evidence over the last 150 years? Assessment of the evidence suggests no association of MS onset with physical trauma, and the data are so limited that no convincing association of MS with psychological stress can be established "with reasonable medical certainty."

Environmental Factors

An early proponent of an environmental cause for MS was Hermann Oppenheim.[377,378] The favorite assistant to Westphal at the University of Berlin, he was interested in environmental toxins early in his career. His initial publications included observations on lead intoxication and alcohol. His monograph on traumatic neurosis, in which he suggested that psychic disturbances had an organic basis, initiated an acrimonious debate; one of his major critics was Charcot.* Reviewing possible exogenous toxins in 1922, Lewellys Barker did not accept the suggestion of Oppenheim of lead, arsenic, and tin, and of von Jaksch of manganese as causes of MS; he said that any neurological disorders they caused were unlike MS.[379] Using the same logic as Risien Russell had some 30 years before, Barker argued that if metal poisoning were the culprit, then MS would be a disease of men, as they were commonly exposed to such agents; but he thought MS occurrence was about equal in the sexes, as many researchers did. Also, the disease often occurred early in life before men could have much chance for occupational exposure. Finally, it would hardly be credible that repeated attacks were repeated bouts of poisoning. In his series of 44 cases from the records of Johns Hopkins Hospital and his own practice, there were no cases of metal poisoning. Barker also rejected Jelliffe's suggestion that alcohol might be a factor in MS, based on his finding that eight percent of his MS cases were inebriates. Barker argued that MS was not common in alcoholics. He also dispensed with the implication of carbon monoxide as a cause, even though scientists recognized that it could cause damage to the nervous system. He then outlined reasons why trauma, thermal injury, and electrical injury were also not reasonable suspects. Barker concluded:

> *"If multiple sclerosis is a disease entity due to a single cause that acts early in life, it may be due to some specific infection, but the evidence available is strongly against it being caused by any of our well-known infections, by any ordinary intoxication (organic or inorganic), or by electrical, thermal or traumatic influences. If the exogenous factors mentioned play any role at all in the etiology of the disease, they must act either as predisposing influences for the true cause, or as aggravators of a disease already started by the true cause."*

---

*Hermann Oppenheim (1858–1919) seemed always at the center of controversy, but he did not accept criticism well. When he was not confirmed as Westphal's successor, he started his own successful neurological clinic that gained an international reputation from its many publications. It was Oppenheim's diagnosis that enabled Koehler to carry out the first brain tumor removal. He wrote a monograph on brain tumors and coined the term dystonia musculorum deformans, which for a time was named Oppenheim's disease, and his description of amyotonia congenita is still called by that eponym.

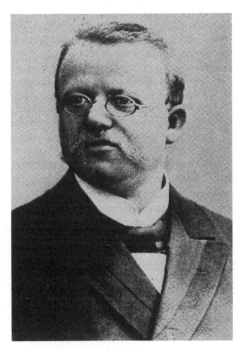

Figure 11.22 Hermann Oppenheim (1858–1919) made many contributions to neurology, but was often at the center of controversy. His theory of an environmental cause of multiple sclerosis was opposed by many French and English for decades, and his belief that post-trauma "neurosis" had an anatomical basis was opposed by Charcot. He took such attacks personally and when rejected for Professor Extraordinarius, he left the academy and set up his own private clinic, which produced an impressive flood of publications and became the internationally known center of neurology in Berlin. He had an interest in brain tumors, and his diagnosis in one patient led to the successful removal by R. Koehler, the first surgical removal of a brain tumor. (Courtesy of the Library of the Northwestern School of Medicine.)

Vaccinations

There has long been a concern about the possibility that vaccinations could precipitate MS. Some patients even worry that vaccinations might cause the disease. Could an immune disease like MS have the immune system stimulated by vaccines and so aggravate the disease process? Could vaccines actually cause MS? Without much except anecdotes and speculation to go on, physicians for generations warned MS patients to avoid vaccines (as they warned against anesthetics and surgery). There has not been convincing evidence that vaccines are harmful (beyond the small transient fever in some after a vaccine), but with millions of people receiving vaccinations each year, some cases of MS could be expected to occur coincidentally, since young adults often get flu and hepatitis vaccines or take other vaccines for travel. This is a serious issue because vaccinations are important for the public health. They are vital as a preventive measure in MS patients who often feel worse during infections and may have exacerbations from infections that could be prevented. In France, a few cases of MS developed during the years of a campaign to vaccinate for hepatitis B, and in October 1998, the French government suspended the school program for hepatitis B vaccination because of concern about MS, even though two preliminary studies, one French and one American, showed an insignificant increase in MS in those vaccinated. Despite the negative studies and a report from the World Health Organization that said there was no causal link between vaccines and MS, the concern prevailed and the program ceased.

The first large group to be assessed for this risk was studied during the swine flu scare in the 1970s, and no convincing relationship to MS or of aggravation of MS was noted. Recently, Christian Confavreaux and the Vaccines in Multiple Sclerosis Study Group reviewed 19 publications (1962–1997) that indicated a possible link, and these discussed mostly single cases.[380] Their study of 643 patients from the European Database for Multiple Sclerosis who had relapses of MS showed no increased risk of relapse because of vaccination. This applied to influenza, hepatitis B, and tetanus vaccines.

REFERENCES

1. Huth E, Murray TJ. *Medicine in Quotations*. Philadelphia: American College of Physicians; 2000:311.
2. Allbutt TC. On the ophthalmoscopic signs of spinal cord disease. *Lancet*. 1870;1: 76-78.
3. Gray LC. *A Treatise on Nervous and Mental Diseases*. London: HK Lewis; 1893:373-378.
4. Ibid, p. 376.
5. Huth E, Murray TJ. *Medicine in Quotations*. Philadelphia: American College of Physicians; 2000:206.
6. Boyd W. *Pathology for the Physicians*. London: Henry Kimpton; 1958:753.
7. Miller H, Smith M. The cost of drug treatment. *Lancet*. 1960;i:45-47.
8. Dumonde DC. The Paradox of Immunity and Infection in Multiple Sclerosis. In: *Clinical Neuroimmunology*. Rose E, Clifford F. Oxford: Blackwell; 1979:275.
9. Paty DW, Ebers GC, eds. *Multiple Sclerosis*. Philadelphia: FA Davis; 1998.
10. Kuhn T. *The Structure of Scientific Revolutions*. 2nd edition. Chicago. University of Chicago Press; 1970.
11. Rindfleisch E. Histologische Detail zu der Grauen Degeneration von Gehirn and Rückenmark. *Virchow Arch Path Anat Physiol*. 1863;26:474-483.
12. Leyden E. Ueber graue Degeneration des Rückenmarks. *Deutsche Klin*. 1863;15:121-128.
13. Moxon W. Eight cases of insular sclerosis of the brain and spinal cord. *Guy Hospital Reports*. 1875;20:437-478.
14. Hamilton AM. *Nervous Diseases: Their Description and Treatment*. London: J&A Churchill; 1878:346-351.
15. Ibid 346-351.

16. Marie P. *Lectures on Diseases of the Spinal Cord*, trans. Lubbock M. London: New Sydenham Society; 1895;153:134-136.

17. Gowers WR. *A Manual of Diseases of the Nervous System*, 2nd ed. London: J & A Churchill; 1893:vol 2:544, 557-558.

18. Gowers WR. *A Manual of Diseases of the Nervous System*. Vol 2: Diseases of the brain and cranial nerves. (2nd ed). Philadelphia: P Blakiston, Son; 1893.

19. Russell JSR. Disseminated sclerosis. In Albutt TC, ed. *A System of Medicine*. London: Macmillan; 1899:50-94.

20. Krafft-Ebing R. *Die Progressive Allgemeine Paralyse*. Wein: Ch Russer and M Werthner. 1894.

21. Wilson SAK. *Neurology*. London: Edward Arnold; 1940:148-178.

22. Gray LC. *A Treatise on Nervous and Mental Diseases*. London: HK Lewis; 1893:373-378.

23. Oppenheim H. *Text-book of Nervous Diseases for Physicians and Students*, trans Bruce A. Edinburgh: Otto Schulze, 1911.

24. Beevor CE. *Diseases of the Nervous System*. London: H. K. Lewis; 1898:272-278.

25. Association for Research in Nervous and Mental Disease. *Multiple Sclerosis (Disseminated sclerosis)*. New York: Paul B. Hoeber; 1922:22-26.

26. Marburg O. Die Sogenannte akute multiple sklerose (encephalomyelitis periaxialis scleroticans). *Jahrb Psychiat V Neurol*. 1906;27:1.

27. Association for Research in Nervous and Mental Disease. *Multiple Sclerosis (Disseminated sclerosis)*. New York: Paul B. Hoeber; 1922:144-165.

28. Brickner R. Studies of the pathogenesis of multiple sclerosis, II. Evidence of the presence of an abnormal lipase in the blood in multiple sclerosis. *Bull Neurol Inst NY*. 1931;1:105.

29. Barker LF. *The Nervous System and its Constituent Neurons*. New York: Appleton; 1899.

30. Barker LF. *Time and the Physician*. New York: Putnam; 1942.

31. Association for Research in Nervous and Mental Disease. *Multiple Sclerosis (Disseminated sclerosis)*. New York: Paul B. Hoeber; 1922:26.

32. Association for Research in Nervous and Mental Disease. *Multiple Sclerosis (Disseminated sclerosis)*. New York: Paul B. Hoeber; 1922:43-48.

33. Jelliffe SE. Emotional and psychological factors in multiple sclerosis. In: *Multiple Sclerosis: An investigation by the Association for Research in Nervous and Mental Disease*. New York: Paul B. Hoeber; 1921:82-90.

34. Association for Research in Nervous and Mental Disease. *Multiple Sclerosis (Disseminated sclerosis)*. New York: Paul B. Hoeber; 1922:197-207.

35. Spiller WG, Camp CD. Multiple sclerosis, with a report of two additional cases with necropsy. *J Nerv Ment Dis*. 1904;31:433-445.

36. Leiner JH. An investigation of the axis cylinder in its relation to multiple sclerosis. In: *Multiple Sclerosis and Disseminated Sclerosis*. Proceedings of the Association for Research in Nervous and Mental Diseases. New York: Paul B. Hoeber; 1922: p. 197-207.

37. Chevassut K. The etiology of disseminated sclerosis. *Lancet*. 1930;552-559.

38. Purves-Stewart J. Treatment of disseminated sclerosis. *Lancet*. 1930;560-562.

39. Talley C. *A History of Multiple Sclerosis and Medicine in the United States, 1870–1960*. PhD dissertation. San Francisco: University of California; 1998.

40. Schumacher GA. Multiple sclerosis and its treatment. *JAMA*. 1950;143:1059-1065, 1146-1154, 1241-1250.

41. McAlpine D, Compston ND, Lumsden CE. *Multiple Sclerosis*. Edinburgh: E&S Livingston; 1955.

42. Reese HH. Multiple Sclerosis and the Demyelinating Diseases. Critique of theories concerning multiple sclerosis. *JAMA*. 1950;143:1470-1473.

43. Curtius F. *Multiple Sklerose and Erbanlage*. Leipzig: G. Thieme; 1933.

44. McAlpine D, Compston ND, Lumsden CE. *Multiple Sclerosis*. Edinburgh: E&S Livingston; 1955.
45. McAlpine D, Compston ND and Lumsden CE. *Multiple Sclerosis: a reappraisal,* 2nd ed. Edinburgh: E & S Livingston; 1972.
46. Putnam TJ. Studies in Multiple Sclerosis. *Arch Neurol Psych*. 1936;35:1289-1308.
47. Rivers TM, Schwentker F. Encephalomyelitis accompanied by myelin destruction experimentally produced in monkeys. *J Exp Med*. 1935;61:698-702.
48. Kabat EA, et al. An electrophoretic study of the protein components in cerebrospinal fluid and their relationship to the serum proteins. *J Clin Invest*. 1942;21:571-577.
49. Arnason B. (personal communication).
50. Leyden E. Ueber graue Degeneration des Rückenmarks. *Deutsche Klin*. 1863;15:121-128.
51. Batten FE. Two cases of a family disease: the symptoms of which closely resemble disseminated sclerosis. *Proc Roy Soc Med*. 1908-09;35-37.
52. Association for Research in Nervous and Mental Disease. *Multiple Sclerosis (Disseminated sclerosis)*. New York: Paul B. Hoeber; 1922:8-19.
53. Association for Research in Nervous and Mental Disease. *Multiple Sclerosis (Disseminated sclerosis)*. New York: Paul B. Hoeber; 1922:47-48.
54. Curtius F. *Multiple Sklerose and Erbanlage*. Leipzig: G. Thieme; 1933.
55. MacKay RP. The familial occurrence of multiple sclerosis and its implications. In: *Multiple Sclerosis and the Demyelinating Diseases*. Proceedings of the Association for Research in Nervous and Mental Diseases. (Dec. 10–11, 1948). Baltimore: Williams & Wilkins; 1950.
56. MacKay RP, Myrianthropoulos NC. Multiple sclerosis in twins and their relatives: preliminary report on a genetic and clinical study. *Arch Neurol Psychiat*. 1958;80:667-674.
57. Larner AJ. Aetological role of viruses in multiple sclerosis: a review. *J Royal Soc Med*. 1986;79:412-417.
58. Popper K. *The Logic of Scientific Discovery*. New York: Basic Books; 1959.
59. Kuhn T. *The Structure of Scientific Revolutions*. 2nd ed. Chicago: University of Chicago Press; 1970.
60. Marie P. *Lectures on Diseases of the Spinal Cord*, trans M. Lubbock. London: New Sydenham Society; 1895:134-136.
61. Association for Research in Nervous and Mental Disease. *Multiple Sclerosis (Disseminated sclerosis)*. New York: Paul B. Hoeber; 1922:144-164.
62. Marie P. *Lectures on Diseases of the Spinal Cord*, p. 134-136.
63. McDonald WI. Attitudes to the treatment of multiple sclerosis. *Arch Neurol*. 1983;40:667-670.
64. Bullock WE. The experimental transmission of disseminated sclerosis to rabbits. *Lancet*. 1913;Oct 25:1185-1186.
65. Gye NE. The experimental study of disseminated sclerosis. *Brain*. 1921;44:213-222.
66. Buzzard EF. The treatment of disseminated sclerosis: A Suggestion. *Lancet*. 1911;1:98.
67. Kuhn P, Steiner G. Über die Ursache der multiplen Sklerose. *Med Klin*. 1917;13:1007.
68. Kuhn P, Steiner G. Multiplin Sklerose. *Stschr Hyg Infections*. 1920:90:417-422.
69. Bullock WE. The experimental transmission of disseminated sclerosis to rabbits. *Lancet*. 1913:Oct 25;1185-1186.
70. Gye NE. The experimental study of disseminated sclerosis. *Brain*. 1921;44:213-222.
71. Association for Research in Nervous and Mental Disease. *Multiple Sclerosis (Disseminated sclerosis)*. New York: Paul B. Hoeber; 1922:121-131.
72. Ibid, p. 43.
73. Adams DK, Blacklock JWS, Dunlop EM, et al. An investigation into the pathogenesis of disseminated sclerosis. *Q J Med*. 1924;17:129-150.
74. Chevassut K. Aetiology of disseminated sclerosis. *Lancet*. 1930;1:522-560.

75. Purves-Stewart J. A specific vaccine treatment in disseminated sclerosis. *Lancet.* 1930;1:560-564.
76. Purves-Stewart J. The etiology and treatment of disseminated sclerosis. *J Nerv Ment Dis.* 1930;72:652-660.
77. Ibid, p. 597.
78. Ibid, p. 598.
79. Carmichael EA. The aetiology of disseminate sclerosis: Some criticisms of recent work especially with regard to the "Spherula insularis." *Proc R Soc Med.* 1931;34:591-599.
80. Murray TJ. The history of MS in *Multiple Sclerosis: Diagnosis, Medical Management and Rehabilitation.* Jack Burks, Ken Johnson, editors. New York: Demos. 2000: p. 1-20.
81. Purves-Stewart, Sir James. *Sands of Time: Recollections of a Physician in Peace and War.* London: Hutchinson; 1939.
82. Kuhn P, Steiner G. Über die ursache der multiplen Sklerose. *Med Klin.* 1917;13:1007.
83. Kuhn P, Steiner G. Multiplen Sklerose. *Ztschr Hyg Infections.* 1920;90:417-422.
84. Steiner G. Acute Plaques in Multiple Sclerosis, Their Pathogenetic Significance and the Role of Spirochetes as Etiological Factor. *J Neuropath Exp Neurol.* 1952;11:343-372.
85. Steiner G. Multiple Sclerosis. *J Michigan State M Soc.* 1950;49:939-940.
86. Steiner G. Multiple sclerosis. I. The etiological significance of the regional and occupational incidence. *J Nerv Ment Dis.* 1938;88:42-66.
87. Innis JRM, Kurland LT. Is multiple sclerosis caused by a virus? *Am J Med.* 1952;12:574-585.
88. McAlpine D, Compston ND, Lumsden CE. *Multiple Sclerosis.* Edinburgh: E&S Livingston; 1955.
89. Ichelson RR. Cultivation of spirochetes from spinal fluids of multiple sclerosis cases and negative controls. *Proc Soc Exp Biology.* 1957;95:57-58.
90. Kurtzke JF, Martin A, Myerson RM, Lewis JI. Microbiology in multiple sclerosis: Evaluation of Ichelson's organism. *Neurology.* 1962;12:915-922.
91. McAlpine D, Lumsden CE, Acheson ED. *Multiple Sclerosis: A Reappraisal,* 2nd ed. Edinburgh: E & S Livingston; 1972.
92. Le Gac P. Nouvelles données sur la sclérose en plaques. *J Méd Bordeaux.* 1960;137:346.
93. Le Gac P. Le traitement de la sclérose en plaues d'origine rickettsienne et néorickettsienne. *J Méd Bordeaux.* 1960;137:577-589.
94. Gay D, Dick G. Is multiple sclerosis caused by an oral spirochete? The evidence. In: Rose FC, Jones R, eds. *Multiple Sclerosis: Immunological, Diagnostic and Therapeutic Aspects,* London: John Libby; 1987.
95. Shevell M, Evans BK. The "Schaltenbrand experiment." Würzburg, 1940: Scientific, historical and ethical perspectives. *Neurology.* 1994;44:350-356.
96. Shevell MI. Racial hygiene, active euthanasia and Julius Hallervorden. *Neurology.* 1992;42:2214-2219.
97. Adams JM, Imagawa DT. Measles antibodies in multiple sclerosis. *Proc Soc Exp Biol Med.* 1962;111:562-566.
98. Adams JM. *Multiple Sclerosis: Scars of Childhood: New Horizons and Hope.* Springfield: Charles C. Thomas; 1977.
99. Murray TJ, Murray SJ. Characteristics of patients found not to have multiple sclerosis. *Can Med Assoc J.* 1984;131:336-337.
100. Poskanzer DC, Schapiro K, Miller H. Multiple sclerosis and poliomyelitis. *Lancet.* 1963;2:917-921.
101. Sibley WA, Foley JM. Measles antibodies in multiple sclerosis. *Trans Am Neurol Assn.* 1963;88:277-281.
102. Larner AJ. Aetological role of viruses in multiple sclerosis: a review. *J Royal Soc Med.* 1986;79:412-417.
103. Adams JM, Imagawa DT. Measles antibodies in multiple sclerosis. *Proc Soc Exp Biol Med.* 1962;111:562-566.

104. *Multiple Sclerosis: Progress in Research.* Field EJ, Bell TM, Cargegie PR, editors. Amsterdam, London, North Holland. 1972, p. 48.
105. Ibid, p. 68.
106. Larner AJ. Aetological role of viruses in multiple sclerosis: a review. *J Royal Soc Med.* 1986;79:412-417.
107. Kurtzke JF, Hyllested K. Multiple sclerosis in the Faeroe Islands: 1. Clinical and Epidemiological features. *Ann Neurol.* 1979;5:6-21.
108. Kurtzke JF, Hyllested K. Multiple sclerosis in the Faeroe Islands. 2. Clinical update, transmission, and the nature of MS. *Neurology.* 1986;36:307-328.
109. Kurtzke JF, Hyllested K. Multiple sclerosis in the Faeroe Islands. 3. An alternative assessment of the three epidemics. *Acta Neurol Scand.* 1987;76:317-339.
110. Kurtzke JF, Hyllested K. Multiple sclerosis in the Faeroe Islands. II. Clinical update, transmission, and the nature of MS. *Neurology.* 1986;36:307-328.
111. Kurtzke JF, Hyllested K, Heltberg A, Olsen A. Multiple sclerosis in the Faeroe Islands. 5. The occurance of the fourth epidemic as validation of transmission. *Acta Neurol Scand.* 1993;88:161-173.
112. Cook SD, Dowling PC. A possible association between house pets and multiple sclerosis. *Lancet.* 1978;1:980-982.
113. Kurtzke JF, Gurdmundsson KR, Bergmann S. Multiple sclerosis in Iceland: a postwar epidemic. *Neurology.* 1980;30:437.
114. Nathanson N, Palsson PA, Gudmundsson G. Multiple sclerosis and canine distemper in Iceland, *Lancet.* 1978;2:1127-1129.
115. Sylvester DL, Poser CM. Association of multiple sclerosis with domestic animals and household pets. *Ann Neurol.* 1979;5:207-209.
116. Gajdusek DC, Gibbs CJ Jr, Alpers M, eds. *Slow, Latent and Temperate Virus Infections.* Washington, DC: US Dept of Health, Education and Welfare; 1965.
117. Sibley WA, Foley JM. Infection and immunization in multiple sclerosis. *Ann NY Acad Sci.* 1965;122:457-468.
118. Sibley WA, Foley JM. Seasonal variation in multiple sclerosis and retrobulbar aneuritis in Northeastern Ohio. *Trans Am Neurol Assn.* 1965;90:295-297.
119. Sibley WA, Kalter SS, Laguna JF. Attempts to transmit multiple sclerosis to non-human primates: preliminary report. *Excerpta Med.* 1977;427:233-234.
120. Sibley WA, Laguna JF, Kalter SS. Attempts to transmit multiple sclerosis to non-human primates. In: Bauer HJ, Poser S, and Ritter G, ed. *Progress in Multiple Sclerosis Research.* New York: Springer Verlag; 1980.
121. Sibley WA, Bamford CR, Clark K. Clinical viral infections and multiple sclerosis. *Lancet.* 1985;1:1313-1315.
122. Poskanzer DC, Schapiro K, Miller H. Multiple sclerosis and poliomyelitis. *Lancet.* 1963;2:917-921.
123. Murray TJ. An Unusual Occurrence of Multiple Sclerosis in a Small Rural Community. *CJNS.* 1976;3(3):163-166.
124. Compston DAS, Vakarelis BN, Paul E, McDonald WI, Batchelor JR, Mims CA. Viral infection in patients with multiple sclerosis and HLA-DR matched controls. *Brain.* 1986;109:325-344.
125. Gilden DH, Devlin ME, Burgoon MP, Owens GP. The search for virus in multiple sclerosis brain. *Multiple Sclerosis.* 1996;2:179-183.
126. Carp RI, Licursi PC, Merz PA, Merz GS. Decreased Percentage of Polymorphonuclear neutrophils in Mouse Peripheral Blood After Innoculation with Material from MS Patients. *J Exp Med.* 1972;136:618.
127. Challoner P, et al. Plaque-associated expression of human herpesvirus 6 in multiple sclerosis. *Proc Natl Acad Sci USA.* 1995;92:7442-7444.

128. Hunter SF, Hafler DA. Ubiquitous pathogens: Links between infection and autoimmunity in MS? *Neurology*. 2000;55:164-165.
129. Challoner P, et al. Plaque-associated expression of human herpesvirus 6 in multiple sclerosis. *Proc Natl Acad Sci USA*. 1995;92:7442-7444.
130. Noseworthy JG. Progress in determining the cause and treatment of multiple sclerosis. *Nature*. 1999; 399(Suppl):A40-A47.
131. Ross RT, et al. Herpes zoster and multiple sclerosis. *Can J Neurol Sci*. 1999;26:29-32.
132. Marrie RA, Wolfson C, Sturkenboom MCJM, et al. Multiple Sclerosis and anticedent infections. *Neurology*. 2000;54:2307-2310.
133. Bray PF, Bloomer LC, Salmon VC, Bagley MH, Larsen PD. Epstein-Barr virus infection and antibody synthesis in patients with multiple sclerosis. *Arch Neurol*. 1983;37:94-96.
134. Sumaya CV, Myers LW, Willison GW, Ench Y. Increased prevalence and titer of Epstein-Barr virus antibodies in patients with multiple sclerosis. *Ann Neurol*. 1985;17:371-377.
135. Larsen PD, Bloomer LC, Bray PF. Epstein-Barr nuclear antigen and viral capsid antigen antibody titers in multiple sclerosis. *Neurology*. 1985;35:435-438.
136. Marrie RA, Wolfson C, Sturkenboom MCJM, et al. Multiple sclerosis and anticedent infections. *Neurology*. 2000;54:2307-2310.
137. Kurtzke JF, Delasnerie-Lauprêtre N, Wallin MT. Multiple sclerosis in North African migrants to France. *Acta Neurol Scand*. 1998;98:302-309.
138. Ebers GR. Immunology. In Paty DW, Ebers GC, eds. *Multiple Sclerosis*. Philadelphia: FA Davis. 1998;403-421.
139. Prusiner S. Prions and neurodegenerative diseases. *N Engl J Med*. 1987;317:1571-1580.
140. Lorber B. Are all diseases infections? Another Look. *An Intern Med*. 1999;131:989-990.
141. Compston A. The story of Multiple Sclerosis. Chapter 1. *McAlpine's Multiple Sclerosis*. London. Churchill, Livingstone; 1998:3-42.
142. Kurland L T. The evolution of multiple sclerosis epidemiology. *Annals of Neurology*. 1994:36;S2-S5.
143. Rupke NA, ed. Medical Geography in Historical Perspective. *Medical History*, Supplement 20, 2000.
144. Uhthoff, W. Untersuchen über die bei multiplen herdsclerose vorkommenden augerstörungen. *Arch Psychiat*. 1890;21:303-410.
145. Davenport C. Multiple sclerosis: from the standpoint of geographic distribution and race. *Arch Neurol Psychiatry*. 1922; 8:51-58.
146. Bramwell B. Disseminated Sclerosis with Special Reference to the Frequency and Etiology of the Disease. *Clinical Studies*. 1904;2:193-210.
147. Bramwell B. The prognosis in disseminated sclerosis; duration in two hundred cases of disseminated sclerosis. *Edin Med J*. 1917;18:15-23.
148. Church A, Peterson F. *Nervous and Mental Diseases*. London: Ribman: 1899.
149. Dana CL. *Textbook of Nervous Diseases*. 3rd ed. New York: William Wood: 1894.
150. Davenport C. Multiple sclerosis: from the standpoint of geographic distribution and race. *Arch Neurol Psychiatry*. 1922; 8:51-58.
151. Bing R, Reese H. Die multiple Sklerose in der Nordwestschweiz. *Schw med Wchnschr*. 1926;56:30-34.
152. Allison RS. Disseminated sclerosis in North Wales. *Brain*. 1931;53:391-430.
153. Brain WR. Critical review: disseminated sclerosis. *Quart J Med*. 1930;23:343-391.
154. Steiner G. Multiple sclerosis. I. The etiological significance of the regional and occupational incidence. *J Nerv Ment Dis*. 1938;88:42-66.
155. Association for Research in Nervous and Mental Disease. *Multiple Sclerosis (Disseminated sclerosis)*. New York: Paul B. Hoeber. 1922:34-35.

156. Morawitz P. Zurkenntris der multiplen Sklerose. *Deutsches Arch Klin Med.* 1904:151-166.

157. Putnam TJ. The Centenary of Multiple Sclerosis. *Arch Neurol Psych.* 1938;40(4):806-813.

158. Wilson SAK. *Neurology.* Bruce AN, ed. London: Edward Arnold; 1940:148-178.

159. Dean G. Annual Incidence, prevalence and mortality of multiple sclerosis in white South African-born and in white immigrants to South Africa. *Brit Med J.* 1976; 2:724-730.

160. Putnam TJ. The pathogenesis of multiple sclerosis: a possible vascular factor. *N Engl J Med.* 1933;209:786.

161. Limberg CC. The geographic distribution of multiple sclerosis and its estimated prevalence in the United States. In: *Multiple Sclerosis and the Demyelinating Diseases.* Proceedings of the Association for Research in Nervous and Mental Disease (Dec 10–11, 1948). Vol 28. Baltimore: Williams and Wilkins; 1950:15-24.

162. Schumacher GA. Multiple sclerosis and its treatment. *JAMA.* 1950;143:1059-1065.

163. Limberg CC. The geographic distribution of multiple sclerosis and its estimated prevalence in the United States. In: *Multiple Sclerosis and the Demyelinating Diseases.* Proceedings of the Association for Research in Nervous and Mental Disease (Dec 10–11, 1948). Vol 28. Baltimore: Williams and Wilkins; 1950:15-24.

164. Kurland LT. Epidemiologic characteristics of multiple sclerosis. *Am J Med.* 1952;21:561-571.

165. MacLean AR, Berkson J, Woltman HW, Schionneman L. Multiple Sclerosis in a rural community. In: *Multiple Sclerosis and the Demyelinating Diseases.* Proceedings of the Association for Research in Nervous and Mental Disease (Dec. 10–11, 1948). Vol 28. Baltimore: Williams and Wilkins; 1950:25-27.

166. Kurland LT. *The frequency and geographic distribution of multiple sclerosis as indicated by mortality statistics and morbidity surveys in the United States and Canada.* (Thesis submitted to School of Hygiene and Public Health, The Johns Hopkins University, in conformity with requirements for the degree of Doctor of Public Health – May, 1951). Also *Am J Hyg.* 1952;55:457-476.

167. Kurland LT. Epidemiologic characteristics of multiple sclerosis. *Am J Med.* 1952;21:561-571.

168. Kurland LT, Westlund KB. Epidemiologic factors in the etiology and prognosis of multiple sclerosis. *Ann NY Acad Sci.* 1954;58:682.

169. McAlpine D, Compston ND, Lumsden CE. *Multiple Sclerosis.* Edinburgh: E&S Livingston; 1955.

170. Kurland L T. The Evolution of multiple sclerosis epidemiology. *Ann Neurol.* 1994:36; S2-S5.

171. Dean G. Annual incidence, prevalence and mortality of multiple sclerosis in white South African-born and in white immigrants to South Africa. *Brit Med J.* 1976;2:724-730.

172. Kurtzke JF, Dean G, Botha DPJ. A method for estimating the age of immigration of white immigrants to South Africa, with an example of its importance. *S Africa Med J.* 1970;44:663-669.

173. Alter M, Okihiro M. When is multiple sclerosis acquired? *Neurology.* 1971;21:1030-1036.

174. Acheson ED, Bachrach CA, Wright FM. Some comments on the relationship of the distribution of multiple sclerosis to latitude, solar radiation, and other variables. *Acta Psychiat Neurol Scand.* (Suppl 147). 1960;35:132-147.

175. Poser CM. The Dissemination of Multiple Sclerosis: A Viking Saga? A Historical Essay. *Ann Neurol.* 1994;36:S231-243.

176. Bailey P. Incidence of multiple sclerosis in United States troops. *Arch Neurol Psychiatry.* 1922;7:582-583.

177. Davenport C. Multiple sclerosis: from the standpoint of geographic distribution and race. *Arch Neurol Psychiatry*. 1922;8:51-58.
178. Brain WR. Critical review: disseminated sclerosis. *Quart J Med*. 1930;23:343-391.
179. McAlpine D. The problem of disseminated sclerosis. *Brain*. 1946;69:233-250.
180. Steiner G. Multiple sclerosis. I. The etiological significance of the regional and occupational incidence. *J Nerv Ment Dis*. 1938;88:42-66.
181. Ulett G. Geographic distribution of multiple sclerosis. *Dis Nerv Syst*. 1946;9:342-346.
182. Limberg CC. The geographic distribution of multiple sclerosis and its estimated prevalence in the United States. In: *Multiple Sclerosis and the Demyelinating Diseases*. Proceedings of the Association for Research in Nervous and Mental Disease (Dec 10–11, 1948). Vol 28. Baltimore: Williams and Wilkins; 1950;15-24.
183. Bulman D, Ebers G. The geography of multiple sclerosis reflects genetic susceptibility. *J Trop Geog Neurol*. 1992;2:66-72.
184. Alter M. Clues to the cause based on the epidemiology of multiple sclerosis. In: *Multiple Sclerosis: A Clinical Conspectus*, ed. EJ Field. Baltimore: University Park Press; 1977:35-82.
185. Behrend RC. Multiple sclerosis in Europe. *Eur Neurol*. 1969;2:129.
186. McCall MG, Brereton, TL, Dawson A, Millingen K, Sutherland JM and Acheson ED. Frequency of multiple sclerosis in three Australian cities—Perth, Newcastle, and Hobart. *J Neurol Neurosurg Psychiatry*. 1968;31:I.
187. Alter M. Clues to the cause based on the epidemiology of multiple sclerosis. In: *Multiple Sclerosis: A Clinical Conspectus*, EJ Field ed. Baltimore: University Park Press; 1977.
188. McDonald WI. Multiple Sclerosis. In: *Cambridge World History of Human Disease*. Kipple K, ed. New York: Cambridge University Press; 1993; (vii.91) 883-887.
189. MacDonald BK, Cockerall OC, Sander JWAS, Showon SD. The incidence and lifetime prevalence of neurological disorders in a prospective community-based study in the UK. *Brain*. 2000;123:665-676.
190. Kurland LT. Personal communication.
191. Alter M. Personal communication.
192. Bulman D, Ebers G. The geography of multiple sclerosis reflects genetic susceptibility. *J Trop Geog Neurol*. 1992;2:66-72.
193. Wynn DR, Rodriquez M, O'Fallon WM, Kurland LT. Update on the Epidemiology of Multiple Sclerosis. *Mayo Clin Proc*. 1989;64:808-817.
194. Wynn D. Rodriguez M, O'Fallon W, Kurland L. A reappraisal of the epidemiology of multiple sclerosis in Olmsted County, Minnesota. *Neurology*. 1992;40:780-786.
195. Poser CM. The Dissemination of Multiple Sclerosis: A Viking Saga? A Historical Essay. *Ann Neurol*. 1994;36:S231-243.
196. Sutherland JM. Multiple Sclerosis: Fifty Years On. *Clin Exp Neurol*. 1983;19:1-12.
197. Davenport C. Multiple sclerosis: from the standpoint of geographic distribution and race. *Arch Neurol Psychiatry*. 1922;8:51-58.
198. Skegg DCG, Corwin PA, Craven RS, et al. Occurrence of multiple sclerosis in the north and south of New Zealand. *J Neurol Neurosurg Psychiatry*. 1987;50:134-139.
199. Compston A. Risk Factors for Multiple Sclerosis: Race or Place? *J Neurol Neurosurg Psychiatry*. 1990;53:821-823.
200. Ebers GC, Bulman DE, Sadovnick AD, et al. A population-based study of multiple sclerosis in twins. *N Engl J Med*. 1986;315:1638-1642.
201. Swingler RJ, Compston DAS. The distribution of MS in the United Kingdom. *J Neurol Neurosurg Psychiatry*. 1986;49:1115-1124.
202. Dean G. Annual incidence, prevalence and mortality of multiple sclerosis in white South African-born and in white immigrants to South Africa. *Brit Med J*. 1976;2:724-730.
203. Rosman KD, Jacobs HA, VanDerMerwe CA. A new multiple sclerosis epidemic? A pilot survey. *South Africa Med J*. 1985;68:162-163.

204. Elian M, Nightingale S, Dean G. Multiple sclerosis among the United Kingdom born children of immigrants from the Indian Subcontinent, Africa and the West Indies. *J Neurol Neurosurg Psychiatry*. 1990;53:906-911.
205. Compston A. Risk Factors for Multiple Sclerosis: Race or Place? *J Neurol Neurosurg Psychiatry*. 1990;53:821-823.
206. Granieri E, Casetta I, Govoni V, et al. The increasing incidence and prevalence of MS in a Sardinian province. *Neurology*. 2000;55:842-847.
207. Alter M. Clues to the cause based on the epidemiology of multiple sclerosis. In: *Multiple Sclerosis: A Clinical Conspectus*, Field EJ, ed. Baltimore: University Park Press; 1977: 35-82.
208. Alter M, Hallpern L, Kurland LT, Bornstein B, Leibowitz U, Silberstein J. Multiple sclerosis in Israel. Prevalence among immigrants and native-born inhabitants. *Arch Neurol*. 1962;7:253.
209. Alter M. Clues to the cause based on the epidemiology of multiple sclerosis. In: *Multiple Sclerosis: A Clinical Conspectus*. Field EJ, ed. Baltimore: University Park Press; 1977: 35-82.
210. Kuroiwa Y. History of Multiple Sclerosis Studies in Japan. In: *Multiple Sclerosis in Asia: Proceedings of the Asian Multiple Sclerosis Workshop*, Kuroiwa Y, ed. Tokyo: University of Tokyo Press; 1977;3-5.
211. Campbell AMG, Daniel P, Porter RJ, Russell WR, Smith HV, Innes FRM. Disease of the nervous system occurring among research workers on swayback in lambs. *Brain*. 1947;70:50-59.
212. Campbell AMG, Herdan G, Tatlow WFT, Whittle EG. Lead in relation to disseminated sclerosis. *Brain*. 1950;73:52-71.
213. Dean G. Motor neuron disease and multiple sclerosis among immigrants to Britian. *Brit J Prevention and Social Medicine*. 1997;31:141-147.
214. Sutherland JM. Multiple Sclerosis: Fifty Years On. *Clin Exp Neurol*. 1983;19:1-12.
215. Deacon WE, Alexander L, Siedler HD, Kurland LT. Multiple sclerosis in a small New England community. *N Engl J Med*. 1959;261:1059-1061.
216. Kurland LT. The evolution of multiple sclerosis epidemiology. *Ann of Neurol*. 1994: 36;S2-S5.
217. Eastman R, Sheridan J, Poskanger DC. Multiple sclerosis clustering in a small Massachusetts community with possible common exposure 23 years before onset. *N Engl J Med*. 1974;289:793-794.
218. Koch MJ, Reed D, Stern R, et al. Multiple sclerosis: A cluster in a small northwestern United States community. *JAMA*. 1974;228:1555-1557.
219. Murray TJ. An Unusual Occurrence of Multiple Sclerosis in a Small Rural Community. *CJNS*. 1976;3(3):163-166.
220. Poskanzer DC, Schapiro K, Miller H. Multiple sclerosis and poliomyelitis. *Lancet*. 1963;2:917-921.
221. Kurtzke JF, Hyllested K. Multiple sclerosis in the Faeroe Islands: 1. Clinical and Epidemiological features. *Ann Neurol*. 1979;5:6-21.
222. Kurtzke JF, Hyllested K. Multiple sclerosis in the Faeroe Islands. 2. Clinical update, transmission, and the nature of MS. *Neurology*. 1986;36:307-328.
223. Kurtzke JF, Hyllested K. Multiple sclerosis in the Faeroe Islands. 3. An alternative assessment of the three epidemics. *Acta Neurol Scand*. 1987;76: 317-339.
224. Kurtzke JF, Hyllested K. Multiple sclerosis in the Faeroe Islands. II. Clinical update, transmission, and the nature of MS. *Neurology*. 1986;36:307-328.
225. Kurtzke JF, Hyllested K, Heltberg A, Olsen A. Multiple sclerosis in the Faeroe Islands. 5. The occurrence of the fourth epidemic as validation of transmission. *Acta Neurol Scand*. 1993;88:161-173.
226. Kurtzke JF, Hyllested K. Multiple sclerosis in the Faeroe Islands: 1: p. 6-21.

227. Kurtzke JF, Gurdmundsson KR, Bergmann S. Multiple sclerosis in Iceland: a postwar epidemic. *Neurology*. 1980;30:437.

228. Cook SD, Dowling PC. A possible association between house pets and multiple sclerosis. *Lancet*. 1978;1:980-982.

229. Shatin R. The geography of multiple sclerosis. *Med J Aust*. 1963;50:30-31.

230. Carlyle IP. Multiple sclerosis: a geographical hypothesis. *Medical Hypothesis*. 1997;477-486.

231. Ryle.

232. Myrian TN. Genetic aspects of multiple sclerosis. In: *Handbook of Clinical Neurology*. Vinken PJ, Bruyn, GW, eds. Amsterdam, North Holland. 1970;9:85-106.

233. Prineas JW. The etiology and pathogenesis of multiple sclerosis. In: *Handbook of Clinical Neurology*. Vinken PJ, Bruyn GW, eds. Amsterdam, North Holland. 1970;9: 107-159.

234. Charcot JM. *Oeuvres complètes. Leçons sur les maladies du système nerveux*. Paris: Vol. 1.; 1894:269.

235. Gowers WR. *A Manual of Diseases of the Nervous System*, Vol. 2. London: J&A Churchill; 1893:544, 557-558.

236. Murray TJ. The history of multiple sclerosis. In: *Multiple Sclerosis: Diagnosis, Medical Management, and Rehabilitation*. Burks J, Johnson K, eds. New York: Demos: 2000; 1-20.

237. Eichhorst H. Über infantile und hereditäre multiple Sklerose. *Virchow's Arch path Anat Berl*. 1896;146:173-192.

238. Dana CL. *Textbook of Nervous Diseases*. 3rd ed. New York: William Wood; 1894.

239. Talley C. *A History of Multiple Sclerosis and Medicine in the United States, 1870–1960*. PhD dissertation. San Francisco: University of California; 1998.

240. Holland JW. Disseminated sclerosis of the spinal cord: 3 cases in one family. *Louisville Med News*. 1882;14:283.

241. Reynolds ES. Some cases of family disseminated sclerosis. *Brain*. 1904;27:163-169.

242. Curshmann H. Ueber familiäre multiple Sklerose. *Dtsch Z Nervenheilk*. 1920;66:225-230.

243. Davenport C. Multiple sclerosis: from the standpoint of geographic distribution and race. *Arch Neurol Psychiatry*. 1922;8:51-58.

244. Brain WR. Critical review: disseminated sclerosis. *Quart J Med*. 1930;23:343-391.

245. Curtius F. *Multiple Sklerose and Erbanlage*. Leipzig: G. Thieme; 1933.

246. Ibid, p. 48.

247. Thums K. Neurologische Zwillingsstudien. I. Zur Erbpathologie der multiplen Sklerose. Eine Untersuchung an 51 Zwillingspaaren. *Z ges Neurol Psychiat*. 1936;155: 185-253.

248. McAlpine D. The problem of disseminated sclerosis. *Brain*. 1946;69:233-250.

249. MacKay RP. The familial occurrence of multiple sclerosis and its implications. In: *Multiple Sclerosis and the Demyelinating Diseases*. Proceedings of the Association for Research in Nervous and Mental Diseases. (Dec 10-11, 1948). Baltimore: Williams & Wilkins; 1950.

250. Ebers GC, Sadovnick AD. Succeptibility: genetics in multiple sclerosis. In: *Multiple Sclerosis*. DW Paty, GC Ebers, editors. Philadelphia: FA Davis. 1998;29-47.

251. Aird RB. *Foundations of Modern Neurology*. New York: Raven Press; 1994.

252. Pratt RT, Compston ND, McAlpine D. The familial incidence of multiple sclerosis and its significance. *Brain*. 1951;237:286-289.

253.

254.

255. Myrian TN. Genetic aspects of multiple sclerosis. In: *Handbook of Clinical Neurology*. VinkenPJ, Bruyn GW, eds. Amsterdam, North Holland. 1970;9:85-106.

256. Dausset J, Svejgaard A, eds. *HLA and Disease*. Copenhagen and Baltimore: Munksgaard, William and Wilkins. p. 9-11.

257. Naito D, Tabira T, Kuroiwa Y. HLA studies of multiple sclerosis in Japan. In: Duroiwa Y, Kurland LT, eds. *Multiple Sclerosis East and West*. Basel: Karger; 1982;215-222.

258. Jersid C, Fog T, Hansen GS, Thomsen M, Svejgaard A, Dupont B. Histocompatibility determinants in multiple sclerosis, with special reference to clinical course. *Lancet*. 1973;2:1221-1225.

259. Klein J, Sato A. The HLA System. *N Engl J Med*. 2000;343:702-708.

260. McDonald WI. The mystery of the origin of multiple sclerosis. Gowers Lecture. *J Neurol Neurosurg Psychiatry*. 1986;49:113-123.

261. Ebers GC. Immunology, Chapter 11. In: *Multiple Sclerosis*. Paty DW and Ebers GC, eds. Philadelphia: FA Davis; 1999;403-426.

262. Compston DAS, Batchelor JR, McDonald WI. B lymphocytes alloantigens associated with multiple sclerosis. *Lancet*. 1976;2:1261-1265.

263. Noseworthy JH, Lucchinetti C, Rodriguez M, Weinshenker BG. *Multiple Sclerosis*. N *Engl J Med*. 2000;343:938-952.

264. Compston A. The Story of Multiple Sclerosis. Chapter 1. In *McAlpine's Multiple Sclerosis*. London: Churchill Livingstone; 1998:3-42.

265. Ebers GC, Bulman DE, Sadovnick AD, et al. A population-based study of multiple sclerosis in twins. *N Engl J Med*. 1986;315:1638-1642.

266. Rindfleisch E. Histologische Detail zu der Grauen Degeneration von Gehirn and Rückenmark. *Virchow Arch Path Anat Physiol*. 1863;26:474-483.

267. Ribbert H. Ueber Multiple Sclerose des Gehirns und Rückenmarks. Archiv. für pathologische. *Anatomie und Physiologie und für Klinsche Medicin*. 1882;90:243-260.

268. Marie P. *Lectures on Diseases of the Spinal Cord*, trans. Lubbock M. London: New Sydenham Society; 1895;153:134-136.

269. Dana CL. *Textbook of Nervous Diseases*. 3rd ed. New York: William Wood; 1894.

270. Putnam TJ. The pathogenesis of multiple sclerosis: a possible vascular factor. *New Engl J Med*. 1933;209:786.

271. Putnam TJ. Studies in Multiple Sclerosis. *Arch Neurol Psych*. 1936;35:1289-1308.

272. Hurst EW, Cooke BT, Melvin P. Experimental demyelination. *Austral J Exper Biol and Med Sci*. 1943;21:115-120.

273. Putnam TJ, Chiavacci LV, Hoff H, et al. Results of treatment of multiple sclerosis with dicoumarin. *Arch Neurol*. 1947;57:1-13.

274. Association for Research in Nervous and Mental Disease. *Multiple Sclerosis and the Demyelinating Diseases*. Baltimore: Williams and Wilkins; 1950.

275. McAlpine D. The problem of disseminated sclerosis. *Brain*. 1946;69:233-250.

276. Talley, Colin. *A History of Multiple Sclerosis and Medicine in the United States, 1870–1960*. PhD dissertation. San Francisco: University of California; 1998.

277. Brickner RM. Multiple Sclerosis. *Med Clin North America*. 1948;32:743-750.

278. Swank RL. Multiple sclerosis: a correlation of its incidence with dietary fat. *Am J M Sc*. 1950;220:421-430.

279. Swank RL, Lerstad O, Ström A, Backer J. Multiple sclerosis in rural Norway: its geographic and occupational incidence in relation to nutrition. *N Engl J Med*. 1952;246:721-728.

280. Swank RL. Plasma and multiple sclerosis—past and present. In: *Multiple Sclerosis: Immunological, diagnostic and therapeutic aspects*. Rose FC and Jones R, eds. *Current Problems in Neurology* Vol 3. London: John Libbey Eurotext; 1987:217-220.

281. Swank RL, Duncan BB. *The Multiple Sclerosis Diet Book*. New York: Doubleday; 1987.

282. Courville CB, Courville DA. Multiple sclerosis as a possible manifestation of cerebral embolism related to disturbance in lipid metabolism. *J Loma Linda Univ Sch Med*. 1966:20:99-114.

283. Paty DW, Ebers GC, eds. *Multiple Sclerosis*. Philadelphia: FA Davis; 1998: p. 410.
284. Dawson JD. *The Histology of Disseminated Sclerosis*. Trans Royal Soc Edin. 1916;50:517-740.
285. Dawson JD. The Histology of Disseminated Sclerosis. *Rev Neurol and Psychiat*. 1917;15:47-166; 369-417, 1918; 16:287-307.
286. Lumsden CE. The neuropathology of multiple sclerosis. In: *Multiple Sclerosis and Other Demyelinating Diseases*. Vinken PJ and Bruyn GW, eds. *Handbook of Clinical Neurology* Vol 9. North Holland. Amsterdam. 1970:217-309.
287. Prineas JW. The neuropathology of multiple sclerosis. In: *Handbook of Clinical Neurology*, Vol 3(47). Koestsier JC, Vinken PJ, Bruyn GW, and Klawans HL, eds. Amsterdam: Elsevier; 1985:213-257.
288. Raine CS, Wu E. Multiple Sclerosis: remyelination in acute lesions. *J Neuropthol Exp Neurol*. 1993;52:199-204.
289. Prineas JW, McDonald WI. Demyelinating Diseases. In: *Greenfield's Neuropathology*, 6th ed. Graham DI and Lantos PL, eds. New York: Oxford University Press; 1997:813-896.
290. Waksman BH. Multiple Sclerosis. In: *Clinical Aspects of Immunology*, eds. PJ Lachman, K Peters, FS Rosen, MJ Walport. 5th ed. Boston: Blackwell Scientific; 1993:2153-2175.
291. Waksman BH. Historical Perspective and Overview. In: *Clinical Neuroimunology*. Antel J, ed. London: Blackwell; 1998:391-404.
292. Waksman BH. The Way Things Were: The discovery of experimental "allergic" neuritis. In: *Immunology and Infectious Diseases of the Peripheral Nerves*. Lator N, Wokke JHJ, and Kelly JJ, eds. Cambridge: Cambridge University Press; 1998:xiv-xviii.
293. Waksman BH. Demyelinating Disease: Evolution of a Paradigm. *Neurochemical Research*. 1999;24:(4)491-495.
294. Glanzmann FL. Die nervosen Komplikationen von Varizellen, Variole Vakzine. *Schweiz med Wschr*. 1927;57:145.
295. Van Bogaert L. Essai d'interprétation des manifestations nerveuses au cours de la vaccination, de la maladie sérique et des maladies éruptives. *Rev Neurol*. 1932;2:12.
296. Rivers TJ, Sprunt DH, Berry GP. Observations on attempts to produce acute disseminated encephalomyelitis in monkeys. *J Exp Med*. 1933;58:39-53.
297. Rivers TM, Schwentker F. Encephalomyelitis accompanied by myelin destruction experimentally produced in monkeys. *J Exp Med*. 1935;61:698-702.
298. Ferraro A. Pathology of demyelinating diseases as an allergic reaction in the brain. *Arch Neurol Psychiat*. 1944;52:443-483.
299. Lumden C. The pathology and pathogenesis of multiple sclerosis. In: *Scientific Aspects of Neurology*. Garland H, ed. Edinburgh: Livingstone. p. 16.
300. Ferraro A. Pathology of demyelinating diseases as an allergic reaction in the brain. *Arch Neurol Psychiat*. 1944;52:443-483.
301. Medawar P. Personal Papers of Sir Peter Brian Medawar FRS, OM (1915–1987, Medical Scientist, Nobel Laureate, Collected by Dr. Robert Reid. Wellcome Archives and MSS, PP/PBM).
302. McAlpine D. The problem of disseminated sclerosis. *Brain*. 1946;69:233-250.
303. McAlpine D, Compston ND, Lumsden CE. *Multiple Sclerosis*. Edinburgh: E&S Livingston; 1955.
304. McAlpine D, Compston ND, Lumsden CE. *Multiple Sclerosis: a reappraisal*. 2nd ed. Edinburgh: E & S Livingston; 1972:512-597.
305. Waksman BH. The Way Things Were: The discovery of experimental allergic neuritis. In: *Immunology and Infectious Deseases of the Peripheral Nerves*. Lator N, Wokke JHJ, and Kelly JJ, eds. Cambridge: Cambridge university Press; 1998:xiv-xviii.
306. Waksman BH. Historial perspective and overview. In: *Clinical Neuroimunolgy*. Antil J, ed. Blackwell Science Inc. 1988, chapter 26;391-404.

307. Waksman BH. *The Way Things Were*: p. xiv-xvii.
308. Paty DW, Ebers GC, eds. *Multiple Sclerosis*. Philadelphia: FA Davis; 1998:29-47.
309. Poskanzer DC, Schapiro K, Miller H. Multiple sclerosis and poliomyelitis. *Lancet*. 1963;2:917-921.
310. Waksman BH. Historial perspective and overview. In: *Clinical Neuroimmunology*. Antil J, ed. Blackwell Science Inc. 1988, chapter 26;391-404.
311. Murray TJ. An Unusual Occurrence of Multiple Sclerosis in a Small Rural Community. *CJNS*. 1976;3(3):163-166.
312. Lisak RP. Overview of the rationale for immunomodulating therapies in multiple sclerosis. *Neurology*. 1988;38(suppl 2):5-8.
313. McDonald WI, Miller DH, Barnes D. The pathological evolution of multiple sclerosis. *Neuropath and Applied Neurobiol*. 1992;18:319-334.
314. McDonald WI. The pathological and clinical dynamics of multiple sclerosis. *J Neuropath Exp Neurol*. 1994;53:338-343.
315. Trapp BD, Peterson J, Ransohoff RM, Rudick R, Mörks, Bö L. Axonal transections in the lesions of multiple sclerosis. *N Engl J Med*. 1998;338:278-285.
316. Broadly SA, Deans J, Sawcer SJ, Clayton D, Compston DAS. Autoimmune disease in first-degree relatives of patients with multiple sclerosis. *Brain*. 2000; 123:1102-1111.
317. Ebers GC. Immunology of MS. Chapter 11. In: *Multiple Sclerosis*. Eds. Donald W. Paty and George C. Ebers. Philadelphia: FA Davis; 1999:403-426.
318. Noseworthy JH, Lucchinetti C, Rodriguez M, Weinshenker BG. *Multiple Sclerosis*. *N Engl J Med*. 2000;343:938-952.
319. Anon. *At Home with Multiple Sclerosis*. Multiple Sclerosis Society of Great Britain and Northern Ireland; 1970.
320. Rindfleisch E. Histologische Detail zu der Grauen Degeneration von Gehirn and Rückenmark. *Virchow Arch Path Anat Physiol*. 1863;26:474-483.
321. Leyden E. Ueber graue Degeneration des Rückenmarks. *Deutsche Klin*. 1863;15:121-128.
322. Hammond WA. A treatise on diseases of the nervous system. Ch. VII, in *Multiple Cerebro-spinal Sclerosis*. New York: D. Appleton; 1871:637-653.
323. Bastian HC. An anomalous case of cerebrospinal sclerosis. *Med Times and Gazette*. London. 1883;2:451.
324. Clevenger SV. *Spinal Concussion*. London: FA Davis. 1889.
325. Mendel K. Tabes and multiple Sklerose in inhren Beziehungen zum Trauma. *Neurol Ctrbl*. 1897;16:140-141.
326. Church A, Peterson F. *Nervous and Mental Diseases*. London: Rebman Publishing; 1899:434-442.
327. Klausner I. Ein Beitrag zur Aetiologie der multiplen Sklerose. *Arch Psychiatr Nervenk*. 1901;34:841-868.
328. Hoffmann J. Die multiple Sklerose des Centralnervensystems. *Dtsch Zts Nervenheilk*. 1902;21:1-27.
329. Association for Research in Nervous and Mental Disease. *Multiple Sclerosis (Disseminated sclerosis)*. New York: Paul B. Hoeber; 1922:48.
330. Brain WR. Critical review: disseminated sclerosis. *Quart J Med*. 1930;23:343-391.
331. Wilson SAK. *Neurology*, Bruce AN, ed. London: Edward Arnold; 1940:148-178.
332. Harris W. The traumatic factor in organic nervous disease. *Br Med J*. 1933;4:955-960.
333. von Hoesslin R. *Ueber multiple Sklerose: Exogene Aetiologie, Pathogenese, und Verlauf*, Munich: J.F. Lehmanns; 1934:68-74.
334. Keschner M. The effect of injuries and illness on the course of multiple sclerosis. *Res Publ Assoc Nerv Ment Dis*. 1950;28:533-547.
335. Brickner RH, Simons DJ. Emotional stress in relation to attacks of multiple sclerosis. In: *Multiple Sclerosis and the Demyelinating Diseases*. Proceedings of the Association for

Research in Nervous and Mental Disease (Dec. 10–11, 1948). Vol 28. Baltimore: Williams and Wilkins; 1950:471-511.

336. McAlpine D. The problem of disseminated sclerosis. *Brain.* 1946;69:233-250.

337. McAlpine D, Compston ND. Some aspects of the natural history of disseminated sclerosis. *Quart J Med.* 1952;21:135-167.

338. Kurland LT, Westlund KB. Epidemiologic factors in the etiology and prognosis of multiple sclerosis. *Ann NY Acad Sci.* 1954;58:682.

339. Ridley A, Schapira K. Influence of surgical procedures on the course of multiple sclerosis. *Neurology.* 1961;11:81-82.

340. Kelly R. Clinical aspects of multiple sclerosis. In: *Handbook of Clinical Neurology.* Vinken PJ, Bruyn GW, Koestier C, eds. Amsterdam: Elsevier; 1985:47:49-78.

341. Alter M, Speer J. Clinical evaluation of possible etiologic factors in multiple sclerosis. *Neurology.* 1968;18:109-115.

342. Sibley WA, Bamford CR, Clark K. A prospective study of physical trauma and multiple sclerosis. *J Neurol Neurosurg Psychiat.* 1991;54:584-589.

343. Sibley WA. Physical trauma and multiple sclerosis (Editorial). *Neurology.* 1993;43:1871-1874.

344. Sibley WA. Risk factors in multiple sclerosis. In: *Multiple Sclerosis: Clinical and Pathogenic Basis*, eds CS Raine, HF McFarland, WW Tourtellotte. London: Chapman and Hal; 1997:141-148.

345. Sibley WA. Risk factors in multiple sclerosis: implications for pathogenesis. In: Crescenzi GS, ed. *A Multidisciplinary Approach to Myelin Diseases.* NATO Advanced Research Series. New York: Plenum: 1988:227-232.

346. Sibley WA, Bamford CR, Clark K, Smith MS, Laguna JF. A prospective study of physical trauma and multiple sclerosis. *J Neurol Neurosurg Psychiat.* 1991;54:584-589.

347. Sibley WA. A prospective study of physical trauma and multiple sclerosis. A reply. *J Neurol Neurosurg Psychiat.* 1992;55:524. Letter.

348. Siva A, Radhakrishnan K, Kurland LT, O'Brien PC, Swanson JW, Rodriguez M. Trauma and multiple sclerosis from Olmsted County, Minnesota. *Neurology.* 1993;43:1878-1882.

349. Gusev E, Boiko A, Lauer K, et al. Environmental risk factors in MS: a case-control study in Moscow. *Acta Neurol Scand.* 1996;94:386-394.

350. American Academy of Neurology. *Report of the Therapeutics and Technology Assessment Subcommittee on MS and Trauma.* Minneapolis. 1999.

351. Firth D. The Case of Augustus d'Este (1794-1848): the first account of disseminated sclerosis. *Proc Royal Soc Med* 1940-41;34:499-52.

352. Firth D. *The Case of Augustus d'Esté.* Cambridge. Cambridge University Press; 1948:21.

353. Charcot JM. *Lectures on the Diseases of the Nervous System.* Trans. by G. Sigerson. London: The New Sydenham Society. 1877, vol. 1: 220.

354. MoxonW. Eight cases of insular sclerosis of the brain and spinal cord. *Guy Hospital Reports.* 1875;20:437-478.

355. Russell JSR. Disseminated sclerosis, in Albutt TC, ed. *A System of Medicine.* London: Macmillan;1899:50-94.

356. Bramwell B, The prognosis of disseminated sclerosis. *Edin Med J.* 1917;18:16-19.

357. McAlpine D. The problem of disseminated sclerosis. *Brain.* 1946;69:233-250.

358. Adams JM. *Multiple Sclerosis: Scars of Childhood: New Horizons and Hope.* Springfield, IL: Charles C. Thomas; 1977.

359. Wilson SAK. *Neurology.* Bruce AN, ed. London: Edward Arnold; 1940:148-178.

360. Selye H. *The Physiology and Pathology of Exposure to Stress: a Treatise on the Concepts of the General-Adaptation-Syndrome and the Diseases of Adaptation.* Montreal: Acta; 1950.

361. Randt CT, Trager CH, Merritt HH. A clinical study of the effect of ACTH on chronic neurological disorders in seven patients. *Proc 1st Clin ACTH Conf.* Mohr JR, ed. Philadelphia: Blakiston; 1950:595.

362. Brickner RH, Simons DJ. Emotional stress in relation to attacks of multiple sclerosis. In: *Multiple Sclerosis and the Demyelinating Diseases*. Proceedings of the Association for Research in Nervous and Mental Disease (Dec. 10–11, 1948). Vol 28. Baltimore: Williams and Wilkins; 1950:471-511.

363. Pratt RTC. An investigation of the psychiatric aspects of disseminated sclerosis. *J Neurol Neurosurg Psychiat*. 1951;14:326-335.

364. Philippopoulos GS, Wittkower ED, Cousineau A. The etiologic significance of emotional factors in onset and exacerbations of multiple sclerosis. *Psychosom Med*. 1958;20:458-474.

365. Pratt RTC. An investigation of the psychiatric aspects of disseminated sclerosis. *J Neurol Neurosurg Psychiat*. 1951;14:326-335.

366. Baldwin MV. A clinico-experimental investigation into the psychologic aspects of multiple sclerosis. *J Nerv Ment Dis*. 1952;115:229-342.

367. Malmbren R, Detels R, Visscher B, Chen S, Clark V. The effect of stress on the course of multiple sclerosis. Presentation to 10th Scientific Meeting of the International Epidemiological Association, Vancouver, BC; 1984.

368. Rabins PV, Brooks BR, O'Donnell, et al. Structural brain correlates of emotional disorder in multiple sclerosis. *Brain*. 1986;109:585-597.

369. Franklin GM, Nelson LM, Heaton RK, et al. Stress and its relationship to acute exacerbations in multiple sclerosis. *J Neurol Rehab*. 1988;2:7-11.

370. Grant I, Brown GW, Harris T, et al. Severely threatening events and marked life difficulties preceding onset or exacerbation of multiple sclerosis. *J Neurol Neurosurg Psychiat*. 1989;52:8-13.

371. Warren S, Greenhill S, Warren KG. Emotional stress and the development of multiple sclerosis: Case control evidence of a relationship. *J Chron Dis*. 1982;35:821-831

372. Warren W, Warren KG, Cockerill R. Emotional stress and coping in multiple sclerosis (MS) exacerbations. *J Psychosomat Res*. 1991;35:37-47.

373. Nisipeanu P, Korczyn AD. Psychological stress as a risk factor for exacerbation in multiple sclerosis. *Neurology*. 1993;43:1311-1312.

374. Sibley WA. Risk factors in multiple sclerosis. In: *Multiple Sclerosis: Clinical and Pathogenic Basis*. Raine CS, McFarland HF, Tourtellotte WW, eds. London: Chapman and Hal; 1997:141-148.

375. American Academy of Neurology. Report of the Therapeutics and Technology Assessment Subcommittee on MS and Trauma. 1999.

376. Mohr DC, Goodkin DE, Bacchetti P, et al. Psychological stress and the subsequent appearance of new brain MRI lesions in MS. *Neurology*. 2000;55:55-61.

377. Oppenheim H. *Zur Pathologie der disseminierten Sklerose*. Berlin: klin. Wschr. 1887:904-907.

378. Oppenheim H. *Text-book of Nervous Diseases for Physicians and Students*, trans. A. Bruce. Edinburgh: Otto Schulze; 1911.

379. Barker L. Exogenous causes of disseminated sclerosis. *ANP*. 1922;8:47-50.

380. Confavreux C, Suissa S, Saddier P, et al. and the Vaccines in Multiple Sclerosis Group. Vaccinations and the risk of relapse in multiple sclerosis. *New Engl J Med*. 2001;344:319-326.

12

Classifying and Measuring MS

W hen MS was first defined, the diagnosis was based on the presence of certain clinical findings and sometimes confirmed by autopsy. Charcot, Marie, and others also classified the patients according to anatomical involvement, as reflected in the clinical findings and supported by later autopsy examination. Charcot recognized four variations of MS: a spinal form, a cerebral form, a cerebrospinal form, and "abortive" forms, which he referred to as *formes frustes*.

Marie classified cases as spastic, cerebellar, and cerebro-spastic and later into the type of course as chronic progressive; chronic course with intermittent attacks, chronic remitting course, and increased improvement with apparent cure.

In 1906, Marburg tried to classify MS patients according to the course of the disease, separating patients into acute, rapidly progressive, chronic progressive without symptoms, typical remitting type with attacks and remissions, and a stationary type.[1] With modification, this approach has been used by most clinicians since. Curschmann in 1908 added a type he regarded as a benign form of MS.[2] In 1943, McIntyre and McIntyre tried to simplify the classification into three types: acute; remittent; and chronic progressive,[3] and in 1950, Allison used this classification in his epidemiological studies.[4] Others simplified classification further to two forms: remitting type and progressive type (Birley and Dudgeon, 1921,[5] Putnam et al., 1947,[6] Schumacher, 1950[7]).

Bramwell, writing the section in later editions of Osler's textbook, divided cases into various types: classical with the Charcot triad, cerebrospinal, intermittent or hysterical, spinal, cerebral, and sacral type.[8] Oppenheim first tried to classify MS according to localization of the pathology, but the rigorous allocation to areas of neuroanatomy based on clinical features was not practical since the patients did not often have such clearly defined anatomical levels, or they displayed many, which changed from attack to attack. Spitzka referred to the bulbar form as "Oblongata type" of MS. Another impractical approach was that of Marquézy, who divided all cases into monsymptomatic and oligosymptomatic.[9] Purves-Stewart had a classification system for the assessment of the cases treated with his *Spirula insularis* vaccine, dividing them into light, moderately advanced, and severe cases.[10]

Other attempts at classification by Guillain in 1924 and Barré in 1948 were no more helpful or practical. Even in their own hands, the system devised by Carter, Sciarra, and Merritt in 1950[11] with a six-level classification: spinal, spinal-cerebellar, brain stem, brain stem-spinal, spinal-optic, and mixed, was impractical in practice. It had the problems of the earlier Oppenheim classification, and was not adopted by other authors. At the end of five years, 56 percent of the MS cases were susceptible to the Carter classification, but by 15 years only 22 percent were, as most cases had fallen into the mixed type.*[12]

The simple line diagrams of the many courses MS patients could take throughout their disease published in the first edition of McAlpine's *Multiple Sclerosis* (1955) became the way clinicians saw and classified the disease.[13] This diagram continues to be shown to illustrate the courses of the disease. In 1952, McAlpine and Compston classified MS into *those with relapses and remission* and those with a *chronic progression*, either from onset or after a number of relapses. By 1955, they had changed the chron-

---

*While clinicians were separating the disease into types, Ferraro argued in 1944 that all demyelinating diseases could be included under one large umbrella pathologically.

ic progressive form to *those with progression after a number of relapses*, or *progression from the beginning*.[14] In 1954, Allison and Miller classified *early*, *probable*, *possible*, and *discarded* in their assessment of cases epidemiologically.[15]

In his review of the status of MS in 1950, George Schumacher divided patients into the remittent form and the steadily progressive form.[16] Schumacher later headed a committee to develop criteria for the classification of MS to be used in clinical practice, but particularly for clinical trials. The principles used by John Kurtzke in evaluating American veterans were codified by the Schumacher panel in 1965 after three years of argument.[17,18] Later, the concept of "definite MS" was added. Criteria since then have built upon the work by Kurtzke and the Schumacher criteria. Further modifications were made by Rose in 1976.[19] In 1977, McDonald and Halliday developed a criteria that was used in many clinical trials and studies for a number of years.[20] (A discussion of the criteria and the outline of each are in the 1988 Kurtzke paper mentioned above.)

The Schumacher criteria were later replaced by criteria developed at the Washington Conference (1983), convened by Dr. Charles Poser; these are now referred to as the Poser criteria.[21,22]

Schumacher Criteria

1. There must be clinical evidence for lesions indicating primarily white matter dysfunction disseminated in time and space in a patient in the expected age range of 10–50 years.
2. There must be objective abnormalities in the neurological examination.
3. The time period for dissemination of lesion should be either:
   a. At least two clear-cut episodes of functionally significant symptoms, each lasting more than 24 hours and being separated by at least one month; or
   b. Slow, progressive development of the same disseminated pattern evolving over at least six months.
4. The diagnosis must be made by a competent clinician and there must be no better explanation for the diagnosis.

The Schumacher classification was a clinical criteria and was useful in the postwar era of clinical trials, but the Poser criteria included many of the clinical criteria of Schumacher as well as new diagnostic testing to help confirm the diagnosis. The Poser criteria grouped patients according to how well the features complied with the criteria: clinically definite MS, laboratory-supported definite MS, probable MS, laboratory-supported probable MS, or possible MS. Each category was accompanied by an explanation.

Only the clinically definite and probable MS cases were included in therapeutic clinical trials.* In the 1990s, patients have been classified according to their initial course, beginning as relapsing-remitting (85 percent) and primary-progressive (15 percent). The later course of MS may be relapsing-remitting, secondary-progressive (relapsing-progressive), primary-progressive, or benign. Other variants are malignant-progressive, optic-neuritis, and transverse myelitis. The terminology has not yet been standardized, a state necessary for clinical trials and treatment decisions and prognosis.

Schumacher defined the age range as 10–50, although confirmed cases are seen outside of this range. Hanefield et al. reviewed the reported cases of childhood MS[23] and Duquette, Murray, et al. collected a large series of cases in Canada from MS clinics and showed they differed little from the adult pattern.[24]

Donald Paty has been concerned with the accuracy of diagnosis in MS and the development of better criteria for diagnosis and classification. He has mentioned (Paty, personal communication) some researchers had wondered why he was so preoccupied with accuracy in a disease for which there was no therapy; his answer was always that if the background work were not done, there would be serious confusion when new therapies did appear. New therapies are now here, and the lack of clear classification has caused problems. It is evident that certain patterns of MS respond to these therapies and others do not.

In 1996, the Advisory Committee on Clinical Trials of the National Multiple Sclerosis Society[25] sought consensus on definitions and found that

---

*In an age of MRI, "laboratory-supported definite MS" is taken to mean supported by a positive MRI, but this originally referred to positive oligoclonal banding in the CSF.

there was agreement on the classification of relapsing-remitting, second-ary-progressive, and primary progressive disease courses, but not on relaps-ing-progressive; they recommended this term be abandoned, and the term progressive-relapsing be established for the occasional case with progression with relapses, with or without recovery. This has not ended the discussion, however, as new MRI studies and therapeutic responses will cause the criteria to change further and the definition becomes useful. The definition of benign MS needs clarification, as does the concept of progression. Progression of one point on the Kurtzke scale on two assessments a month apart has been taken as the measure of progression in some clinical trials.

Benign MS is much more difficult to define and is perhaps the type with the least clarity. Everyone knows there is a benign form, but at what point is it possible to say it is benign? What are the predictors that might allow one to say that a patient's MS would likely turn out to be benign? Or is it a form that can only be diagnosed in retrospect, after 10, or 15, or 20 years with minimal disability? (Neurologists do not agree on the time period). And is it really benign since it may be seen to progress much later in the disease?

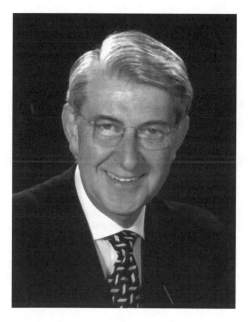

Figure 12.1 Professor W. Ian McDonald made substantial contributions to many aspects of MS over 40 years of clinical investigations at the National Hospital, Queen Square. In the 1960s he characterized the pattern of demyelination and remyelination. In the 1970s he pioneered laboratory techniques and understanding of conduction in normal and abnormal nerves. Since the 1980s he has led the use of MRI technology to understand the underlying mechanisms in MS and how MRI can be used to assess therapies. He has been a leader in collaborations and organizations committed to MS research and care. He currently is Harverian Librarian at the Royal College of Physicians, London. (Courtesy of Professor W. Ian MacDonald.)

A new set of diagnostic criteria was formulated in 2001 by an international committee convened by the National MS Society and the MS International Federation chaired by Professor W. Ian McDonald.[26]

RATING THE DISABILITY

Until 1950, the evaluation of clinical change and the change with therapy was general and subjective and required a decision by the physician and the patient about whether things were better, the same, or worse. In 1950, Arkin et al.[27] attempted a more objective measure in a clinical trial of tetraethylammonium chloride in MS and in 1951, Leo Alexander[28] went further in attempting to devise a scale that could be applied to any clinical therapeutic trial. This was an important concept that moved away from a general subjective decision to a more systemized approach. Although it was a clumsy scale, with a complex system of 30 neurological signs and disabilities, with variable numerical values, some repetitions, and a score that came from adding the 30 numbers, it opened the door to the development of better measures. The refinement of such measures continues to evolve with experience in continuing clinical trials.

In 1955 and 1961, Kurtzke put forward a "new scale for evaluating disability in multiple sclerosis," which he developed for a study of the effect of isoniazid as a therapy initiated in 1953.*[29] The Disability Status Scale (DSS) became widely used, and in 1983, this evolved into the Expanded Disability Status Scale, which is used in virtually all clinical trials.[30] There were some problems with the original DSS scoring, with insensitivity in the mid-range of functional changes, so Kurtzke proposed the Expanded Disability Status Scale (EDSS), which allowed the steps to be further subdivided (1; 1.5; 2; 2.5; 3 instead of just 1 and 2 and 3).[31–34]

The EDSS scale of John Kurtzke measures function in the patient and is based on the neurological examination. The scale goes from normal examination (0) to death (10) and is heavily based on clinical findings,

---

*It is interesting to note the nature of clinical research, seeking more accurate answers to questions. The first isoniazid trial by Kurtzke was positive, but when he organized the first multicenter, randomized, placebo-controlled trial of MS therapy, the final results did not confirm the initial results. Such is the nature of clinical research.

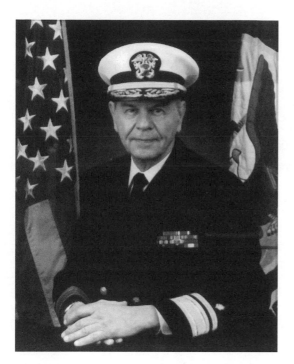

Figure 12.2 Dr. John F. Kurtzke coupled a career of contributions to MS research and epidemiology with a career of clinical neurology, residency training in the Veterans Administration and at Naval Hospital, Bethesda, rising from a pharmacist mate during WWII to Rear Admiral when he retired from the Naval Reserve in 1986. He continues a very active career in the epidemiology of MS. He has been awarded the Charcot Prize and the Dystel Prize for contributions to MS research. (Courtesy of Dr. John Kurtzke.)

with little attempt to assess subjective symptoms. Later a functional scale with eight groups was added; the groups were mostly rated from 0 to 5 or 6, but were independent measures, and the results were not added up to a score.

Although reasonably reproducible in inter-rater and intra-rater studies, the EDSS has been criticized for being focused on mobility, for ignoring many features of the disease that are significant to the patient (e.g., fatigue, pain, quality of life), and for being bimodal in assessment of groups of MS patients. When a large population of MS patients is assessed by the EDSS, the scores are not evenly distributed through the scale, either by numbers or by time at various phases. There are large numbers at EDSS 1–3 and 6–8, with fewer patients in the 4–5 stages. Seen another way, patients spend more time getting from EDSS 0 to EDSS 3, move quickly through EDSS 4 and 5 and then have more years in stages EDSS 6 and 7 and beyond.

Despite these concerns, the scale devised by Kurtzke was a practical and reproducible system that, with modifications, remains the standard in all trials almost a half a century later. It can be argued, and was argued by Kurtzke, that the more lesions, the more signs, and that symptoms are unreliable. His scale was based primarily on objective neurological signs and was essentially a modification of the standard neurological examination familiar to all clinicians. Although relatively simple and structured, it had the great advantage of achieving reasonably similar results if the tests were done over time, and by different examiners. This was important, as trials were already getting bigger, involving many clinicians in many centers, and the scoring by different examiners should be the same, whether in Baltimore, Toronto, or Athens.

There have been mumblings by those who have used the scale for 40 years, but without much evidence of a better way to rate MS. The most notable critics have been Willoughby and Paty,[35] but the EDSS continues to be the international standard. Kurtzke likened the scale, with all its deficiencies, to democracy, which has been called the worst form of government—except for all the others.

There have been other scales. The Scripps Neurologic Rating Scale (NRS),[36] the Troiano Scale (TS),[37] the Quantitative Examination of Neurological Function (QENF) 1,[38] and the Hauser Ambulatory Index[39] have all attempted to capture the global involvement of MS in an objective and reproducible way.*[40] Measures of disability have included the Incapacity Status Scale (ISS)[41] and the Functional Independence Measure (FIM).[42] Measures of handicap include the Environmental Status Scale (ESS) and the Minimal Record of Disability (MRD).[43] There are also various measurements of the quality of life (QOL), some general for any disease and some specifically designed for MS.

Recently, the NMSS task force recommended the use of a quantative functional scale using three functional tests: the timed 25-foot walk, the 9-hole peg test, and the paced auditory serial addition test (PASAT), combined into the MS Functional Composite (MSFC).[44] In the next few years, these methods of measuring multiple sclerosis effects will evolve and undoubtedly combine what the neurologist measures with what the patient experiences.

---

*All the various neurological rating scales are reviewed by Robert N. Herndon.

RELAPSE RATE

Judging the effect of therapy requires an understanding of the frequency of attacks of MS and the eventual prognosis. In 1947, Putnam et al. found there was an attack every 2.3 years in his study of patients prior to therapy with dicoumerol.[45] In an extensive statistical study of 3,797 attacks in 810 patients over an average observation period of 9.7 years, Müller found an attack occurred once every two years.[46] Current understanding is that the attack rate is extremely variable, but averages one attack every 1.25 years.

There has been some confusion about what features indicated a poor prognosis. In 1921, Birley and Dudgeon found the most favorable prognosis in those who were having acute attacks.[47] This was confirmed by Misch-Frankl (1931), Brain (1936), and Miller (1949). In 1950, MacLean et al. calculated that patients with recurrent attacks of MS became disabled at a rate of four percent per year.[48] Coates noted in 1930 that patients with a gradual onset of MS were unlikely to have remissions.[49] Thygesen found from his cases that of those with a progressive onset in the first year, 43 percent were dead at 15 years, while of those with relapses and remissions in the first year, only 21 percent were dead at 15 years.[50] It was accepted that those with signs of cerebellar disease had a poor prognosis (Misch-Frankl 1931, Brown and Putnam 1939, Thygesen 1949), and those with a spinal form of MS had a better prognosis (Brain 1936, Sciarra, and Carter 1950). Thygesen felt that in his MS cases, and in many published series, onset later in life had a better prognosis, and Brain (1936), and McAlpine (1946) agreed. In contrast, others found a better prognosis for MS if the onset was earlier (Miller 1949, Müller 1949).

Müller felt that the discrepancies in prognosis and other features in the disease were:

> *"artificial, caused by 'statistics,' and a result of the different prognostic criteria and extremely varying interpretation of 'slowly progressive disease,' 'rapidly progressive course,' 'persistent progression of symptoms,' 'progressive bouts, etc. The inaccuracy of retrospective evaluation, moreover, contributes to increase the confusion."*
>
> R. Müller, 1949[51]

These disease criteria continue to evolve and the definitions of attacks have been increasingly refined by clinical trials that used relapses as a primary outcome measurement. These clinical trials have also repeatedly noted that the number of relapses or attacks decrease over time, so even in a trial of an ineffective therapy, the number of relapses goes down over the years the patients are assessed.

FORMES FRUSTES

Charcot indicated we would learn more about the variations and variants of MS with more experience and this would increase the recognition and diagnosis of the disease. He called these variations *formes frustes*. Today

Demyelinating Syndromes

- Acute variants
  - Acute disseminated encephalomyelitis
  - Acute necrotizing transverse myelitis
  - Marburg-type malignant multiple sclerosis
  - Baló's concentric sclerosis
  - Schilder's sclerosis
  - Devic's neuromyelitis optica
  - Concentric lacunar leucoencephalopathy
  - Transitional sclerosis
- Chronic variants (multiple sclerosis)
  - Relapsing remitting
    - Secondary-progressive
    - Primary-progressive
    - Progressive-relapsing
    - Benign
- Isolated Syndromes
  - Optic neuritis
  - Transverse myelitis
- MS diagnosed on biopsy or autopsy or MRI
  - Large tumor-like areas of demyelination
  - Asymptomatic demyelination

some of the later defined variations are included in the diagnosis of MS; others are defined separately and tenuously related to multiple sclerosis; still others are regarded as separate conditions.

Poser clarified the array of disorders affecting the myelin sheath by classifying them into three categories: 1) the myelinoclastic diseases including MS and disseminated encephalomyelitis; 2) the dysmyelinating diseases with inborn errors of metabolism such as the leukodystrophies; and 3) inflammatory conditions such as subacute sclerosing panecephalitis.[52]

As the disease became better defined, more and more forms, variations, and subtle presentations became recognized as MS. Initially, only a florid case that had progressed to significant involvement would be diagnosed as MS, when many of the characteristic features were present. For instance, the "Charcot triad," thought to useful in the early years (ophthalmoplegia, ataxia, and scanning speech), was present in as few as 10 percent of the cases recognized as MS by neurologists by the late 19th century. Initially, other variants such as the combination of optic neuritis with myelitis (Devic's disease) were thought to be coincidences; later, they were regarded as variants of MS. More recently, they have been seen as separate diseases.

Acute diffuse demyelination cases have been called by a number of terms: acute MS, acute encephalomyelitis disseminata, Marburg's disease, or Schilder's disease. These were reviewed by Sigrid Poser, who presented five cases in young adults.[53]

ACUTE DISSEMINATED ENCEPHALITIS (ADEM)

Initially, there were comparisons of multiple sclerosis, especially in acute presentations, with allergic disseminated encephalmyelitis. Dawson, Turnbull, Putnam, Lumsden, and Müller felt ADEM was only quantitatively different from MS. Van Bogaert described five of 19 cases who progressed to MS, but today we might call many of those cases acute MS. McAlpine and Miller differentiated ADEM from MS and regarded the conditions as separate. Henry Miller used ACTH to treat ADEM and from this promising experience, suggested it might be a useful therapy in MS. Initially thought to be an acute form of MS, ADEM now is seen as a separate disorder, a postinfectious CNS inflammation mostly in children.[54]

MARBURG'S DISEASE

In 1906, Marburg published a series of 19 cases of MS from the literature and three of his own, of a condition of acute demyelination that he called "encephalomyelitis periaxialis scleroticans,"[55] an analogy to the acute demyelination described in the peripheral nervous system by Gombault as "neuritis periaxialis." Many of the patients had a dramatic onset and rapid progression to death. Bitsch recently reviewed the pathological changes of demyelination in cases of Marburg's disease.[56]

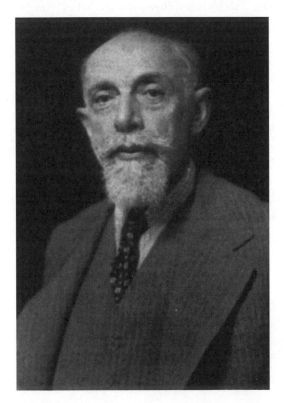

Figure 12.3 Otto Marburg (1874–1948) was a prominent neuropathologist and director of the Neurological Institute of Vienna when the Nazi regime forced him to escape to the United States, where he became Clinical Professor of Neurology at Columbia University, and continued his neuropathological research at Montefiore Hospital and the Neurological Institute of New York. Although he wrote over 200 original papers and many books, when he wrote his own obituary, to save his friends the trouble, he mentioned that his work on MS was an important step in the study of the disease. (From the collection of Mrs. Malvine Marburg.)

SCHILDER'S DISEASE

Schilder's initial case was a 14-year-old girl who had an acute onset of raised intracranial pressure, bilateral optic nerve involvement, and at autopsy, widespread demyelination throughout the centrum ovale bilaterally. It was called myelinoclastic diffuse sclerosis and, later, "Schilder's disease."[57] Schilder presented two further cases in 1913 and 1924, but these are now regarded as adrenoleukodystrophy and subacute sclerosing panencephalitis. Charles M. Poser reviewed the concept of Schilder's disease and gave a set of criteria for its diagnosis.[58] He described two additional cases of a transitional type that shared features of Schilder's disease and of multiple sclerosis, which he called "diffuse disseminated sclerosis." Later, he described two new cases of Schilder's disease, and he described cases with smaller plaques in addition to the large hemispheric lesions, as were classified as *transitional sclerosis*.[59]

BALÓ'S CONCENTRIC SCLEROSIS

Although noted by Marburg in 1906 and Barré in 1926, the pathological picture of concentric bands of demyelination alternating with bands of myelin was named after Baló, who published case reports in 1927 and 1928. József Mátyas Baló (1895–1979) was born in Budapest and after medical training, which involved time in the United States, he became chairman of the pathology department at Budapest. In 1927, he examined the brain of a 23-year-old man who had died of a rapidly progressive disease. He had signs interpreted as a brain tumor and had a craniotomy, but died the next day. Baló's report in 1927 described the unusual ring pattern of demyelination in the white matter of the hemispheres. The paper was translated into English the next year in the *Archives of Neurology and Psychiatry* as Encephalities Periaxialis Concentrica.[60] The rings of demyelination indicate varying ages, as tree rings do, with more recent changes at the periphery. These startling-looking lesions can be seen anywhere in the central nervous system (CNS). Sometimes MS-like plaques are seen elsewhere in the CNS, supporting the view that this condition is a variant of MS. A variant on this variant is concentric lacunar leukoen-

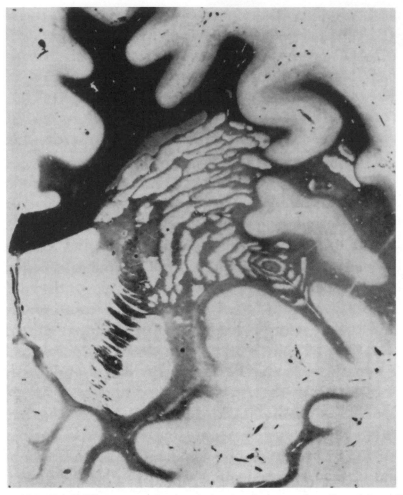

Figure 12.4 Balo's diffuse concentric sclerosis showing the layers of myelin and demyelination. (Davison, 1948.)

cephalopathy, which shows extensive axonal loss in the areas of demyelination. The reason for the peculiar ring formation in these cases is not clear.

DEVIC'S DISEASE

The first clinical presentation of the syndrome of optic neuritis with acute myelitis was by T. Clifford Allbutt, in an 1870 review of many spinal syndromes with optic nerve involvement.[61] Two cases were also described by Erb, and three by Sequin. There were pathological presentations of the disease by Dreschfeld (1882), Sharkey and Lawford (1884), Achard and Guinon (1889), and Fuch (1893). It was clarified as a distinct syndrome of myelitis associated with acute or subacute optic nerve neuritis by Devic and his student Gault in 1894, and the findings at autopsy were published a year later.[62,63] Gault wrote his thesis in Lyon on the syndrome in 1895 and described 16 cases, of which seven recovered, seven died and two had an unknown outcome. The disorder became known as neuromyelitis optica or Devic's disease, even though there were many earlier descriptions of the disorder, cited by Greenfield.[64] Arguments have continued over whether Devic's disease is a form of MS or a distinct entity. A group of cases in Edinburgh reported by Scott after a follow-up of 30 years showed that none of them developed MS, indicating that this was a separate disease.[65] Although it continues to be included in discussions of MS, justified as part of the differential diagnosis, the most recent pathologic, CSF, and MRI evidence suggests that this is a distinct disease entity. Recent MRI and magnetization transfer imaging again confirms that Devic's syndrome is probably a distinct entity from MS.[66] Alternatively, there may be a number of forms, one of which is MS; these cases have lesions elsewhere than in the regions responsible for the eye and cord symptoms.

TRANSVERSE MYELITIS

Transverse myelitis can occur as a severe acute necrotizing myelopathy or any acute demyelinating myelitis. Türck was aware of the relationship between myelitis and the condition we have come to know as multiple sclerosis, even before Charcot's description. The risk for developing MS after an acute episode varied in different series in the 20th century from 3 to 72 percent. It would appear that patients with severe acute myelopathy have a low risk for developing MS, but partial and mild transverse myelopathy patients have a higher risk. More recently, it has been demonstrated that transverse myelitis without MRI evidence of demyelination elsewhere has a low likelihood of developing into clinically definite MS, whereas the presence of multiple lesions elsewhere in the nervous system indicates a high likelihood of the development of clinically definite MS, even within a year.

SINGLE OR SILENT MS

A variation that is of great interest appears in the patient who develops an acute episode indicative of MS and never has another episode. Even stranger is the increasingly recognized subclinical case of MS, found on MRI but without symptoms or signs, and MS found at autopsy, with no prior history indicative of MS. Sir William Osler diagnosed a case of MS who was symptom-free for 50 years until Parkinson's disease. The autopsy showed the accuracy of Osler's earlier diagnosis.[67]

REFERENCES

1. Marburg O. Sie Sogenannte akute mulltiple sklerose (encephalomyelitis periaxialis scleroticans) *Jahrb Psychiat Neurol.* 1906;27:1.
2. Curshmann H. *Ueber familiäre multiple Sklerose.* Dtsch Z Nervenheilk. 1920;66:225-230.
3. MacIntyre HD, MacIntyre AP. Prognosis of Multiple Sclerosis. *Arch Neurol & Psychiat.* 1943;50:431-438.
4. Allison RS. Survival in disseminated sclerosis: a clinical study of a series of cases first seen twenty years ago. *Brain.* 1950;73:103-120.
5. Birley JL, Dudgeon LS. A clinical and experimental contribution to the pathogenesis of disseminated sclerosis. *Brain.* 1921;44:150-212.
6. Putnam TJ, Chiavacci LV, Hoff H, et al. Results of treatment of multiple sclerosis with dicoumarin. *Arch Neurol.* 1947;57:1-13.
7. Schumacher GA. Multiple sclerosis and its treatment. *JAMA.* 1950;143:1059-1065, 1146-1154, 1241-1250.
8. Osler W. *The Principles and Practice of Medicine.* New York: D. Appleton; 1892.
9. Marquezy R. These de Paris. 1924.
10. Purves-Stewart J. A specific vaccine treatment in disseminated sclerosis. *Lancet.* 1930;1:560-564.
11. Carter S, Sciarra D, Merritt HH. The course of multiple sclerosis as determined by autopsy proven cases. In: *Multiple Sclerosis and Demyelinating Diseases.* Proceedings of the Association for Research in Nervous and Mental Disease, (Dec. 10-11, 1948). Vol 28. Baltimore: Williams and Wilkins; 1950:471-511.
12. Ferraro A. Pathology of demyelinating diseases as an allergic reaction in the brain. *Arch Neurol Psychiat.* 1944;52:443-483.
13. McAlpine D, Compston ND, Lumsden CE. *Multiple Sclerosis.* Edinburgh: E&S Livingston; 1955.
14. Ibid.
15. Allison RS, Miller J. Prevalence and familial incidence of disseminated sclerosis: A report to the Northern Ireland Hospitals Authority on the results of a three year survey. *Ulster Med J.* 1954;23(suppl 2):1-92.
16. Schumacher GA. Multiple sclerosis and its treatment. *JAMA.* 1950;143:1059-1065, 1146-1154, 1241-1250.

17. Schumacher GA. Whither research in demyelination disease? In: Research in Demyelinating Diseases. *Annals New York Acad Sci.* 1965:569-570.
18. Kurtzke JF. Multiple sclerosis: what's in a name? *Neurology.* 1988;38:309-316.
19. Rose AS, Ellison GW, Myers LW, Tourtellotte WW. Criteria for the clinical diagnosis of multiple sclerosis (Abstract). *Neurology.* 1976;26(suppl):20-22.
20. McDonald WI, Halliday AM. Diagnosis and classification of multiple sclerosis. *Brit Med Bull.* 1977;33:4-8.
21. Kurtzke JF. Multiple sclerosis: what's in a name? *Neurology.* 1988;38:309-316.
22. Poser CM, Paty DW, Scheinberg L, et al. New diagnostic criteria for multiple sclerosis: *Ann Neurol.* 1983;13:227-231.
23. Hanefield F, Christen H-J, Krusse B, Bauer HJ. Childhood and juvenile multiple sclerosis. In: *Multiple Sclerosis: Its impact from childhood to old age.* Bauer HJ, Hanefeld FA, eds. London: WB Saunders; 1993:14-52.
24. Duquette P, Murray TJ, et al. Multiple Sclerosis in Childhood: Clinical Profile in 125 Patients. *J Pediatrics.* 1987;111(3):359-363.
25. Advisory Committee on Clinical Trials of the National Multiple Sclerosis Society (USA). *Neurology.* 1996; 46:970-911.
26. McDonald WI, Comston A, Edan G, et al. Recommended Diagnostic Criteria for Multiple Sclerosis: Guidelines from the International Panel on the Diagnosis of Multiple Sclerosis. *Ann Neurol.* 2001;50:121-127.
27. Arkin H, Sherman IC, Weinberg SL. Tetraethylammonium chloride in the treatment of multiple sclerosis. *Arch Neurol Psychiat.* 1950;64:536-545.
28. Alexander L. New concept of critical steps in the course of chronic debilitating neurologic disease in evaluation of therapeutic response. *Arch Neurol Psychiat.* 1951;66:253-258.
29. Kurtzke JF. A new scale for evaluating disability in multiple sclerosis. *Neurology.* 1955;5:580-583.
30. Kurtzke JF, Berlin L. The effects of isoniazid on patients with multiple sclerosis: preliminary report. *Ann Rev Tuberc.* 1954;70:577-592.
31. Kurtzke JF. Rating neurologic impairment in multiple sclerosis: an expanded disability scale status (EDSS). *Neurology.* 1983;33:1444-1452.
32. Kurtzke JF. Further notes on disability evaluation in multiple sclerosis, with scale modifications. *Neurology.* 1965;15:654-661.
33. Kurtzke JF. Multiple sclerosis: what's in a name? *Neurology.* 1988;38:309-316.
34. Kurtzke JF. On the evaluation of disability in multiple sclerosis. *Neurology.* 1961;11:686-694. This classic article was reprinted in *Neurology.* 1998;50:317-321
35. Willoughby EW, Paty DW. Scales for rating impairment in multiple sclerosis: a critique. *Neurology.* 1988;38:309-316.
36. Sipe JC, Knobler RL, Braheny SL, et al. A neurological rating scale (NRS) for use in multiple sclerosis. *Neurology.* 1984;34:1368-1372
37. Cook SD, Troiano R, Zito G, et al. Effect of total lymphoid irradiation in chronic progressive multiple sclerosis. *Lancet.* 1986;1:1405-1409.
38. Syndulko, K, Tourellotte WW, Baumhefner RW, Ellison GW, Myers LW, Belendiuk G, Kondraske GV. Neuroperformance evaluation of multiple sclerosis disease progression in a clinical trial: implications for neurological outcomes. *J Neuro Rehab.* 1993;7:153-176.
39. Hauser SL, Dawson DM, Lehrich JR, Beal MF, Kevy SV, Propper RD, Millis JA, Weiner HL. Intensive immunosuppression in progressive multiple sclerosis. *N Engl J Med.* 1983;308:173-180.
40. Herndon RM. *Handbook of Neurologic Rating Scales.* New York: Demos Vermande; 1997.
41. Haber A, LaRocca N, eds. *Minimal Record of Disability for Multiple Sclerosis.* New York: National Multiple Sclerosis Society; 1985.

42. Granger CV, Hamilton BB, Sherwin FS. *Guide for the Use of the Uniform Data Set for Medical Rehabilitation*. Buffalo, NY: Uniform Data System for Medical Rehabilitation Project Office, Buffalo General Hospital; 1986.

43. Haber A, LaRocca N, eds. *Minimal Record of Disability for Multiple Sclerosis*. New York: National Multiple Sclerosis Society; 1985.

44. Rudick RA, Antel J, Confavreau C, et al. Recommendations from the National Multiple Sclerosis Society Clinical Outcomes Assessment Task Force. *Ann Neurol.* 1997;42:379-382.

45. Putnam TJ, Chiavacci LV, Hoff H, et al. Results of treatment of multiple sclerosis with dicoumarin. *Arch Neurol.* 1947;57:1-13.

46. Müller R. Studies on disseminated sclerosis. *Acta med Scand.* 1949;133(suppl 222):1-214.

47. Birley JL, Dudgeon LS. A clinical and experimental contribution to the pathogenesis of disseminated sclerosis. *Brain.* 1921;44:150-212.

48. MacLean AR, Berkson J, Woltman HW, Schionneman L. Multiple Sclerosis in a rural community. In: *Multiple Sclerosis and the Demyelinating Diseases*. Proceedings of the Association for Research in Nervous and Mental Disease (Dec. 10–11, 1948). Vol 28. Baltimore: Williams and Wilkins; 1950:25-27.

49. Coates. 1930

50. Thygesen P. Prognosis in initial stage of disseminated primary demyelinating disease of the central nervous system. *Arch Neurol (Chicago).* 1949;61:339.

51. Müller R. Studies on disseminated sclerosis. *Acta med Scand.* 1949;133(suppl 222):1-214.

52. Poser S, et al. Acute demyelinating disease. Classification and non-invasive diagnosis. *Acta Neurol Scand.* 1992; 86:579-585.

53. Poser S, et al. Acute demyelinating disease. Classification and non-invasive diagnosis. *Acta Neurol Scand.* 1992;86:579-585.

54. Dale RC, et al. Acute disseminated encephalo-myelitis, multiphasic disseminated encephalomyelitis and multiple sclerosis in children. *Brain.* 2000;123:2407-2422.

55. Marburg O. Die Sogenannte akute mulltiple sklerose (encephalomyelitis periaxialis scleroticans) *Jahrb Psychiat Neurol.* 1906;27:1.

56. Bitsch A, Wegener C, da Costa C, et al. Lesion development in Marburg's type of acute multiple sclerosis from inflamation to demyelination. *Multiple Sclerosis.* 1999;5:138-146.

57. Schilder P. Zur Kenntoris der sogenannten diffusen Sclerose (über Encephalitis periax-ialis diffusa). *Z Neurol.* 1912;10:1-60.

58. Poser CM. Diffuse disseminated sclerosis in the adult. *J Neuropath Exper Neurol.* 1957;16:61-78.

59. Poser CM. Myelinoclastic diffuse sclerosis. In: *Handbook of Clinical Neurology*. Vinken PJ, Bruyn GW, Klawans HL, eds. Amsterdam: North Holland Publishing; 1985:419-424.

60. Baló J. Encephalitis periaxialis concentrica. *Archives Neurol Psychiat.* 1928;19:242-264.

61. Allbutt, T. Clifford. On the ophthalmoscopic signs of spinal cord disease. *Lancet.* 1870;1:76-78.

62. Devic E. Myelite subaigue compliquée de nervite optique. *Bull Med.* 1894;8:1033-1034.

63. Devic E. Myelite aigue dorse-lombaire avec nervite optique, autopsie. *Congress Francais Medicine* (Premiere Session, Lyon). 1995;1:434-439.

64. *Greenfield's Neuropathology*, 2nd ed. Blackwood W, McMenemey WH, Myer A, Norman RM, Russell. DS, eds. London: Edward Arnold; 1963.

65. Scott GI. Ophthalmic aspects of demyelinating diseases. *Proc R Soc Med.* 1961;54:38-42.

66. Filippi M, Rocca MA, Moiola L, et al. MRI and magnetization transfer imaging changes in the brain and cervical cord of patients with Devic's neuromyelitis optica. *Neurology.* 1999;53:1705-1710.

67. Risse W, Jones GL, East IE, Beamer-Maxwell E, Davis HE. Disseminating demyeli-nating process of over 50 years duration first seen by Dr. William Osler. *Confina Neurologia.* 1952;12:113-120.

13

The Nature of the MS Plaque

O ne of the recognizable characteristic features of multiple sclerosis, evident to the first observers in Germany, France, and Austria was the scattered lesions throughout the white matter of the central nervous system. Charcot called them plaques, and even though Greenfield indicated later that this word refers to something that is flat, rather than ovoid, spherical, or the many other shapes that these lesions take, the term has held.[1]

Virchow described neuroglia of the nervous system and named myelin in 1858. He suggested neuroglia provided mechanical support and repair functions. In 1883, Golgi suggested the neuroglial cells also provide nutritional support and in 1897, Bevan and Lewis noted the cells' role in removal of debris. Early users of microscopes noted a marked loss of myelin in the plaques of MS, with relative sparing of axons. The oligo-dendrocyte was first described by Robertson in 1899. It was further defined in 1921 by Rio Hortega, who named, characterized, and typed these cells. In 1932, Penfield suggested the cells were involved in the production and maintenance of myelin. Classic descriptions of the pathology of the plaques have been given by Bielschowsky (1903, 1904); Marinesco and Minea (1909); Siemerling and Raecke (1911); Dawson (1916); Jacob

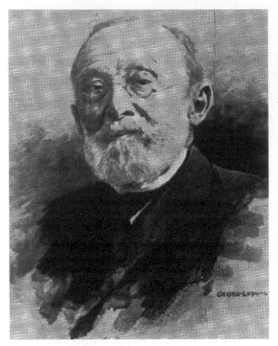

Figure 13.1 Rudolph Ludwig Carl Virchow (1821–1902) changed the concept of disease by his book *Die Cellularpathologie* (1858). His cellular concepts of disease, along with his many publications on the brain and neurological disease influenced those who studied MS, including Vulpian and Charcot. Although capable of visionary reductionist science of the cells in disease, he was also capable of a broad community vision and was throughout his career a left wing activist and politician, believing that politics was just medicine on a grand scale. (From the collection of Dr. Hans Schlumberger.)

(1929); and Steiner (1931). Important reviews of the field have been presented by Brain (1930); Ferraro (1937 and 1944); Schaltenbrand (1943); and Hurst (1952).

The earliest writers speculated little on the nature of the grey softening they saw and felt as they ran their fingers over spinal cords at the autopsies of their MS patients. However, in 1863, Rindfleisch indicated that the basis might be in an inflammatory process in the small veins seen in the center of the grey lesions.[2] Charcot felt that an overgrowth of glia was the specific abnormality, damaging the myelin sheaths and sometimes the axons. The local vascular changes would be secondary to glial overgrowth and the breakdown of nerve tissue that was followed by macrophage removal of the lipid products of myelin, a process Charcot observed under his microscope and illustrated in his careful drawings. His student Joseph Babinski[3,4] also felt the changes were a demyelinating process, even though Compston[5] had pointed out that one of the illustrations to his thesis showed the appearance of remyelination, with thin layers of myelin surrounding the axon and fat granule cells removing the myelin debris. Strümpell[6] and Müller[7] agreed with Charcot that the defect was an inborn disease of neuroglia. Another Charcot student, Pierre Marie, argued strongly (and he did argue the point with his detractors) that these changes were the result of an infection.[8] This was later supported by the observation that viral infections could cause scattered areas of perivascular demyelination, also seen in postvaccinal encephalomyelitis, and postinfectious encephalitis.

The lesions in MS are scattered, some small and some large, and some coalescing into other lesions to form even larger areas of demyelination. They can be anywhere in the white matter, and even extend into the grey matter in some instances.[9] They tend to be in characteristic areas, especially in the periventricular region.*[10,11] Cruvielhier[12–16] showed lesions in the corpus callosum,† and Gowers felt the lesions were more numerous posteriorly.[17]

Charcot and other early writers noted the relative preservation of the axons in the MS plaques. Charcot felt that repair could occur after myelin breakdown. His student Babinski agreed, but described a process of nerve regeneration rather than remyelination, even though some of the fibers in the illustrations of his 1885 thesis on multiple sclerosis showed thin myelin around some axons, which is now recognized as remyelination.[18] In 1903, Bielschowsky was impressed that the axons were preserved within the plaques, but also noted some axonal shrinkage, and he suggested that the picture may convey a false impression of normality. Greenfield and King[19] used Bielschowsky's method on frozen sections to examine 125 cerebral plaques; they noted that only 10 percent had severe loss of axons, retaining only 15–20 percent, but of the remaining 90 percent, half the plaques had moderate loss, and the rest had little change. They concluded that axons do not pass intact through a plaque. They and others found some evidence of sprouting and some "retraction bulbs," but cautioned that this should not be interpreted as attempts at regeneration.

---

* S.A. Kinnier Wilson referred to the periventricular location of lesions as the "Wetterwinkel of Steiner."

† In 1940, Hallervorden said they were so characteristic of MS that the diagnosis should be questioned if they were not present.

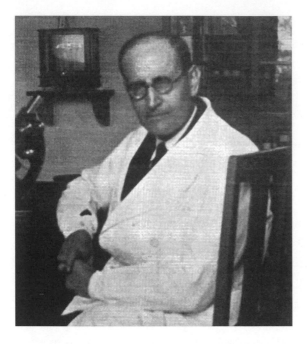

Figure 13.2 The famed Spanish investigator Pio Del Rio Hortega advanced the understanding of the CNS glia through his microscopic studies of microglia and oligodendrocytes. He was able to discern the relationship of oligodendrocytes to myelin. (Courtesy of Dr. William Gibson.)

Marburg,[20] Dawson,[21,22] and Hassin[23] also believed that the process occurring in the shadow plaques was demyelination; but Dawson felt the vascular change shown by Rindfleisch[24] could be the primary change. Rindfleisch, Rossilimo, and Church and Peterson also commented on the vessel at the center of a plaque and felt the appearances were of an embolism or thrombosis, which sets up vascular lesions that produce irritative sclerosis of the adjacent neuroglia. Marie admitted the importance of vascular changes in the plaque, but felt the cause was infection, or as he emphasized, infections.[25] Combining the vascular and demyelinating features, Bielschowsky thought a lipolytic substance passed through the vessel wall to damage the myelin.[26] Early on, there was significant focus on the glia and even Charcot considered the glia change as primary, with everything else being secondary. In Charcot's view, the axon which had lost its myelin sheath could conduct, but would do so "irregularly in a broken or jerky manner." This would, in turn, cause irregular tremulous motor movements when the limbs were in use.

In his autobiography, *No Man Alone*, the Canadian neurosurgeon Wilder Penfield (1891–1976) wrote of his early interest in the oligoden-

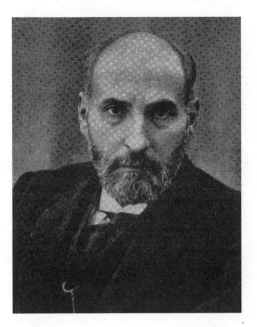

Figure 13.3   Santiago Ramon Y. Cajal made many advances in the understanding of the peripheral and central nervous system by his remarkable microscopic and staining techniques. (Courtesy of the National Library of Medicine.)

droglial cells when he was working in the Madrid lab of Pio del Rio-Hortega in 1924.[27] There was controversy at the time about the non-nervous cells in the brain that formed the supporting structure. There were astrocytes, often referred to as neuroglia (from the Greek, meaning "nerve glue"), and there was a "third element" made up of oligodendrocytes ("few-branching glue cells") and microglia ("small glue cells").*[28] Some researchers, including the famed neurohistologist Ramón y Cajal, also in Madrid, did not agree that oligodendrocytes were part of the neuroglia, because this could not be demonstrated in his stains. Trying out tissue stains in Rio-Hortega's lab, Penfield saw an oligodendrocyte that was particularly well stained; it was not "few branching," but had many branches. He made a note of the details of his staining technique, did ink drawings of the cells he observed, and sent a paper off to the journal *Brain*, pointing out that the oligodendrocyte was confirmed as a cell that made up a third of the neuroglia.[29] The 33-year-old Penfield was not hesitant to chide the famous Cajal in the paper, indicating that the Nobel

---

* The Germans called microglia Hortega cells. Del Rio-Hortega first described oligodendroglia and microglia.

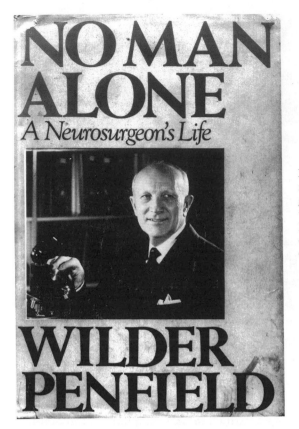

Figure 13.4 Wilder Penfield, famous Canadian neurosurgeon, published on glial cells while studying with Rio-Hortega early in his career. (Courtesy of Little Brown and Company Publishers.)

laureate rejected the presence of oligodendrocytes because he could not find them in his stains. Penfield emphasized that it was Cajal who had previously said it was dangerous to assign value to negative results.

Penfield had brought some microscopic sections from New York that he hoped to review in Madrid and one was from a man who died of a malignant brain tumor. When looking at the neurologlial cells, he saw something that amazed him, and he suddenly understood what happens when the brain reacts to damage. Penfield had made another discovery of importance for the understanding of changes in the plaques of MS: the recognition that microglia were in one form when "at rest" in the brain, but change into "amoeba-like scavenger cells that wander through the tissue and devour the broken parts of the dead cells and their branches." Soon he was sending off his second paper. The first had been based on the observation of a few cells, and the second was based on a single slide. The view that macrophages were scavenger cells persisted until Prineas examined their function further in recent years.

In 1936, J.G. Greenfield and Lester King described the histopathology of lesions in 13 cases of MS, describing the early changes in fresh plaques with intense wall formation by gitter cells packed against the normal myelin.[30] In the secondary stage, they saw perivascular accumulation of gitter cells with lymphocytes, plasma cells, and pale mononuclear cells. Some cells contained fat granules and these phagocytic cells were thought to be of connective tissue origin. In the third stage, the fat disappeared and the gitter cells were fewer. They described the staining characteristics of the myelin breakdown and the products of this destruction. They stated that the persistence of the axons in MS is only relative, and there is loss in many cases. Extreme loss, however, as reported by Putnam, was not common in the 125 plaques they examined.

Greenfield and King noted that the changes seen in the axons have been ignored in the English literature, but were well-described in the French and German literature. There were nerve sprouts, nerve bulbs and loops, and *boules de retraction* interpreted as regenerative phenomena. Some of these changes, particularly the *boules de retraction,* were probably changes representing degeneration and they pointed out illustrations of this degenerative change in the works of Cajal.

They then discussed gliosis, noting that it was one of the six stages in the natural history of MS (the fourth) noted by Dawson, and that in the English literature, it was regarded as a secondary phenomenon, whereas in the Continental literature it was regarded as a primary process, even though the view of glial change as the primary cause put forward by Strümpell and Müller was not tenable. They asked if gliosis is an initial process or a reaction and concluded it was too early and intense to be just a secondary process.

The vessel changes were thought to be common by Dawson and others, but Bielschowsky and Greenfield felt that this was not a constant finding, seen mostly in small plaques, but obscured in larger ones where coalescence of many plaques occurred. The perivascular nature of the pathology was also less definite, as in postinfectious encephalomyelitis.[31]

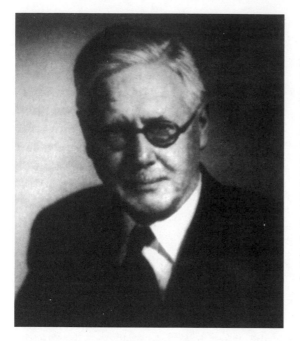

Figure 13.5 Joseph Godwin Greenfield (1884–1958) was the dean of "neuropathology" in the early half of the 20th century, known to all neurologists by his influential and comprehensive textbook of *Neuropathology* published in 1958. He died prior to the publication of the second edition in 1963. When in Edinburgh, the young James Walker Dawson worked under Greenfield and produced the definitive work on the pathology in 1916. Greenfield contributed to the pathology of MS over four decades.

Greenfield described the centrifugal spread of plaques as a "wall formation" of inflammatory cellular activity at the periphery of the plaque, with more complete demyelination in the center, forming a "shadow plaque." Shadow plaques (*Markshattenherde*) have been interpreted differently by different writers. Marburg thought they were areas of demyelination. Alzheimer (1910) thought they were young plaques in the making, but Greenfield said he found them mostly in chronic cases of MS, where there was little activity. Prineas later showed they were older areas that had remyelinated fibers.

Dr. William G. Spiller initially wondered in 1904 whether the primary change was in the "noble tissues" using the French term referring to the nerve fibers, or whether it was primarily in the neuroglia, and he concluded the latter.[32] He concluded that MS was probably an acute disease caused by some circulating toxin, partly inflammatory, and probably dependent on vascular supply to the area of the plaques. In 1922, Joshua H. Leiner indicated that the axis cylinder could be involved in the lesion, although it might survive.[33] Studies on the proliferative progenitor oligodendrocyte are summarized by Compston.[34]

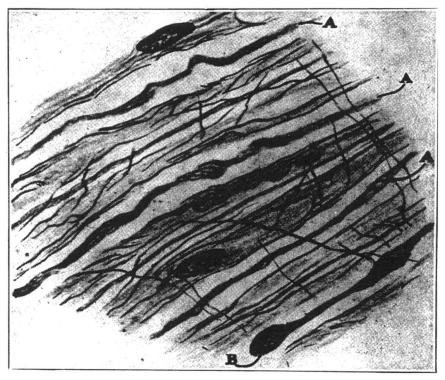

Figure 13.6   Illustration used by Joshua Leiner to illustrate pathological changes in MS in his paper to the ARNMD in 1921. The myelin has disappeared, leaving naked axons surrounded by glial fibres (A). The axons show irregular calibre, vacuolization, and with an enlarged end bulb (B). (ARNMD, 1922.)

By 1937, Schmidt used polarized light analysis and x-ray diffraction to demonstrate that the structure of myelin was made up of concentric layers of lipid and protein. Reviews of the pathology of plaques were extensive in the first 40 years of the 20th century, leading Tracy Putnam to suggest in 1938 that it was unlikely that anything substantial could be learned further about the process of breakdown and repair. Such predictions are always risky and we are still learning important new information as we enter a new century.

Putnam had done experiments in 1931, injecting cod liver oil into the carotids of eight cats and seven dogs, and caused demyelination that he felt resembled MS.[35,36] He later blocked cerebral vessels by oil injection. However, his presentation of this work was criticized by neuropathologists, who were not impressed with his interpretation of the areas of demyelination. One other experiment of interest in the discussion of the current vogue among MS patients for subcutaneous injections of bee venom, and actual bee stings as a form of therapy, was the work of Cornil in 1939 producing demyelination with subcutaneous injections of bee venom in mice and guinea pigs. Continuing the experiments on vascular induction of demyelination, Hurst injected olive oil and egg yolk in a solution he called a "mayonnaise" into one carotid of animals and got changes of demyelination but concluded these were not related to the changes in MS; he felt they looked more like those of Binswanger's disease.[37]

Hans Reese gave a critique of the various theories of etiology of MS at the ARNMD meeting on MS in 1948 and in a later publication.[38,39] He indicated that various theories have come from the interpretation of the morphology of the MS plaque, the scattered nature of the plaques, the role of blood vessels, heredity, the constitution of the patient, immunization, geographic distribution, racial differences, and whether there may be both intrinsic and extrinsic causes working together. He felt that the Strümpell-Müller theory of glial dysplasia and myelin dysplactic theories were now discounted, but work on tissue changes resulted in fruitful knowledge of the process of the disease. He was unconvinced by the familial studies and the twin data and the resulting theories of neuropathic traits, which he thought led only to confusion and argument. The myelinolytic theory of Marburg (1906) and the lipolytic theory of Brickner (1930) were equally unconvincing as was Weil's theory of an abnormal esterase activity, or impaired inorganic phosphorous balance in MS. Reese was more impressed that the problems MS patients noted during menstruation, pregnancy, and the postpartum period suggested an abnormality of hormonal or lipid metabolism.

Reese asked the central question: if there is something that affects the central nervous system and causes the plaques repeatedly, how does it get there? A clinician would immediately suggest the vascular system as route, and although this idea appealed to some, others disagreed. Reese felt there were four possible scenarios: the cause was an infection, a venular thrombosis as postulated by Putnam, a spasm of the vessels, or diffusion into the CNS by antigenic substances. He related the supporting data for each and the contradictory evidence for each theory, and concluded with the verdict of "not proven." However, he suggested further research should be in four directions: myelin metabolism and the things that could affect it, neuroallergy, a search for specific antigens and antibodies, and psychological assessment of the total personality of the MS patient.

Fog reviewed the literature on the relationship of the vessels to plaques from Rindfleisch's observations in 1863 to 1947. Noting the theory of Putnam (1930–1939 reports) that thrombosis of small veins may be the underlying mechanism of plaque formation, and the studies on this by Dow and Berglund (1942), Zimmermann and Netsky (1950), and his own work (1948, 1950), Fog concluded that there may be some small vessel changes, but these are intermittent and variable. His subsequent study of 51 plaques from two cases of typical MS, making thin sections of the plaques and following their shape and course with direct drawings of each section, showed that most (39/51) were prolongations of periventricular plaques, and that the plaques did follow the course of the venous system.[40]

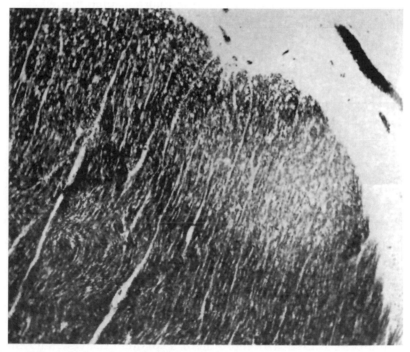

Figure 13.7   A shadow plaque. (Zimmermann, 1948.)

In a detailed assessment of the pathology of 50 cases of MS by H.M. Zimmerman and Martin Netsky at the ARNMD meeting in 1948, there was no evidence to support an intimate relationship of plaque with blood vessels shown by others and no evidence of the thrombosis postulated by Putnam.[41]

H.H. Reese said that in areas of demyelination, there were some fibers denuded (naked axis cylinders), others with fragmented myelin, and others with destruction of both myelin and the axons.[42,43] Adams felt the earliest change noted was perivascular cuffing of small venules by lymphocytes, followed by macrophage recruitment with exocytosis of macrophage enzyme causing demyelination.[44] In 1978, John Prineas noted that in the MS plaque, where an immunological reaction was known to occur, there was involvement by macrophages, plasma cells, and microglia, necessary for the digestion of myelin.[45,46] He showed that the chronic lesion demonstrated continued expression and processing of antigen in the absence of new lesions.

In 1979, Prineas and Connell showed that remyelination was part of the process in MS,[47] and Lassmann noted that the thin fibers thought by earlier studies to be partially demyelinated fibers were fibers that had thin myelin, formed by oligodendrocytes.[48] The new myelin sheath was thinner and the shadow plaques thought previously to be demyelination are in actuality areas of remyelination, and McDonald showed, slower in conducting impulses.[49] Prineas felt that the inflammatory process that removed the debris after myelin breakdown was crucial to the remyelination process.[50]

Can conduction occur in the denuded axons where demyelination has occurred? Charcot thought it could, but in an irregular manner that resulted in tremor, for instance. Although working with peripheral nerves, Derek Denny-Brown at Harvard showed that a nerve lesion that caused myelin to break down would stop conduction. In a simple but elegant demonstration, he showed that stimulation above an area of pressure-induced demyelination did not produce muscle contraction distally, but stimulation below the area of demyelination did, and he concluded that an area of demyelination produced a conduction block. McDonald showed that this occurred in the dorsal root ganglia of cats injected sys-

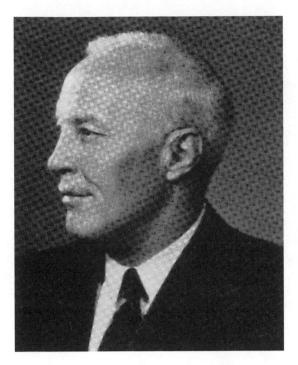

Figure 13.8 Derek Denny-Brown, a native of New Zealand, trained with Sherrington at Oxford, and then became a physician at the National Hospital, Queen Square. On the retirement of Tracy Putnum in 1939, he was appointed at Harvard. His careful experiments with peripheral nerves showing the effects of demyelination and conduction block were influential to McDonald and others learning about the process in the central nervous system. (Courtesy of the Royal College of Physicians, London.)

tematically with diphtheria toxin; a block developed abruptly where demyelination began. In single nerve fibers, conduction through a demyelinating lesion was slowed. If this occurred in the central nervous system, it would explain the major functional disruption to conduction in a disease like MS, which was characterized by patchy areas of demyelination. During the 1970s, McDonald, Tom Sears, and their colleagues defined the characteristic of remyelination in the central nervous system and showed that this helped explain the clinical phenomena in MS.

Studies of remyelination in MS gained momentum in 1961 with the studies of Bunge and Bunge[51] and later with the work of Prineas in the 1970s.[52–55]

The first electron microscope pictures of a plaque in MS by Perier and Gregoire in 1965 showed thin myelin; they concluded this was evidence of remyelinated fibers. This conclusion was confirmed by the studies of McDonald's group at Queen Square on cats with spinal cord compression, and by Prineas. McDonald then showed that this allowed restoration of function as well.

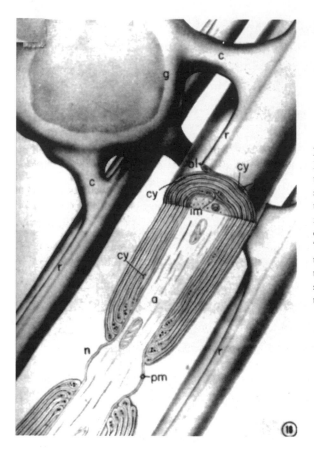

Figure 13.9 Richard and Mary Bunge demonstrated that shadow plaques represented areas of remyelination. They demonstrated remyelination using a model of cats given CSF barbtage. Their illustration of the relationship of the oligodendryte to myelin is a classic image still used in lectures on multiple sclerosis. (Bunge, 1961.)

Work by Martin Halliday, Ian McDonald, and others at Queen Square showed that the delay in conduction seen in the peripheral nervous system could also occur in the central nervous system in MS.[56,57] They showed that demyelinated nerves could not consistently transmit long trains of impulses at high frequency, due to an increased refractory period over the damaged area, and that this relative block could be made complete by increases in temperature, often very small increases of half a degree. Conversely, the conduction time could be improved by cooling. Remyelination could occur, but the renewed conduction was slower than normal, and this might be due to conduction in the axons that persisted but were still demyelinated, as predicted by Charcot.

McDonald suggested to Martin Halliday that they might use evoked potentials to distinguish demyelination from degeneration, because of the characteristic of slowing in demyelinated fibers. With their first three cases, they were able to confirm this.[58,59] This finding led to the application of evoked potentials in MS; and the next year, they published the frequency of delays in cases of MS. The mechanism of slowing is probably not due to conduction in remyelinated nerves, but conduction in the persistently demyelinated axon is mediated by the increase in new sodium channels. McDonald demonstrated that the remyelinated axon had distinct morphological features.[60,61] The diagnostic tests developed on the basis of the slowing of central nerves fibers, were visual, auditory, and sensory evoked potential studies. McDonald suggested that conduction could be restored in demyelinated nerves by conduction in the demyelinated nerve, or by remyelination. Perhaps both occur. Restoration of function might depend on increased numbers of sodium channels in demyelinated nerves, as shown by Waksman and Ritchie in 1985. The experiments of Bunge, Bunge, and Ris had indicated that the oligodendrocyte was responsible for myelination and remyelination.[62] Others raised the possibility of strategies to enhance remyelination in MS.[63,64]

"The persistence of axons is such a cardinal point in the pathologic picture that many articles on the subject leave the impression that all are intact in all sclerotic plaques. This is certainly not the case, and modern pathologists who have made intensive studies of the disease (for example Dawson, Speilmyer, Jakob, Atassin and Bertrand) all agree that axons are seldom undamaged and are often completely destroyed and that secondary degeneration is common."

T.J. Putnam, 1936[65]

Though it became understood that nerves could demyelinate in MS, but could remyelinate again, the question of why the disease progressed remained. Even if nerves had thin myelin and conducted slowly, reasonable function should continue. There must be some other factor that limits the process and causes the disease eventually and sometimes primarily, to progress. Evidence is accumulating that the key is an observation made over and over by even the earliest workers such as Charcot, that axons are often damaged even early in the process.[66] He noted globules at the end of axons in the plaque. Even if this damage were a minor part of an acute demyelinated plaque, repeated events in the area and in other connecting areas would add up and more irreparable axonal damage would accumulate. It is conceivable that the axon requires the presence of myelin to continue to be viable. However, understanding the processes of axonal degeneration will be crucial in understanding the nature of the progression of MS and may allow us to focus our therapeutic efforts more effectively.

Axonal loss had been noted by Charcot, Babinski, Dejerine, Frommann, Bielschowsky, Williamson, Marie, Marburg, Dawson, Symonds, Greenfield, and others.[67] Charcot had observed in 1868 that axonal swellings and axonal loss can occur and in 1878, Frommann carried out detailed studies of the axonal damage in multiple sclerosis. Babinski and Bielschowsky also noted that the axons that were demyelinated but not lost could remyelinate.[68] As early as 1906, Marburg emphasized that axonal preservation in the face of evident demyelination must be regarded as relative; he noted extensive axonal loss, more than others were reporting. In 1936, Putnam noted large axonal loss in his study of plaques, but Greenfield and King the same year found only 10 percent of plaques had some destruction, by which they meant the numbers were reduced by one fifth or one seventh. Greenfield and King speculated that axons that were damaged might regenerate. By 1951, Russell Brain pondered the possibility that axonal damage may be important and questioned whether myelin was really the target of MS.[69] Axonal loss had not been emphasized in the face of the more obvious widespread demyelination that seemed to offer a reasonable explanation for the disease. However, the fate of the axon may be an important determinant in the progression of the disease, as predicted by McDonald in 1991.[70] Konek and Lassmann have reviewed the history of observations on axonal involvement in MS.[71]

Although axonal involvement appeared in microscopic examination of MS brain material by the earliest writers, only in the last decade has it been noted that axonal damage may be the key to understanding the progressive nature of MS. Since the mid-1980s, McDonald has asked whether the axon loss was substantially contributing to disability in MS, and in 1995, his group published a study designed to answer that question that showed that there was a strong correlation between persistent dis-

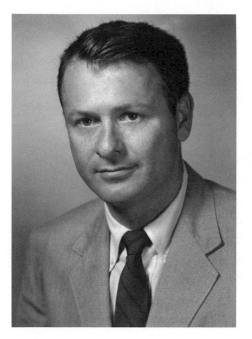

Figure 13.10 Dr. Cedric Raine. (Courtesy of Dr. C Reine. H. Boudakian, Illustration Service, Rockefeller Institute.)

ability and a persistent reduction in the concentration of NAA.[72] Trapp later showed elegant illustrations of the nature of that axonal loss.[73]

The hope that drugs that modify and reduce the inflammatory response would encourage remyelination has not been borne out by studies so far, perhaps because we have poor methods to assess remyelination. However, newer strategies are being developed.[74] With the development of MRI and clear evidence of widespread plaques, as well as some evidence of a more general abnormality, there has been an effort to correlate the images with the changes seen pathologically. This work is continuing. Pathologically, the plaque shows inflammation and demyelination with some degree of axonal loss and gliosis or scarring. The plaques are classified according to the degree of activity present into acute, chronic-active, and chronic-silent lesions. The acute lesion has an area of acute inflammation with uniform hypercellularity throughout and with evidence of both demyelination and remyelination. In the chronic-active lesion, there are chronic changes in the center, but inflammatory changes at the periphery with demyelination by macrophages along the border, but also increased oligodendrocytes and remyelination. The chronic-silent plaque has a more abrupt edge with evidence of demyelinated axons, some axonal loss and gliosis, and little evidence of remyelination.

Gliosis in the plaque is a major contributor to the changes seen on the T1 MRI scan. Van Walderveen et al. have shown that parenchymal damage, particularly axonal loss, is the basis of the hypotense areas on T1-weighted images.[75] Chronic lesions are easily visible on MRI. The basis of the T2-prolongation that is characteristic of MS plaques is unclear, but probably is related to increased water in the plaque. Contrast enhancement may represent breakdown in the blood–brain barrier, which indicates activity in the plaque, and it can be one of the initial changes in MS. As techniques of MRI scanning advance, so do efforts to make clear correlations among pathophysiological changes in the plaque. The distribution of MRI lesions may relate in some way to structures involved in olfaction, and Gowers said that the olfactory "nerve," or as McDonald corrects, the olfactory tract, is often involved.[76] Scarvelli and McDonald have shown "dégéneration grise" in the olfactory tract where demyelination is present, and recent studies have shown olfactory abnormalities in patients with MS.

Douglas Arnold in Montreal showed axonal loss on MR spectroscopy in 1994.[77] Bruce Trapp and others have noted that although it is clear there is an inflammatory process resulting in demyelination underlying MS, which might be an autoimmune phenomenon, there is increasing evidence that along with this process, there is also a progressive and increasing transection of axons that results in the irretrievable loss of function in those axons.[78]

Using a rapid autopsy-retrieval system in Cleveland, Trapp was able to carry out MRIs and autopsies on MS patients soon after death and to examine the brain and spinal cord using various immunochemical techniques. His studies showed that terminal axonal ovoids or axonal retractions were prominent in areas of demyelination, and counted 11,236 per mm^2 of brain tissue in a plaque. These axonal ovoids were seen in the core of the plaque, at the edge, and even in smaller numbers in the areas of "normal" tissue. It is also possible that the oligodendrocytes later are affected and the supportive function of these cells may later be lost as well. This would compound the problem, accounting for the relentless

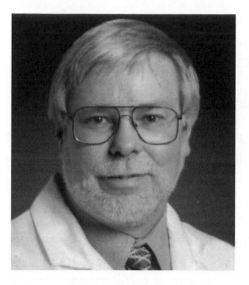

Figure 13.11 Bruce Trapp, Cleveland Clinic, carried out important work on the widespread axonal loss in MS. Following studies of axonal degeneration in transgenic mice with the myelin associated glycoprotein (MAG) was removed from the mouse genome, Bruce Trapp and his colleagues Richard Rudick and Richard Ransohoff developed a rapid autopsy protocol to obtain MS brains within five hours of death, and found substantial axonal transection in the early stages of lesion formation as well as in chronic lesions. Although axonal loss had been noted for a century and a half, there is recent focus on this as a possible basis for the progressive aspect of the disease. (Courtesy of Dr. Bruce Trapp.)

disease progression that might occur even when attacks are no longer happening. Trapp wondered if this could be due to immune attack on the neurons, vulnerability of the demyelinated axons to the inflammatory environment, or because demyelinated axons may be prone to degenerate. What is clear, however, is that once transected, the axon ceases to function and may later have proximal degeneration as well.

Further studies on the spinal cord showed that the axonal loss was remarkable in its extent. A triangulated section of the cord of MS patients compared to normal cord showed a loss of axons up to 75 percent. As in ALS, where 50 percent of motor neurons may be lost before the patient seeks medical attention, or 80 percent of substantia nigra cells in Parkinson's disease may be lost before the patient complains of significant symptoms, there is a lot of silent axonal loss in MS patients before many clinical disease features appear. The capacity of the brain to compensate for cell loss is great, but these findings argue for the earliest possible therapeutic intervention, since much damage has likely occurred well before the patient notes the first symptom. It remains to be seen if reducing attacks of MS by suppressing the inflammatory lesions will result in a reduction in late progression.

This research not only helps explain how progression is occurring in MS, but alters our views on therapy and monitoring of patients. In the future, we will need techniques that allow monitoring of inflammation, demyelination, axonal loss, and general atrophy to understanding how patients are faring; these techniques should also benefit development of therapies.

There is now evidence from immunochemical staining and measurements of n-acetylaspartate (NAA) using MR spectroscopy (MRS) or high-performance chromatography (HPLC) that there is axonal loss, not only in lesions, but in normal appearing white matter, and even in grey matter.[79] Arnold has shown by magnetization transfer that a normal-appearing brain may have axonal damage going on before a lesion occurs.[80] Grey matter lesions were occasionally reported by early investigators but, like axonal damage, are less obvious than inflammation and demyelination.

John Prineas of Australia did much of his neurology training in England, but his subsequent career has been in the departments of pathology and neurosciences at the medical school of the University of Medicine and Dentistry of New Jersey. His studies of demyelination, remyelination, and the immunological and pathological changes in the plaque of MS have advanced the knowledge of the process and aided later attempts to find ways to alter the changes therapeutically.*[81]

Prineas has been a careful student of the changes in and around the MS plaque, the role of the various cells involved in the process, the resultant demyelination of the nerves, and the attempts to remyelinate.

"I would say that the neuroimmunologists more than any other group have brought us to the present point in an understanding of MS. Amongst these I would single out as having the greatest effect on the direction of MS research during the past three decades are Byron Waksman, Barry Arnason, Bill Norton, Wallace Tourtellotte, Cedric Raine, Henry Wisniwski, Peter Lambert, Margaret Esiri, Louise

---

*John Prineas, winner of the 2001 Dystel Prize for contributions to MS research, is a graduate of the University of Sydney. After neurology training in London, he moved to the United States in 1967 as a NMSS postdoctoral fellow, influenced by his mentors Labe Scheinberg and Robert Terry. He spent the next 25 years in MS research at the University of Medicine and Dentistry, of New Jersey Medical School. He recently returned to Australia to continue his research at the Institute of Clinical Neurosciences in Sydney. His work has shown how macrophages and antibody are involved in the MS plaque and how remyelination can occur.

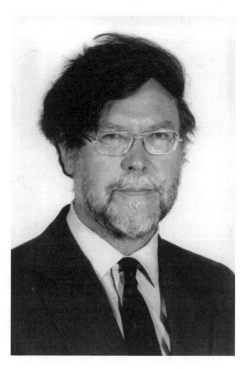

Figure 13.12   John Prineas of Australia did much of his neurology training in England, but much of his career has been in the departments of pathology and neurosciences at the New Jersey Medical School. His careful studies of the demyelination, remyelination, and the immunological and pathological changes in the plaque of MS has advanced the knowledge of the process and aided later attempts to find ways to alter the changes therapeutically. (Courtesy of Dr. John Prineas.)

Cuzart, Chris Livingston, Hans Lassman, Wolfgang Brüch, plus many others.... The contributions that pathologists have made are generally not that well-known or understood by the clinicians."

John Prineas, 2001
(Personal Communication)

Prineas listed seven main developments since the review by Lumsden in 1970 in the *Handbook of Neurology,* Vol. 9, on demyelinating diseases:[82]

1. The view that the macrophages are scavenger cells that remove the myelin debris has altered so that we now see them as the main effectors of myelin breakdown by phagocytosis and by secreting toxic molecules. How they are directed to the myelin and recognize it remain open questions. Prineas made an important contribution to this understanding by his electron microscopic studies of MS and the macrophage destruction of myelin in Guillain-Barré syndrome and chronic inflammatory demyelinating polyradiculopathy.

2. Remyelination can occur and the oligodendrocytes may persist. Prineas showed that myelin internodes at the edge of plaques were thin, short remyelinated internodes. This was the first demonstration that nerves could remyelinate. Using specific oligodendrocyte markers, he was able to demonstrate in Marburg-type acute MS that oligodendrocytes had an abrupt and dramatic loss, but the areas were soon repopulated by large numbers of these cells and that remyelination could begin, leaving the "shadow plaques" commonly seen in acute MS.

3. Acute MS is not a variant of acute disseminated encephalomyelitis but is related to classic patterns of MS; Marburg's severe and acute variant is a *forme fruste* of the relapsing-remitting pattern of MS.

4. The disease is probably autoimmune in nature, and the autoantigen is still an unidentified component of myelin and/or oligodendrocytes.

5. Axonal loss might also be a very important aspect of MS according to Prineas, Barnes, and McDonald.

6. Despite the many variations in MS, and attempts to suggest the syndrome of MS may contain different conditions, the process is probably a singular one with an underlying process.

7. Promising HLA studies have not yet helped identify the antigen nor have interesting epidemiological studies shown convincing clues to the underlying cause of MS.

In recent years, there have been attempts pathologically to demonstrate activity stages of various plaques. It had long been known that some lesions were acute, with great cellular infiltrate and inflammatory changes and perivascular reaction. There were also chronic lesions with signs of activity, usually at the periphery, and others with little sign of activity.[83] There were also shadow plaques in some areas. Bo and Trapp, van der Valk, Buicke and Lassmann, and The Vienna Consensus Conference all attempted to define stages of the plaque. Their definitions are similar, with the exception of the Vienna classification, which seems more complex and impractical. They essentially define the features of active, chronic-active, and chronic-inactive plaques. More important than the specific components of each classification is the definition, as each study attempts to outline similar features.

Lucchinetti has proposed four patterns of MS lesions.[84] Patterns 1 and 2 have features of immune-mediated disease. Patterns 3 and 4 resemble oligodendroglial disease with a dying-back pneumonia. Patients tend to have lesions of the same pattern and these observations may have implications for future therapy.

The clinical symptoms of MS and deficits manifested by the patient are likely due to conduction block resulting from demyelination that follows inflammation. The inflammation causes local production of nitric oxide by macrophages prominent in the lesions. Nitric oxide causes graded, dose-dependent conduction block in nerve fibers.[85]

REFERENCES

1. Greenfield JG, King LS. Observations on the histopathology of the cerebral lesions in disseminated sclerosis. *Brain*. 1936;59:445-458.
2. Rindfleisch E. Histologische Detail zu der Grauen Degeneration von Gehirn and Rückenmark. *Virchow Arch Path Anat Physiol*. 1863;26:474-483.
3. Babinski J. *Etude Anatomique et Clinique sur la Sclérose en Plaques*. Paris: G Masson; 1885.
4. Babinski J. Recherches sur l'anatomie pathologique de la sclérose en plaques et étude comparative des diverses variétés de scléroses de la moelle. *Arch Physiol Norm Pathol*. 1885;5(series 3):186-207.
5. Compston A. Remyelination in multiple sclerosis: a challenge for therapy. The 1996 European Charcot Foundation Lecture. *Multiple Sclerosis*. 1997;3:51-70.
6. Strümpell A. Über diffuse hirnsklerose. *Arch f Psychiat*. 1879;9:268-285.
7. Müller R. Studies on disseminated sclerosis. *Acta med Scand*. 1949;133(suppl 222):1-214.
8. Marie P. *Lectures on Diseases of the Spinal Cord*, trans. M Lubbock. London: New Sydenham Society; 1895;153:134-136.
9. McDonald WI. The mystery of the origin of multiple sclerosis. The Ninth Gowers Memorial Lecture. *J Neurol Neurosurg Psychiat*. 1986;49:113-123.
10. Greenfield JG, King LS. Oberservations on the histopathology of the cerebral lesions in disseminated sclerosis. *Brain*. 1936;59:445-458.
11. Wilson SAK. *Neurology*. Bruce AN, ed. London: Edward Arnold; 1940:148-178.
12. Cruveilhier J. *Medical Tracts*. Wellcome Library. 1828; 621.4.
13. Cruveilhier J. *Anatomie pathologique du corps humain, ou descriptions avc figures lithographiees et coloriées, des diverses alterations morbides dont le corps humain est suceptibles*. Vol 2. Paris: J. B. Baillière; 1835-1842.
14. Cruveilhier J. *Anatomie Descriptive*. 4 Vols. on the nervous system with illustrations. Paris: Béchet; 1836-1841.
15. Cruveilhier J. *Anatomia Pathologica del corpo umano*. Trans. Pietro Banchelli. Florence: Vincenzo Batelli; 1837-1841.
16. Murray TJ. The history of MS. In: *Multiple Sclerosis: Diagnosis, Medical Management and Rehabilitation*. New York: Demos. 2000;1-20.
17. McDonald WI. The mystery of the origin of multiple sclerosis. The Ninth Gowers Memorial Lecture. *J Neurol Neurosurg Psychiat*. 1986;49:113-123.

18. Compston A. Remyelination in multiple sclerosis: a challenge for therapy. The 1996 European Charcot Foundation Lecture. *Multiple Sclerosis*. 1997;3:51-70.

19. Greenfield JG, King LS. Observations on the histopathology of the cerebral lesions in disseminated sclerosis. *Brain*. 1936;59:445-458.

20. Marburg O. Die Sogenannte akute mulltiple sklerose (encephalomyelitis periaxialis scleroticans) *Jahrb Psychiat Neurol*. 1906;27:1.

21. Dawson JD. The Histology of Disseminated Sclerosis. *Trans Royal Soc Edin*. 1916;50:517-740.

22. Dawson JD. The Histology of Disseminated Sclerosis. *Rev Neurol Psychiat*. 1917;15:47-166; 369-417; 1918;16:287-307.

23. Hassin GB. Pathological studies in the pathogenesis of multiple sclerosis. In: *Multiple Sclerosis: Association for Research in Nervous and Mental Diseases*. Vol 2. New York:. Paul B. Hoeber; 1922:144-175.

24. Rindfleisch E. Histologische Detail zu der Grauen Degeneration von Gehirn and Rückenmark. *Virchow Arch Path Anat Physiol*. 1863;26:474-483.

25. Marie P. *Lectures on Diseases of the Spinal Cord*, trans. M Lubbock. London: New Sydenham Society; 1895;153:134-136.

26. Bielschowsky M. Die marklosen Nervenfasern in den Herden der multiplen Sklerose. *Neurol Centralbl*. 1904;23:59-62.

27. Penfield W. *No Man Alone: A Neurosurgeon's Life*. Boston: Little Brown; 1977.

28. Ibid, p. 103-106.

29. Penfield W. Oligodendroglia and its relation to classical neuroglia. *Brain*. 1924;47:430-452.

30. Greenfield JG, King LS. Observations on the histopathology of the cerebral lesions in disseminated sclerosis. *Brain*. 1936;59:445-458.

31. *Greenfield's Neuropathology*, 2nd ed. Blackwood W, McMenemey WH, Myer A, Norman RM, Russell DS. eds. London: Edward Arnold; 1963:488.

32. Spiller WG, Camp CD. Multiple sclerosis, with a report of two additional cases with necropsy. *J Nerv Ment Dis*. 1904;31:433-445.

33. Leiner JH. An Investigation of the axis cylinder in its relation to multiple sclerosis. In: *Multiple Sclerosis and Disseminated Sclerosis. Proceedings of Association for Research in Nervous and Mental Diseases*. New York: Paul B. Hoeber; 1922:197-208.

34. Compston A. Remyelination in multiple sclerosis: a challenge for therapy. The 1996 European Charcot Foundation Lecture. *Multiple Sclerosis*. 1997;3:51-70.

35. Putnam TJ. The pathogenesis of multiple sclerosis: a possible vascular factor. *N Engl J Med*. 1933;209:786.

36. Putnam TJ, McKenna JB, Morrison LR. Studies in multiple sclerosis: the histogenesis of experimental sclerotic plaques and their relation to multiple sclerosis. *JAMA*. 1931;97:1591.

37. Hurst EW. A review of some recent observations on demyelination. *Brain*. 1944;67;103-125.

38. Reese HH. Critique of theories concerning the etiology of multiple sclerosis. In: *Multiple Sclerosis and the Demyelinating Diseases. Proceedings of the Association for Research in Nervous and Mental Disease* (Dec. 10-11, 1948). Vol 28. Baltimore: Williams and Wilkins; 1950.

39. Reese HH. Multiple Sclerosis and the Demyelinating Diseases. Critique of theories concerning multiple sclerosis. *JAMA*. 1950;143:1470-1473.

40. Fog T. On the vessel-plaque relations in the brain in multiple sclerosis. *Acta Psychiat Neurol Scand*. 1963;39;suppl 4:258.

41. Zimmerman HM, Netsky MG. The pathology of multiple sclerosis. In: *Multiple Sclerosis and the Demyelinating Diseases. Proceedings of the Association for Research in Nervous and Mental Diseases*. (Dec. 10-11, 1948). Vol 28. Baltimore: Williams and Wilkins; 1950:271-312.

42. Reese HH. Disseminated Sclerosis and Dicoumerol Therapy. *Tran Am Neurol Assoc.* 1944;70:78.
43. Reese HH. Disseminated Sclerosis and Dicoumerol Therapy. *Tran Am Neurol Assoc.* 1944;70:78.
44. Adams CWM. The onset and progression of the lesion in multiple sclerosis. *J Neurol Sci.* 1975;25:165-182.
45. Prineas JW, Connell F. Remyelination in multiple sclerosis. *Ann Neurol.* 1979;5:22-31.
46. Prineas JW, Wright RG. Macrophages, lymphocytes, and plasma cells in the perivascular compartment in chronic multiple sclerosis. *Lab Med.* 1978;38:409-421.
47. Prineas JW, Connell F. Remyelination in multiple sclerosis. *Ann Neurol.* 1979;5:22-31.
48. Lassmann H. *Comparative Neuropathology of Chronic Experimental Allergic Encephalomyelitis and Multiple Sclerosis.* Berlin, Heidelberg, New York: Springer; 1983.
49. McDonald WI, Sears TA. The effects of experimental demyelination on conduction in the central nervous system. *Brain.* 1970;93:583-598.
50. Prineas JW, Barnard RO, Kwon EE, Sharer LR, Cho ES. Multiple sclerosis: remyelination of nascent lesions. *Ann Neurol.* 1993;33:137-151.
51. Bunge MB, Bunge RP, Ris H. Ultrastructural study of remyelination in an experimental lesion in the adult cat spinal cord. *J Biophys Biochem Cytol.* 1961;10:67-94.
52. Prineas JW, Connell F. The fine structure of chronically active multiple sclerosis plaques. *Neurology.* 1978;28:68-75.
53. Prineas JW, Wright RG. Macrophages, lymphocytes, and plasma cells in the perivascular compartment in chronic multiple sclerosis. *Lab Med.* 1978;38:409-421.
54. Prineas JW, Connell F. Remyelination in multiple sclerosis. *Ann Neurol.* 1979;5:22-31.
55. Noseworthy JG. Progress in determining the cause and treatment of multiple sclerosis. *Nature.* 1999;399(suppl):A40-A47.
56. Halliday AM, McDonald WI, Mushin J. Delayed visual evoked response in optic neuritis. *Lancet.* 1972;I:982-985.
57. Halliday AM, McDonald WI, Mushin J. Delayed pattern-evoked responses in optic neuritis in relation to visual acuity. *Trans Opthalmol Soc UK.* 1973;93:315-324.
58. Halliday AM, McDonald WI, Mushin J. Delayed visual evoked response in optic neuritis. *Lancet.* 1972;I:982-985.
59. McDonald WI. Chance and Design. *J Neurol.* 1999;246:654-660.
60. McDonald WI. The dynamics of multiple sclerosis: the Charcot lecture. *J Neurology.* 1993;240(1):28-36.
61. McDonald WI. The mystery of the origin of multiple sclerosis. Gowers Lecture. *J Neurol Neurosurg Psychiat.* 1986;49:113-123.
62. Bunge MB, Bunge RP, Ris H. Ultrastructural study of remyelination in an experimental lesion in the adult cat spinal cord. *J Biophys Biochem Cytol.* 1961;10:67-94.
63. Compston A. Remyelination in multiple sclerosis: a challenge for therapy. The 1996 European Charcot Foundation Lecture. *Multiple Sclerosis.* 1997;3:51-70.
64. Prineas JW, Barnard RO, Kwon EE, Sharer LR, Cho ES. Multiple sclerosis: remyelination of nascent lesions. *Ann Neurol.* 1993;33:137-151.
65. Putnam TJ. Studies in Multiple Sclerosis. *Arch Neurol Psych.* 1936;35:1289-1308.
66. Kornek B, Lassman H. Axonal pathology in multiple sclerosis. A historical note. *Brain Pathology.* 1999;9:651-656.
67. Kornek B, Lassman H. Axonal pathology in multiple sclerosis. A historical note. *Brain Pathology.* 1999;9:651-656.
68. Compston A. Remyelination in multiple sclerosis: a challenge for therapy. The 1996 European Charcot Foundation Lecture. *Multiple Sclerosis.* 1997;3:51-70.
69. Compston A. Reviewing multiple sclerosis. *Postgrad Med J.* 1992;68(801):507-515.
70. McDonald WI. *Brain.* 1991/1971.

71. Kornek B, Lassman H. Axonal pathology in multiple sclerosis. A historical note. *Brain Pathol*. 1999;9:651-656.
72. Davie CA, Barker GJ, Webb S, Tofts PS, Thompson AJ, Harding AE, McDonald WI, Miller DH. Persistent functional deficit in multiple sclerosis and autosomal dominant cerebellar ataxia is associated with axonal loss. *Brain*. 1995;118:1583-1592.
73. Trapp BD, Peterson J, Ransohoff RM, Rudick R, Mörks, Bö L. Axonal transections in the lesions of multiple sclerosis. *N Engl J Med*. 1998;338:278-285.
74. Noseworthy JG. Progress in determining the cause and treatment of multiple sclerosis. *Nature*. 1999;399(suppl):A40-A47.
75. Ibid.
76. McDonald WI. The mystery of the origin of multiple sclerosis. Gowers Lecture. *J Neurol Neurosurg Psychiat*. 1986;49:113-123.
77. Arnold DL, Reiss GT, Mathews PM. Use of proton magnetic resonance spectroscopy for monitoring disease progression in multiple sclerosis. *Ann Neurol*. 1994;36:76-82.
78. Trapp BD, Peterson J, Ransohoff RM, Rudick R, Mörks, Bö L. Axonal transections in the lesions of multiple sclerosis. *N Engl J Med*. 1998;338:278-285.
79. Trapp BD, Peterson J, et al. Axonal transections in the lesions of multiple sclerosis. *N Engl J Med*. 1998;338:278-285.
80. Arnold DL, Reiss GT, Mathews PM. Use of proton magnetic resonance spectroscopy for monitoring disease progression in multiple sclerosis. *Ann Neurol*. 1994;36:76-82.
81. Prineas JW, Barnard RO, Kwon EE, Sharer LR, Cho ES. Multiple sclerosis: remyelination of nascent lesions. *Ann Neurol*. 1993;33:137-151.
82. Lumsden CE. The neuropathology of multiple sclerosis. In: Vinken PJ, Bruyn GW, eds. *Multiple Sclerosis and Other Demyelinating Diseases. Handbook of Clinical Neurology*. Vol 9. Amsterdam: North Holland. 1970:217-309.
83. Van der Valk P, De Groot CJ. Staging of multiple sclerosis (MS) lesions: pathology of the time frame of MS. *Neuropathol Appl Neurobiol*, 2000;26:2-10.
84. Lucchinetti C, Bruck W, Parisi J, Scheithauer B, Rodriguez M, Lassmann H. Heterogeneity of multiple sclerosis lesions: implications for the pathogenesis of demyelination. *Ann Neurol*. 2000;47:707-717.
85. McDonald WI. Relapse, remission and progression in multiple sclerosis. *N Engl J Med*. 2000;343:148-1487.

14

Investigations

"It is perhaps true of disseminated sclerosis than of any other chronic nervous disease that the diagnosis is difficult in the earliest stages."
Ashley W. MacKintosh, 1903

During the 19th century, multiple sclerosis was recognized as a distinct neurological entity, separable from other neurological diseases by the clinical and eventually pathological features in the patient. It was evident that multiple sclerosis could look like other disorders at different stages of its progression, but the patient's age, disease course, and clinical features were usually distinctive enough to make a clinical diagnosis in life. Even today, the "gold standard" for MS diagnosis is a clinical diagnosis, as the remarkable new diagnostic tests still only *confirm* the clinical suspicion, but cannot *make* the diagnosis.

A second important point to consider as we discuss the history of diagnostic techniques is that these developments have also allowed clinicians to better understand the disease process and how the nervous system functions in health and disease. There is a tendency to regard techniques developed to help in the diagnosis of MS only in terms of the percentage of positive or negative results and the regretful false-positive and negative results, and to neglect what we have learned from the application of the tests. The CSF tests of the 1940–1985 period told us much about CSF dynamics and the effects of infective and irritative disorders. The evoked potential studies of the 1970s told us much about how the nervous system functions and perceives the world, even though evoked potential is only a moderately good test for MS. The MRI was initially most useful in recognizing the lesions of MS, but has now been developed in ways that show how the disease evolves and changes. New methodologies will show brain functioning and axonal changes not seen by the original MRI "snapshots" of the inflammatory lesions.

MS AS A CLINICAL DIAGNOSIS

Although the clinical features and course of MS allowed it to be diagnosed by a history and physical examination in many instances defined by Charcot and others, a search for a more objective measure became increasingly important when it was clear that there were many cases that did not have established cardinal features, such as Charcot's triad. Also, mild cases and *formes frustes* of the disease were being recognized. Other conditions can look very much like MS so better methods of diagnosis, whether clinical or technological, were needed. Charcot and his followers had some technological methods to record tremor, eye movements, and gait, but these were more for documentation than as an aid in diagnosis.

The clinical diagnosis outlined by Charcot, his colleagues, and students was a rigid one. Using a diagnostic pattern of the fully developed

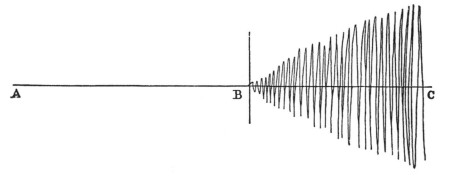

Figure 14.1 A demonstration of the tremor in multiple sclerosis used by Charcot to point out the difference from paralysis agitans (Parkinson's Disease). The straight line is the hand at rest with "absolutely no tremor." When the patient makes a movement (B) the tremor begins and increases as the movement continues.

disease and incorporating features such as the Charcot triad allowed the diagnosis to be made only in very advanced cases. English and American clinicians began to complain about the rigid French approach and comment that the clinical diagnosis must become more refined and broadened to identify earlier and "minor" cases of MS and the increasingly recognized *formes frustes* of the disease.

Charcot and his students did employ some measurement techniques in MS, as they did for other disorders. They had methods of recording hand control by handwriting, muscle strength by dynometer, tremor by sphygmographs originally designed for recording pulses, and gait by foot ink prints, which were used to document disability in the patients and to extend the clinical examination. These tests did not confirm or make the diagnosis. Charcot had a photography studio at the Salpêtrière to document patients and Bramwell was regularly photographing his neurological cases in Scotland. Compston suggested the first photographic representations of MS are in volume 3 of *Nouvelle iconographic* by Blocq and Londe in 1890.[1]

Once clinicians had a recognizable pattern of clinical features to aid in diagnosis, there was further effort to classify the types of patterns seen, either by anatomical area that seemed involved or by the varying clinical course. Charcot noted the disease could occur in many forms and there were no features always present in every case. He said that cephalgic and spinal forms of the disease were distinct patterns. Although he would later be criticized for what others saw as a rigid diagnostic approach, Charcot recognized there were less well-defined cases, and that the incidences of MS would tend to increase as diagnoses reached a higher level of accuracy.[2,3]

By the turn of the century, clinical criteria were better defined and the diagnostic accuracy sought by Charcot was improving, but no diagnostic test had been developed. In practice, patients were often not given the MS "label" until their cases were quite advanced, as occurred in the case of W.N.P. Barbellion.[4]

In the early 20th century, diagnosis was still difficult in the initial stages of MS and when the patterns or symptoms were unusual. As an example, in a survey of the cases of MS from 15 New York and New Jersey metropolitan hospitals between 1930 and 1939, there were 33 cases of MS clinically, but 10 turned out at autopsy to have other diseases.[5] In

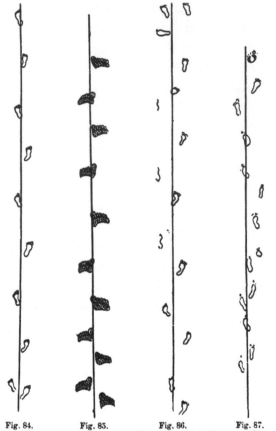

Fig. 84.   Fig. 85.   Fig. 86.   Fig. 87.

Fig. 84.—Sketch of the normal gait according to Gilles de la Tourette. The steps are of equal length, the feet maintain the same direction in the different steps. and the same distance from the line of progress.

Fig. 85.—Diagram representing the gait of a patient suffering from insular sclerosis. Spastic gait. The steps are short; the ball of the foot alone touches the ground, the feet are turned inwards and have a tendency to cross each other (overstepping at times the median line, which represents their progress).

Fig. 86.—Sketch of the gait of a patient suffering from insular sclerosis (after Gilles de la Tourette). Cerebellar gait. The steps are very unequal in length, the direction of the feet varies in the different steps and they do not remain at the same distance from the median line, indicating the direction of their progress.

Fig. 87.—Sketch of the gait of the same patient, as fig. 86 (after Gilles de la Tourette). Cerebellar gait. The irregularity is even more marked than in the preceding sketch.

Figure 14.2 Georges Gilles de la Tourette developed a gait test that recorded the gait of patients with neurological disease, including MS, as seen here, by having them walk on lengths of paper with inked feet.

addition, 11 additional cases were identified at autopsy during that period that were not diagnosed as MS in life. Clearly, an objective test or series of tests was needed to supplement the improving clinical skills of the physician.

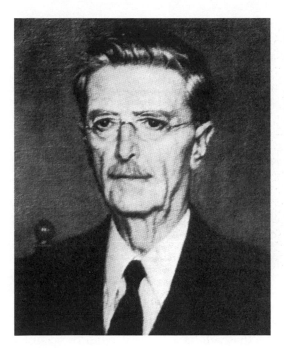

Figure 14.3   Sir Gordon Holmes, a noted teacher and clinician, performed definitive studies on cerebellar function, and established the modern methods of neurological examination.

Even the features that seemed to define the clinical picture were variable and controversial. Ever since Strümpell noted the disappearance of the abdominal reflexes in MS in 1896, this became a defining feature.[6]

Up to the 1960s, many clinicians were reluctant to make a diagnosis if the abdominal reflexes were present, but these reflexes are now disregarded as a sign in MS. Babinski's observation of the upgoing large toe on plantar stimulation in cases with involvement of the pyramidal tract was very helpful in recognizing disturbance in the central nervous system in MS. Even the prognosis was argued with some early writers who indicated many patients lived only 8–12 years, while others described patients who lived for 20 or 30 years, often with little reduction in life expectancy.

In a review of MS in the 1950s, Schumacher felt that to arrive at a diagnosis of MS just on the presence of certain signs such as nystagmus or tremor was using "cookbook medicine," but to do so based on symptoms alone was worse and inexcusable. He tried to apply certain rules to the diagnostic criteria. He discussed the elements of what would later be the Schumacher criteria for diagnosis of MS;[7] these would be further refined first by Kurtzke and later by the Poser committee. Many believe the cur-

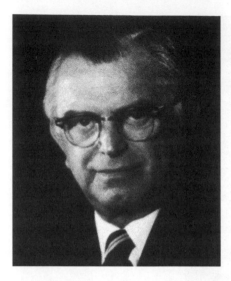

Figure 14.4 Morris Bender clarified the nature and characteristics of many eye signs in neurological disease, among these the internuclear ophthalmoplegia due to a lesion, often from MS, in the medial longitudinal fasciculus of the brain stem. Noting a connectedness among those interested in MS, it is interesting to note that Bender was a student of Spiller, who was a pupil of Gowers, Edinger, Oppenheim, and Schilder, who are also mentioned in these pages. Bender was a master of the neurological examination and devised many signs and techniques of examination. (From the collection of Mrs. Sara Bender.)

rent classifications of MS are not justified and improved technology that allows further refinement of the underlying mechanisms will allow a more realistic classification, one that will have better prognostic accuracy and will influence therapeutic decisions.

Objective measures were also needed to clarify whether all cases of MS are the same, or even the same disease. If there are groupings, they might respond differently to new therapies. Some argued that it was not necessary to have such definitive tests for a disease that had no specific treatment, but others recognized that having such tests in place would be imperative if treatments came along, in order to evaluate results, especially if they applied only to certain features, patterns, or groups of MS patients (Donald Paty, personal communication).

CSF TESTS

The first test that was helpful in confirming the clinical diagnosis of MS was CSF analysis. The work of Heinrich Irenaüs Quincke* and Hans

---

*Heinrich Irenaüs Quincke (1842–1922) was born in Germany but became professor of medicine in Bern, Switzerland. In 1882, he described angioneurotic edema and differentiated *E. coli* and *E. histolytica*. He is remembered for introducing the method of therapeutic lumbar puncture in 1891, but it had been performed for the same reason and by the same method two years earlier by Walter Essex Wynter (1860–1945).

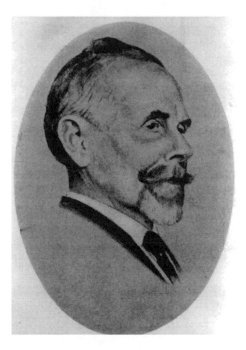

Figure 14.5 Heinrich Irenaeüs Quincke (1842–1922) while an assistant to Frerichs, did studies of CSF in animals and adapted his technique of inserting a fine needle with stylet into the subarachnoid space of an infant with hydrocephalus, and after his presentation of this discovery in 1891, he noted the importance of careful manometric pressure measurements and the ability to examine the CSF for cells, protein, sugar, bacteria and the presence of blood. His technique became important in multiple sclerosis when Lange noted the colloidal gold pattern in syphilis, and it was later found that in MS there were often similar "leutic" and "paretic" patterns. CSF was improved as a confirmatory test hen gamma globulin elevation was noted, and more recently oligoclonal bands. (From the collection of Dr. Frederick Hiller.)

Heinrich Georg Queckenstedt,* on techniques of tapping and sampling the cerebrospinal fluid, noting its appearance and pressure, led to further analysis of CSF in diseases such as syphilis and MS. Although the test was developed initially for therapeutic drainage for hydrocephalus and infections, the ability to examine cerebrospinal fluid became helpful in assessment of changes due to syphilis, meningitis, and other conditions.

The first important observation in MS was the identification by Hinton of abnormal protein precipitation similar to that of syphilis in the CSF of many MS patients.[8] The most characteristic change was visible with the colloidal gold test, often positive in many MS patients. Fifty percent of the MS fluids showed a *paretic curve* and 20 percent a *luetic curve*, in other words, similar to the curves of precipitation seen in those forms of syphilis. Attempts to quantify the colloidal gold reaction helped, but these were still nonspecific. Other conditions such as infections and immunological disorders had the same reactions. There were also variations in dif-

---

*Hans Heinrich George Queckenstedt (1876–1918) of Hamburg showed the method of assessing a block in the spinal canal by compressing the jugular vein (Queckenstedt test). The manometer does not rise as expected.

ferent laboratories from a 20 percent to an 80 percent positive rate,[9] so confidence in a nonspecific and variable test waned. In addition, this was a test developed for syphilis that gave the same responses in MS; a test was needed to separate MS from neurosyphilis, which was still very common; its features often resembled those of MS. The colloidal gold test was helpful in differentiating MS from other diseases of the nervous system, but not from syphilis; the development of serological tests for syphilis were useful in distinguishing that disease more easily. In 1939, Lange[10] introduced a modification of the Pandy colloidal gold test, controlling the size of the colloidal particles and the pH, and the result was the "Lange curve," which had a much higher positive rate in MS. Seventy-three percent of Houston Merritt's cases had a positive result; many others had less-characteristic but still abnormal results. In Merritt's MS cases, the colloidal gold test was abnormal in 33 percent, the Lange D curves in 73 percent, and there was elevated gamma globulin in 91 percent.

Houston Merritt pointed out that the value of the CSF tests in the 1940s was limited by the quality of the laboratory and whether a CSF test was a special interest of the lab, or just another routine test. If the lab just did the CSF assay as a routine test, the accuracy and the number of positive results dropped off. The test seemed deceptively easy to perform. Merritt said it was not worth the expense sending samples to laboratories that did not have special interest in the quality of the CSF test.[11]

Most experienced neurologists emphasize to their students that they used the colloidal gold tests, but would never overturn a diagnosis based on whether the test was positive or negative. In other words, they were happy to have their diagnosis confirmed by the test, but at the end of the day, their clinical acumen was to be relied on in all cases. George Schumacher was emphatic:

> *"I never allow biological tests largely to influence diagnosis. If I make up my mind on clinical grounds that a case is multiple sclerosis, I am willing to have the laboratory corroborate that diagnosis, but I will not allow the negative findings to upset the positive diagnosis."*

This confidence extended to syphilis as well, and he added the statement:

"I still maintain there may be clues in spite of negative findings."

The fear of precipitating an attack of MS made neurologists reluctant to do lumbar punctures on patients suspected of having MS. Early in the 20th century, lumbar punctures were usually done on MS patients to test for syphilis. Only a few brave neurologists used the method of forced CSF drainage as a treatment for MS, and many believed that the procedure of lumbar puncture could cause exacerbations of MS, as reported by Maruézy in 1924. In his reminiscences of a half century as a neurologist, Lord Walton said that in 1946, a lumbar puncture in a patient with multiple sclerosis was thought to be dangerous, and a myelogram was not done, as "the professor" would not permit an LP on anyone suspected of this multiple sclerosis diagnosis.* He commented:

"I now shudder to think how many patients with undiagnosed spinal tumors there were in (the wards) carrying the diagnostic label of disseminated sclerosis."

Lord Walton, 1993[12]

Dr. Elvin Kabat of Columbia University studied the immunological response in the CSF of MS patients using the new technique of electrophoresis.[13] His studies in 1942 and later with Melvin Yahr in 1954 and 1957 established the diagnostic value of quantitative determinations of CSF gamma globulins in clinical neurology, especially in MS.[14] They noticed that the CSF of MS patients contained an increased proportion of gamma globulin. This supported the suggestion that an immunological process occurred in MS. It also sparked an increasing interest in the immunological basis for the development of the MS plaque. In later decades, it directed the therapeutic approach with drugs that modified or suppressed the immune system.

In 1964, Lature used gel electrophoresis to find an oligoclonal pattern in the CSF of MS patients with a discontinuous aspect of the globulin zone, with several fractions.[15] He showed the pattern was more impor-

---

*This was still a lingering concern when I was training in neurology in the 1960s. We had become accustomed to the LP for CSF examination and regarded it as safe, but were still discussing whether a myelogram might precipitate acute relapses.

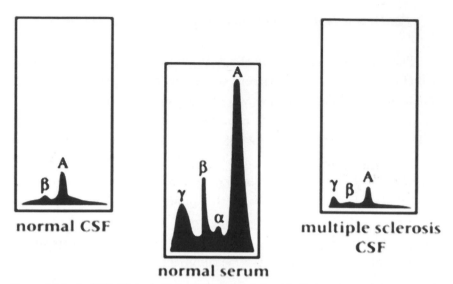

Figure 14.6 In 1942, Elvin A. Kabat (1914–) at Columbia University used the new technique of electrophoresis to study the immunological response in MS. He noted the CSF of MS patients had an increase in gamma globulin.

tant than increased globulin level, as there could be an abnormality of oligoclonal banding when the globulin was normal. The immunoglobulin changes produced characteristic increases of clonally restricted antibodies (IgG) to produce oligoclonal banding. Although this could occur in other immunological diseases affecting the nervous system, it was characteristic of MS and was used by the Poser committee in 1983 as part of the diagnostic criteria, to fulfill the criteria for "laboratory-supported definite MS (LSDMS).[16]

EEG AND EMG

When an investigation becomes available in neurology it will usually be tried in MS. The EEG has been said to be abnormal in half the cases of MS studied, but this did not help in diagnosis, as the changes were not distinctive or abnormal enough to add useful diagnostic or prognostic information. Herbert Jasper of Montreal and Reginald Bickford of the Mayo Clinic cooperated in 1948 to assess the characteristics of the EEG in MS when the EEG was finding a prominent place in clinical neurology.

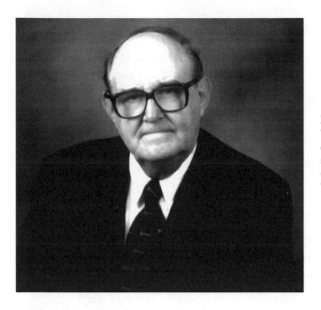

Figure   14.7 Wallace
Tourtellotte clarified the
changes in the cerebro-
spinal fluid in MS.
(Courtesy of Dr. W.
Tourtellotte.)

They found 90 percent of patients had abnormal EEGs in the acute
phase, chiefly in the slow wave forms; 75 percent in the subacute stages;
but only 30 percent in the period of remission. The changes were not
characteristic enough to be useful clinically, but they thought the different levels of activity in the different stages must relate in some way to the
activity of the process. There was interest in a possible peripheral nerve
and myoneural junction abnormality in MS, but again the EMG changes
were too minor to be helpful and might have been mostly secondary
changes.

RADIOGRAPHY

The development of imaging techniques in MS was reviewed by
Ormerod, du Boulay, and McDonald, who showed the remarkable
advances made from the era of pneumoencephalography to the time of
magnetic resonance imaging.[17] The earliest evidence of MS on imaging
was the demonstration on pneumoencephalography, showing ventricular
enlargement and cortical atrophy.[18] Myelography could show expansion
of the cord in an area of transverse myelitis or contraction of the cord
(contracting cord sign in MS) in more chronic cases.[19]

CEREBRAL BLOOD FLOW

Cerebral blood flow studies were attempted in MS patients soon after the technique was developed by Kety and Schmidt in 1948. Within months, W.M. Tucker and his team in Philadelphia presented 30 cases of MS who had cerebral blood flow studies, showing that half had reduction in blood flow, but the results could vary if the studies were repeated.[20]

ISOTOPE BRAIN SCANS

Radionucleide scans (the first "brain scans") depend on the passing of radioactive-labeled material through disruption in the blood–brain barrier; although this occurs in MS, it is not visualized well or often by this technique. The first such scans noted were in a series by Seaman on brain tumors, where one case turned out to be MS. Another single case was found in a survey of non-neoplastic neurological disease.[21] Gize and Mishkin collected 28 cases of active MS over six years and found that five had positive isotope brain scans.[22] Moses found only one patient to have a positive scan in 14 cases scanned during an acute MS attack, and later noted that positivity on the scan could come and go.[23] Antunes et al. showed that only three of 160 scans in MS were positive, demonstrating that although a scan could be positive in MS if the lesion and the breakdown in blood–brain barrier were large enough, it was not positive in most cases and not sensitive enough to be a useful diagnostic technique.[24]

EVOKED POTENTIAL STUDIES

An important advance in adapting a test to the pathophysiology of demyelination came with the work of Ian McDonald and others on the block of conduction in demyelinated fibers and the delay in remyelinated fibers. McDonald suggested to Martin Halliday that measuring conduction block in the visual system might be a useful way to assess changes due to clinical or subclinical optic nerve demyelination. Attempts in the next few years to effectively assess conduction block in the visual system were unsatisfactory in separating the normal from the abnormal in a definitive manner using a flash stimulus. The studies showed greater sensitivity with a rapidly reversing black and white checkerboard pattern in a pilot study of 19 patients with unilateral optic neuritis. Further studies showed this to be a useful technique, particularly when it could demonstrate a second area of involvement in a suspected MS case who had only a spinal cord or brain stem lesion. Studies later showed that up to 90 percent of confirmed MS cases had some delay in the optic nerve, suggesting that this would be a useful test for screening patients for MS and for assessing cases of spastic paraplegia for the possibility that the underlying etiology was MS.[25,26]

The concept of delayed conduction was most useful in assessing the visual system (visual evoked potential studies [VEP]), but it was developed for the auditory system to assess the brain stem (brainstem auditory evoked potential studies [BAER]); and sensory system to assess the spinal cord (sensory evoked potential studies [SEP]). These studies contributed to a developing technology that not only added a group of useful tests, but told something about how the nervous system worked in health as well as in illnesses such as MS.

CAT SCANNING

In the century after Wilhelm Roentgen demonstrated the first radiograph by a method he called X-ray, the methodology was accepted to improve neurological diagnosis with Walter Dandy's ventriculography (1918) and pneumoencephalography (1919) and Egaz Moniz's cerebral arteriography (1927). There was great excitement in the early 1970s when a method was developed using repeated beams of X-rays rotating around the object (originally the head) to measure the density of the tissue (computerized axial tomography [CAT]). This was fed into a computer in layers and the density "dots" recreated a picture of the nervous system as a density portrait, which had remarkable clarity.* William Oldendorf developed the

---

*The consensus was that the development of computerized axial tomography would be the front runner for the 1979 Nobel Prize, but the controversy, as so often happens, was over who should be recognized by the award. No one would disagree with the recognition of Godfrey Hounsfield, the British World War II radar engineer who joined Thorne-EMI in 1952 and

basis of the computerized axial (CAT) scan in 1961; the scan was developed into a working diagnostic model by Godfrey Hounsfield, an engineer, and Alan Cormack, a mathematician and physicist.

William Oldendorf trained in neurology under A.B. Baker in Minneapolis in the 1950s, where neurology residents did all their own arteriograms and ventriculograms on their own patients. Contemplating how the brain could be imaged better, he developed in his basement an elegantly simple method that would become CT scanning. He published the method in 1961 (unfortunately in an obscure journal) and patented the idea in 1963. Standard X-ray equipment manufacturers thought the idea was impractical. One manufacturer wrote Oldendorf:

> *"Even if it could be made to work as you suggest, we cannot imagine a significant market for such an expensive apparatus that would do nothing but make a radiographic cross-section of a head."*[27]

Oldendorf noted that in the past, the importance of an EEG as a replacement for neurological examination had been over emphasized, and it would be foolhardy to overemphasize the CAT or ultrasound, but to ignore the importance of these techniques was just as foolhardy.

The prototype CAT scanner developed by Hounsfield was put in place at the Atkinson-Morley Hospital in London and the first pictures of the brain published were printed on small Polaroid prints. These prints were enough to impress every neurologist and neurosurgeon of the potential to demonstrate the brain and the ventricular system without painful invasive tests.

The first four American sites to have CAT scans were the Massachusetts General Hospital, the Mayo Clinic, Rush-Presbyterian-St. Luke's Hospital in Chicago, and the Dent Neurological Institute in Buffalo. In most instances, as related by Maynard Cohen,[28] radiology departments were uninterested, and the equipment was mostly acquired

---

became director of their research department in 1972. Nor was there disagreement with the award to South African-born American physicist Allan MacLeod Cormack, who did the mathematical computations. The controversy was over the snub to the Chicago neurologist William Oldendorf, who independently developed and published the concept in an obscure journal. The Americans compensated for this by awarding him many honors in subsequent years.

by enthusiastic neurologists and neurosurgeons. Dr. Jack Greenberg's comment when he saw the first CAT images was that he had seen Valhalla!

With the advent of computerized tomography (CT for computerized tomography, or CAT for computerized axial tomography), efforts were made to use this technique in MS; studies showed 9 to 75 percent enhancing lesion, depending on how carefully the cases had been selected.[29] The first demonstration of an MS lesion on a CAT scan was by Davis and Pressman, who showed a positive scan confirmed by biopsy to be an area of demyelination. CAT scanning was such an exciting advance in the 1970s–1980s that most patients with brain disease were scanned, so the experience with MS was extensive.[30–32] It was clear that lesions were not easily identified by computerized tomography, and that most definite cases of MS had normal CAT scans. There was evidence of cerebral atrophy in 45 percent of cases scanned.[33] Cases of very large tumor-like lesions were reported, and biopsy demonstrated demyelination. In 1976, Wuthrich reported the use of enhanced CAT scans in MS, and later experience suggested that MS lesions that appeared on enhanced CAT scans were evidence of active disease.[34] The presence of multiple white matter lesions was highly suggestive of MS, but unfortunately not specific, since there were other conditions that could give the same appearance. Later experience showed that these enhancing lesions might fade and even disappear, and they might clear with steroid use. These low-density lesions were mostly periventricular, and the suspicion that they were areas of demyelination was confirmed by autopsy in a number of instances. The information revealed by scans could be increased by using a double-dose of contrast and delaying the scan for an hour (a high-volume delayed [HVD] CAT),[35] which Ebers showed was positive in 53 percent of scans in those patients who had acute relapsing MS. The positive percentage was lower in stable patients.[36] Paty found as many as 72 percent of cases had multiple enhancing lesions in the acute stage; the percentage diminished as the clinical activity decreased.[37,38] Scattered lesions on the CAT scan could be used to fulfill the criteria for the lesions to be disseminated in space, part of the Poser criteria for the diagnosis of definite MS in research protocols.

An important advantage of the CAT scan in MS in the early years of its use, as today, was the ability to eliminate other diagnoses that could produce the same symptoms manifested by MS patients, especially brain tumors. If there is a delay in the ability to get an MRI scan, a CAT scan will at least provide reassurance that another serious lesion such as a tumor is not being missed.

PET SCANNING

Positron emission tomography (PET) scanning, developed in 1974 by Phelps, Hoffman, and Ter Pogossian, showed the MS patients exhibited some variations of MS patients from a normal group, but this was not a helpful diagnostic method in MS.

MRI SCANNING

A few years ago, it would have been difficult to accept the existence of a test that would have people lie inside a machine, and without any injections, any X-rays, or any other invasion, spin the molecules in their body so that a computer could read the spins to create a remarkable image of the nervous system, equivalent to the black and white photographs in anatomy atlases. Within a short period of time, we moved from the impressive technology of the CAT scan to the amazing technology of the MRI, which soon became the most effective confirmatory diagnostic test in MS.

> *"When the idea of a scanner ... occurred to me, I thought that actually performing the experiments would be running off in a tangent. I had been proceeding nicely down a main highway of research in salt and water biophysics for almost eight years and here I was flirting with an idea that would detour directly into the unknown."*
> Raymond V. Damadian, 1995[39]

In the past, innovators were remembered as heroes of medicine, often with an eponymous technique or disease, but not many will associate one of the amazing scientific innovations of the 20th century with the names

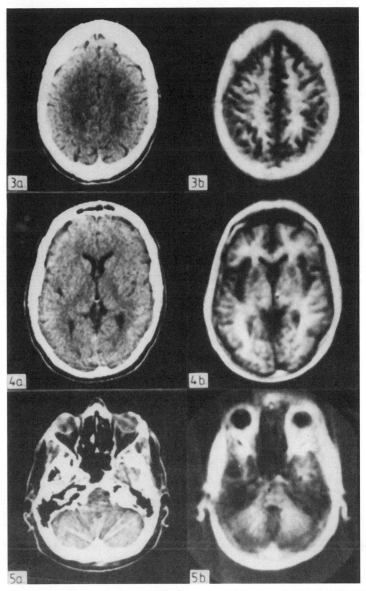

Figure 14.8 A milestone in the history of MS was the publication of the first MRI (NMR) by Doyle and co-workers at the Hammersmith Hospital and Thorne-EMI Limited in London in *The Lancet* of Saturday, 11 July, 1981. They noted the unparalleled differentiation between the grey and white matter within the brain, and although they did not show a case of MS in this paper, postulated that this technique would be valuable in demonstrating demyelinating diseases as well as infective and toxic disorders that affect the white matter. 3ab, 4ab, and 5ab show slices through the normal brain. (Reprinted with permission from Elsevier, *The Lancet*, 1981, 318:53–57.)

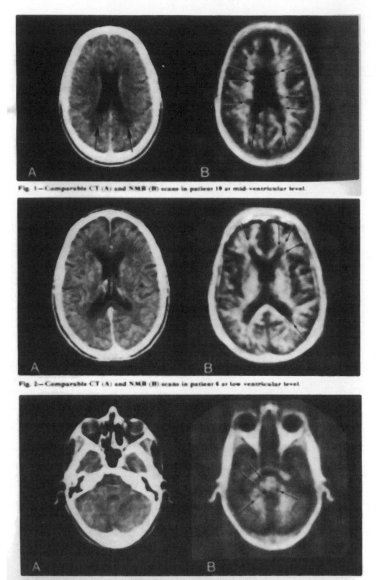

Fig. 1—Comparable CT (A) and NMR (B) scans in patient 10 at mid-ventricular level.

Fig. 2—Comparable CT (A) and NMR (B) scans in patient 6 at low ventricular level.

Fig. 3—Comparable CT (A) and NMR (B) scans in patient 10 at pontine level.

Figure 14.9 The first published MRI scan in MS (called NMR scan for nuclear magnetic resonance) by Ian Young and co-workers at Hammersmith Hospital, London, 1981. Figure 1a shows two posterior periventricular lesions on the CT scan while the MRI in Figure 1b shows the two lesions plus six others not seen on the CT scan. Figure 2a shows a CT in another MS case with normal CT, but the MRI in Fib 2b shows five lesions. Similarly, another MS patient in Figure 1a has a normal CT scan, but four lesions on the MRI. (Reprinted with permission from Elsevier, *The Lancet*, 1981, 318:1063–1066.)

Isidor Rabi, Norman F. Ramsey, Edward M. Purcell, Felix Bloch, Nicholaas Blomembergen, Richard R. Ernst, Raymond V. Damadian, or Paul C. Lauterbur. These are the pioneers of magnetic resonance imaging and the last two particularly made the technology applicable to the diagnosis of human disease. Although arguments continue about who made the major contributions and who was the foremost pioneer, in the end it is the nature of modern innovations that they are made by many individuals from many disciplines who ultimately remain anonymous.[40] The world of radiology and neuroradiology changed dramatically in April 1980 when Damadian, a physician, after years of experimenting with NMR spectrometry on cancer and other tissues, demonstrated the first commercial NMR scanner to the American Roentgen Ray Society.

Magnetic resonance spectroscopy had been employed for many years before methods of display using computerization were developed. The

Who Was Tesla?

Nikola Tesla (1856–1943), the most inventive and brilliant electrical engineer of the 20th century, is credited for "lighting the world" with his invention of alternating current power generation and transmission. Among his hundreds of inventions was the radio. Although Marconi had developed a method of transmission, it was incapable of covering long distances, and he used Tesla's patented method. Only in 1943 would the U.S. Supreme Court affirm Tesla's claims over Marconi. This genius was pushed to the side by many who became rich by his inventions, and by 1916, he declared bankruptcy. This eccentric bachelor died alone in a New York hotel room, forgotten by a society he substantially changed by his inventions. His name has been revived by the imaging power of every MRI. In 1956, the General Conference on Weights and Measures in Geneva incorporated in the System of Units (SI), the scientific "yardsticks," the *Tesla Unit* as the measure of magnetic flux density.[41] Neuroradiologists now talk about their 1.5 Tesla machine, their pride in their 3.0 Tesla machine, and their hope for a 4.0 Tesla in the future.

first images of the brain in eight normal people and 14 patients (none of them with MS) by NMR (nuclear magnetic imaging, later called magnetic resonance imaging [MRI]) using a .15 Tesla machine, were done by F.H. Doyle and his colleagues. Their *Lancet* article on this exciting new technique noted the striking differences between grey and white matter, and they predicted the technique might be useful in diagnosing demyelinating diseases.[42] Within months, another, now classic, article appeared in *The Lancet* showing the first MRI images of multiple sclerosis.

In 1981, Ian Young and A.S. Hall from the Central Research Laboratories of Thorn-EMI in Middlesex, and clinical colleagues Christopher Pallis, G.M. Bydder, Nigel Legg, and R.E. Stener at the Hammersmith Postgraduate Hospital published striking pictures of MS lesions demonstrated by the new technique of nuclear magnetic resonance imaging (NMRI).[43] In the early papers of the 1980s, the abbreviations of NMRI, NMR, and MRI were used for this technique, but MRI is now the convention. Young and his colleagues showed the striking difference between the CAT scan and MRI in the same patient; there was a

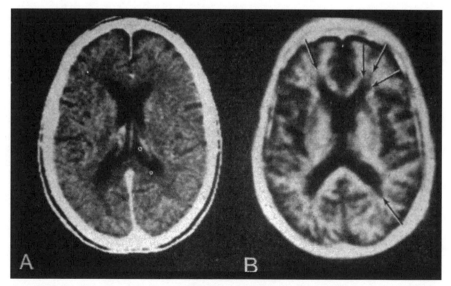

Figure 14.10 This observation that the number of MS lesions that could be seen on MRI was ten fold that of CT, showed the major advantage of MRI as a diagnostic technique in MS. (Reprinted with permission from Elsevier, *The Lancet*, 1981, 318:1063–1066.)

normal CAT scan, but five lesions were visible on the MRI. Young accurately predicted:

"The technique may also prove a measure of the severity of disease …
and thus be used to monitor the effectiveness of therapeutic regimens."

Young's group then compared the lesions seen in 10 patients (eight definite and two possible MS) and saw 19 lesions on CAT scans, but 131 on MRI. The MRI demonstrated all the lesions seen on CAT scans and 121 others. Since then, the characteristics of the lesions in MS have been better defined and the technology of MRI has improved year by year.[44–46] That the MRI signal corresponds to the plaques in the brain was confirmed by MRI-pathologic correlations in formalin-fixed brains by Stewart et al. in 1986 and Ormerod et al.[47,48] The first systemic studies of MRI in MS were carried out in the early 1980s by Paty and Li and their team in Vancouver.[49–51] When MRI machines began appearing in many medical centers, there was an immediate and understandable demand for their use for clinical care, and investigators had difficulty finding time in their schedules to do many of the needed investigational studies. Some investigators, such as Ian McDonald in London and Donald Paty in Vancouver, had MRI machines with major research dedication, and longitudinal studies and responses to therapies could be carried out. During the 1990s, drug studies in MS incorporated MRI assessment as a secondary and sometimes primary outcome measure, providing a great deal of information about the capacity of the technique and the ongoing nature of MS changes. Like the earlier evoked potential studies, the MRI was important in diagnosis, but played a vital role in providing information about the underlying disease.

It was obvious that MRI had the potential to be an effective confirmatory diagnostic tool, better than anything before it. At the same time, researchers increasingly recognized that changes that resemble MS lesions could occur in other conditions, and even in apparently normal healthy people, especially those over the age of 50. Criteria for the acceptance of the lesions characteristic of MS were suggested.[52,53] Experience with frequently repeated MRIs on the same patient over long periods shows that the disease has continuous activity, even when the patient is not experiencing new symptoms.*[54] Computerized methods were developed to measure the "disease burden" by assessing the number and volume of the MRI lesions.

The nature of the primary event in MS had been argued since the earliest reports on the disease. Rindfleisch felt it was an inflammatory event centered around the vessels, but Charcot disagreed, suggesting the defect was in the neuroglia. In recent years, there has been increasing evidence from biopsy examination of acute lesions, the appearance of EAE, and from MRI that the acute lesions were local and acute inflammatory reactions. In 1986, Robert Grossman in Philadelphia showed that the enhancing agent gadolinium-DPTA caused some lesions to enhance while others did not.[55] He indicated that the enhancement identified breakdown of the blood–brain barrier, indicating areas of inflammation. The important point that the blood–brain barrier breakdown and gadolinium (Gd) enhancement was due to an inflammation was demonstrated by McDonald and Clive Hawkins in EAE. In 1993, Katz et al. had the opportunity to study a patient who died unexpectedly ten days after having a Gd-DTPA-enhanced MRI; the enhancing lesions were associated with inflammation, while the non-enhancing lesions were not.[56]

For relapsing-remitting MS and secondary-progressive MS, the combination of triple-dose Gd-DTPA and delayed imaging more than doubled the ability to demonstrate contrast enhancing lesions. This did not apply to primary-progressive MS where no method of enhancement significantly improved sensitivity. Gadolinium enhancement then became a useful technique to demonstrate new and active MS lesions, effectively monitoring disease activity, an important asset in subsequent clinical trials of new drugs for MS.[57]

In a number of papers in the early 1990s, Ian McDonald and his group were able to demonstrate the series of events in the developing lesions of MS.[58–60] The first step is a breakdown in the blood–brain barrier due to inflammation. Edema develops over the next few weeks and then the blood–brain barrier repairs, with reduced edema and a smaller lesion visible on the MRI.

---

*Recently Jack Simon demonstrated the appearance of 63 new lesions in a patient over 18 months in the CHAMPS trial, though the patient did not have a second attack during this time.

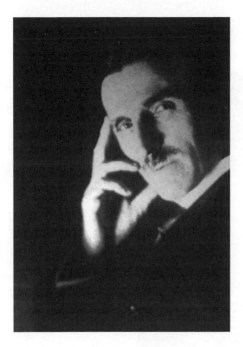

Figure 14.11 Nikola Tesla (1856–1943) transformed the world by the invention of the technology for altering current generation and transmission. A forgotten bankrupt bachelor who profited little from his inventions, which included radio, he died alone in a New York hotel room. He is remembered now for the Tesla units for MRI machines. (Electrical Experimenter cover, 1919.)

In 1989, Wolff and Balaban introduced magnetization transfer (MT) as a technique to improve the contrast of MRI, and this technique has become very useful in clarifying the nature of lesions seen on the conventional MRI. This has aided the visualization and categorization of lesions that are visible and some that are occult on the conventional MRI. (It is an indication of how technology is advancing that we are now speaking of "conventional MRI"). The technique can be directed at individual lesions or to the global brain disease in MS.[61]

During the first years of MRI studies, many groups clarified the nature of the lesions in MS and their differentiation from other neurological diseases. It became clear that the features seen on MRI are not pathognomonic, but are so characteristic that in the presence of a typical clinical history, the MRI is strongly supportive of the diagnosis of MS. The neuroradiologist reporting the MRI, even when it is typical of MS, will not report it diagnostic of MS, but as being in keeping with demyelination, or in keeping with MS. It is the role of the clinician to decide that the clinical features, supported by the MRI, are diagnostic of MS. No test in MS, including MRI, *makes* the diagnosis, but the tests can help *confirm*

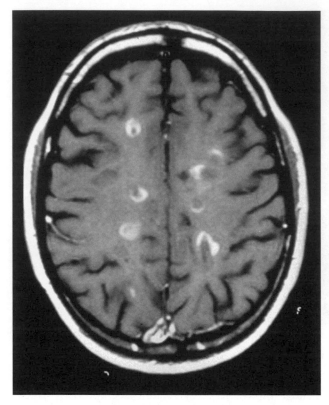

Figure 14.12 MRI was advanced by the technique of enhancement using gadolinium-DPTA by Robert I Grossman in 1986.   Enhancement showed areas of breakdown in the blood–brain barrier, and could be used to demonstrate new and active MS lesions.

the clinical suspicion or clinical diagnosis. It was disconcerting to find how poorly the MRI appearance correlated with the clinical picture of how well or poorly the patient seems to feel. MRI techniques are being continually improved and as more is learned, the technique will undoubtedly be more useful in therapeutic decisions and prognostication.

Although imaging of the CNS in MS, with or without gadolinium enhancement, has been the standard method that gave us a great deal of information on the dynamic nature of MS and allowed greater accuracy in confirming the diagnosis, many new MRI techniques will be used in the future. These include T1-weighted imaging of black holes, T1 gadolinium enhanced imaging, fast MRI, magnification transfer imaging, functional MRI, and magnetic resonance spectroscopy. These technologies are already being used to study MS and will help us to have a new understanding of the process of MS, as they evolve into even better techniques.

AUTOPSY

"In the absence of any specific laboratory test, or diagnostic biopsy techniques, autopsy provides the only means of confirming a clinical diagnosis of multiple sclerosis."

E.D. Acheson, 1972[62]

The final diagnosis of MS is made by autopsy. Earlier in this century, neurologists often argued that the diagnosis was always tentative until confirmed by autopsy. As dissection became permissible, more and more was learned about the human body and the diseases that affect it. In the era of Vulpian and Charcot, it was close observation of clinical phenomena coupled with later findings at autopsy that led to the discovery of so many new conditions and processes. The use of the microscope and the addition of tissue staining techniques rapidly advanced medicine in the 19th century. A person who before received the general diagnoses of "myelitis," "paraplegia," or "creeping paralysis" could now be recognized as having syringomyelia, multiple sclerosis, tumor, or some other specific condition.

One does not think of autopsy as a "test," but for the first century after MS was described, it was the only way to verify that the clinical diagnosis was indeed correct. As mentioned earlier, even in the 1930s many of the clinical diagnoses of MS were shown to be incorrect at autopsy and many cases identified as MS at autopsy were not diagnosed in life.

The characteristic change noted at autopsy was scattered lesions in the white matter, with the features of inflammation, demyelination, some axonal damage, and gliosis. "Internal hydrocephalus" had been noted at autopsy by early investigators, discussed by Merle and Pastine, and by Siemerling and Raecke in their studies of MS and commented on by Brain.[63] Brain felt hydrocephalus could be due to atrophy of the hemispheres, but others had suggested there might be obstruction of the aqueduct of Sylvius by surrounding sclerosis and inflammation. In recent years, Brain's observation has been rediscovered and there is interest in whether interferons may slow the rate of atrophy.

Recently, there have been attempts to clarify plaques seen under the microscope to categories such as active, chronic-active, and chronic-inactive while describing the cellularity and sometimes the surrounding normal-appearing white matter. The systems currently being used were developed by Bo and Trapp, by Bruck and Lassman, by Van der Valk, and a more complex system by the Vienna Consensus Group. Tests for MS have improved in their specificity and sensitivity, but the diagnosis remains a clinical one, which can be strengthened and confirmed by the tests.

REFERENCES

1. Compston A. The Story of Multiple Sclerosis. Chapter 1 in: *McAlpine's Multiple Sclerosis*. London: Churchill Livingstone; 1998:3-42.
2. Guillain GJM. *Charcot (1825–1893): sa vie—son oeuvre*. Paris: Masson; 1955.
3. Guillain G. *JM Charcot 1825–1893. His life—his work*. Ed. and trans. Pierce Bailey. London: Pitman Medical; 1959.
4. Barbellion WNP. (pseudonym for BF Cummings). *The Journal of a Disappointed Man*. London: Chatto and Windus; 1919.
5. Pohlen K. Statistics of clinical and pathological statements on causes of death. *Health and Statistics*. Statistical Bulletin II: Nos. 4/5. Battle Creek, MI: W.K. Kellogg Foundation; 1942.
6. Strümpell A. Zur pathologie der multiplen Sklerose. *Neurol Centralbl*. 1896;15:961-964.
7. Schumacher GA. Multiple sclerosis and its treatment. *JAMA*. 1950;143:1059-1065, 1146-1154, 1241-1250.
8. Hinton WA. CSF in MS. In: Studies in the cerebrospinal fluid and book in multiple sclerosis. Eds. Ayer JB, Foster HE. *Multiple Sclerosis: Association for Research in Nervous and Mental Diseases*. Vol. 2. New York: Paul B. Hoeber; 1922;113-121.
9. Schumacher GA. Multiple sclerosis and its treatment. *JAMA*. 1950;143:1059-1065, 1146-1154, 1241-1250.
10. Lange. Interpretation of findings, techniques, and systematic interpretation of albumin–globulin ratio. *J Lab Clin Med*. 1946;31:552-556.
11. Friedman A. Houston Merritt. In: *Historical Aspects of the Neurosciences: a festschrift for MacDonald Critchley*, Rose FC, Bynum WF, eds. New York: Raven Press; 1982:379-382.
12. Walton J (Lord John Walton of Detchent). *The Spice of Life*. London: Royal Soc Med: 1993.
13. Kabat EA, et al. An electrophoretic study of the protein components in cerebrospinal fluid and their relationship to the serum proteins. *J Clin Invest*. 1942;21:571-577.
14. Cohen M. *The American Academy of Neurology: The First 50 Years—1948–1998*. MN. AAN; 1998.
15. Lature EC. Les proteines du LCR à l'état normal et pathologique. *Arscia*. 1964. Also, *Neurology*. 1970;20:982.
16. Poser CM, Paty DW, Scheinberg L, et al. New diagnostic criteria for multiple sclerosis: *Ann Neurol*. 1983;13:227-231.
17. Ormerod IEC, du Boulay GH, McDonald WI. Imaging in multiple sclerosis. From *Multiple Sclerosis*. McDonald WI, Silberberg DH, eds. London: Butterworths, 1986:11-36.
18. Freeman W, Cohen R. Electroencephalographic and pneumoencephalographic studies of multiple sclerosis. *Arch Neurol Psych*. 1945;53:246-247.
19. Haughton VM, Ho KC, Boe-Decker RA. The contracting cord sign of multiple sclerosis. *Neuroradiology*. 1979;17:207-209.

20. Tucker WM, Donald DC, Farmer RA. Cerebral blood flow in multiple sclerosis. In: *Multiple Sclerosis and the Demyelinating Diseases.* Proceedings of the Association for Research in Nervous and Mental Disease. (Dec. 10–11, 1948). Vol 28. Baltimore: Williams and Wilkins; 1950:203-215.

21. Overton MC III, Haynie TP, Snodgrass E. Brain scans in non-neoplastic lesions: scanning with chlormerodrin Hg 203 and chlormerodrin 197. *JAMA.* 1965;191:431-436.

22. Gize RW, Mishkin FS. Brain scans in multiple sclerosis. *Radiology.* 1970;97:297-299.

23. Moses DC, Davis LE, Wagner HN Jr. Brain scanning with 99mTcO4 in multiple sclerosis. *J Nucl Med.* 1972;13:847-487.

24. Antunes JL, Schlesinger EB, Michelsen WJ. The abnormal brain scan in demyelinating diseases. *Arch Neurol.* 1974;30:269-271.

25. Halliday AM, McDonald WI, Mushin J. Delayed visual evoked response in optic neuritis. *Lancet.* 1972;I:982-985.

26. Halliday AM, McDonald WI, Mushin J. Delayed pattern-evoked responses in optic neuritis in relation to visual acuity. *Trans Opthalmol Soc UK.* 1973;93:315-324.

27. Cohen M. *The American Academy of Neurology: The First 50 Years, 1948–1998.* MN. AAN; 1998:277.

28. Cohen, Maynard. *The American Academy of Neurology: The First 50 Years, 1948–1998.* MN. AAN; 1998.

29. Cala LA, Mastaglia FL. Computerized axial tomography in multiple sclerosis. *Lancet.* 1976;1:689.

30. Paty DW. Multiple sclerosis: assessment of disease progression and effect of treatment. *Can J Neurol Sci.* 1987;14:518-520.

31. Paty DW, Li DKB. Neuroimaging in multiple sclerosis. *Clin Neuroimaging.* 1988:249-278.

32. Paty DW. magnetic resonance imaging in the assessment of disease activity in multiple sclerosis (Olszewski Lecture). *Can J Neurol Sci.* 1988;15:266-272.

33. Wulthrich R, Gigli H, Wiggli U, et al. CT scanning in demyelinating disease. In: *Cranial Computerized Tomography*, eds. Lanksch W, Kafner E. New York: Springer-Verlag. 1976:239-243.

34. Ibid, p. 239-243.

35. Vinuela FV, Fox AJ, Debrun GM, Feasby TE, Ebers GC. New perspectives in computerized tomography of multiple sclerosis. *Am J Rad.* 1982;139:123-127.

36. Ebers GC. A Historical Overview. In: *Multiple Sclerosis.* Paty DW, Ebers G, eds. Philadelphia: FA Davis; 1998:1-4.

37. Paty DE, Oger JJF, Kastrukoff LF, et al. MRI in the diagnosis of MS: A prospective study with comparison of clinical evaluation, evoked potentials, oligoclonal banding, and CT. *Neurology.* 1988;38:180-185.

38. Paty DW, Issac C, Palmer M, et al. Northern lights neuroscience symposium on myelin and demyelination. *Acta Neurol Scand.* 1988;77:242-268.

39. Mattson, James, Merrill, Simon. *The Pioneers of NMR and Magnetic Resonance in Medicine. The Story of MRI.* Jericho, NJ: Bar-Ilan University Press/Dean Books Company; 1996:651.

40. Ibid, p. 651.

41. Cheyney M, Uth R. *Tesla: Master of Lighting.* New York: Barnes and Nobles; 1999.

42. Doyle FH, Gore JC, Pennock JM, et al. Imaging of the brain by nuclear magnetic resonance. *Lancet.* 1981;318:53-57.

43. Young IR, Hall AS, Pallis CA, Bydder GM, Legg N, Steiner RE. Nuclear magnetic resonance imaging of the brain in multiple sclerosis. *Lancet.* 1981;318:1063-1066.

44. Ormerod IEC, Miller DH, McDonald WI, et al. The role of NMR imaging in the assessment of multiple sclerosis and isolated neurological lesions. A quantitative study. *Brain.* 1987;110:1579-1616.

45. Ormerod IEC, Miller DH, McDonald WI, et al. The role of NMR imaging in the assessment of multiple sclerosis and isolated neurological lesions: a quantitative study. *Brain*. 1987;110:1579-1616.

46. Paty DW, Li DKB. Neuroimaging in multiple sclerosis. In: *Clinical Neuroimaging*. Theodore WH, ed. New York: Alan R. Liss; 1988:249-278.

47. Ormerod IEC, Miller DH, McDonald WI, et al. The role of NMR imaging in the assessment of multiple sclerosis and isolated neurological lesions. A quantitative study. *Brain*. 1987;110:1579-1616.

48. Ormerod IEC, Miller DH, McDonald WI, et al. The role of NMR imaging in the assessment of multiple sclerosis and isolated neurological lesions: a quantitative study. *Brain*. 1987;110:1579-1616.

49. Li D, Mayo J, Fache S, Robertson WD, Paty D, Genton M. Early experience in nuclear magnetic resonance imaging of multiple sclerosis. *Ann Y Acad Sci*. 1984;436:483-486.

50. Li D, Mayo J, Fache S, Robertson WD, Paty D, Genton M. Early Experience in Nuclear Magnetic Resonance Imaging of Multiple Sclerosis. *Ann Y Acad Sci*. 1984;436:483-486.

51. Paty DW. Magnetic resonance imaging in the assessment of disease activity in multiple sclerosis (Olszewski Lecture). *Can J Neurol Sci*. 1988;15:266-272.

52. Ibid, p. 266-272.

53. Paty DW, Issac C, Palmer M, et al. Northern lights neuroscience symposium on myelin and demyelination. *Acta Neurol Scand*. 1988;77:242-268.

54. Simon J, Jacobs L, Campion M, et al. and the Multiple Sclerosis Collaborative Research Group. Magnetic resonance studies of intramuscular interferon ß-1a for relapsing multiple sclerosis. *Ann Neurol*. 1998;43:79-87.

55. Grossman RI, et al. Multiple sclerosis: gadolinium enhancement in MR imaging. *Radiology*. 1986:161:721-725.

56. Katz D, Taubenberger JK, Canella B, et al. Correlation between magnetic resonance imaging findings and lesion development in chronic, active multiple sclerosis. *Ann Neurol*. 1993;34:661-669.

57. Paty, DW, Li DKB. Neuroimaging in multiple sclerosis. In: *Clinical Neuroimaging*. Theodore WH, ed. New York: Alan R. Liss Inc.; 1988:249-278.

58. McDonald WI, Miller DH, Barnes D. The pathological evolution of multiple sclerosis. *Neuropath and Applied Neurobio*. 1992;18:319-334.

59. McDonald WI. The dynamics of multiple sclerosis: the Charcot lecture. *J Neurology*. 1993;240 (1):28-36.

60. McDonald WI. The pathological and clinical dynamics of multiple sclerosis. *J Neuropath Exp Neurol*. 1994;53:338-343.

61. Filippi M, Rocca MA, Moiola L, et al. MRI and magnetization transfer imaging changes in the brain and cervical cord of patients with Devic's neuromyelitis optica. *Neurology*. 1999;53:1705-1710.

62. McAlpine D, Compston ND, Lumsden CE. *Multiple Sclerosis: a reappraisal*, 2nd ed. Edinburgh: ES Livingston; 1972:7.

63. Brain WR. Critical review: disseminated sclerosis. *Quart J Med*. 1930;23:343-391.

15

Searching for Therapy

"Multiple sclerosis is often one of the most difficult problems in clinical medicine."

Jean-Martin Charcot, 1894[1]

"The prognosis of disseminated sclerosis is hopeless. I am sorry to say that no case of cure has even been recorded."

Landon Carter Gray, 1883[2]

"I have little doubt, in fact, gentlemen, that in the employment of such a substance as the vaccine of Pasteur or lymph of Koch the evolution of insular sclerosis will someday be rendered absolutely impossible."

Pierre Marie, 1895[3]

"When more is known of the causes and essential pathology of the disease in different cases, more rational methods may brighten the therapeutic prospect."

Sir William Gowers, 1898[4]

"Empiric forms of treatment have encouraged the optimistic but a rational therapy can scarcely be expected before the pathogenesis of the disease is understood."

Tracy Putnam, 1938[5]

"The pharmacopoeia has been ransacked for 'nerve tonics,' which flatter only to deceive."

S.A. Kinnier Wilson, 1940[6]

EARLY ATTEMPTS AT THERAPY

In a disease that fluctuates spontaneously, often showing recovery after an acute worsening, and that may have long periods of remission, any attempts at therapy may appear to be responsible for the improvement. In addition, there is a strong placebo effect in a chronic distressing, unpredictable disease. As a result, all ineffective therapies initially appear to work.

Even in the earliest recognized cases of MS, treatment was attempted in three directions: to ameliorate the acute attacks; to treat the symptoms; and to try to affect the underlying disease.

The early approach to treatment of any patient with a chronic neurological disease was based on how illness was understood. From 500 B.C. to 1750 A.D., the concept of disease, which dominated the approach to health and therapy was the belief that the body required the establishment and maintenance of a balance of the four humors: *blood*, which was associated with heat and moisture; *phlegm*, associated with moisture and cold; *black bile*, associated with cold and dryness; and *yellow bile*, associated with dryness and heat. Galen (A.D. 129–200) related the Hippocratic concept of the *four humors* to the earlier concept of Empedocles of Acragas of the *four elements* of earth, air, fire, and water, which must all be in balance for health. An imbalance led to disease, and therapy was aimed at re-establishing that balance with agents that could affect those characteristics. It should also be noted that prior to the 18th century, there was little need or effort to classify specific disease other than in the general categories (such as fever, paralysis, dropsy, gout, etc.). Within these large categories were many conditions that shared similar general features. Since a general imbalance was at fault, knowing the detailed anatomy of an organ had little relevance, which is why anatomy was such a late scientific interest, and why medical anatomical drawings up to the 18th century were often very primitive. Many of the beautiful anatomical drawings of the 16–18th centuries were by artists and were not applied by physicians to their management of disease.

The solidism theory of Hoffmann, Boerhaave, and Cullen in the 18th century added the idea that the balance between the nervous system and the blood vessels could also be out of alignment. This could lead to hyper-irritability of the system, which could be treated by drugs and therapies to lower the pulse and deplete and sedate the system. Or there could be lowered energy in the system, requiring stimulants and tonics, electricity, and other physical measures. In the 1770s, John Brown of Edinburgh characterized these as hyperexcitable (sthenic) disorders, or lowered excitability (asthenic) disorders. His system had an 80-point scale, which could precisely quantify the degree of the patient's illness. These were the concepts in vogue when Margaret Davis, Heinrich Heine, and Augustus d'Este were being treated for their progressive neurological disorders. Only in the context of these general beliefs can we understand the enthu-siasm for treating neurological disorders with Galvanic and Faradic stim-ulation, or wrapping patients in cold wet sheets and aiming hoses of icy water on them. Bleeding was a logical therapy for thousands of years, as it was thought to rid the body of noxious elements and restore balance. Fever therapy was used for almost a century on MS patients, even when the patients must have felt much worse from the treatment, enthusiasti-cally prescribed by their neurologists because the therapy made sense in the contemporaneous concept of nervous disease.

Treatments in the mid-19th century were general therapies, part of the armamentarium the physician applied to any acute or chronic illness. Prescriptions for multiple sclerosis looked very much like prescriptions for any chronic neurological disease. The body was seen as a mechanistic, homeostatic physiological system, which could be rebalanced by thera-peutic measures. Later, there were efforts to measure the imbalance in the laboratory. Many of the remedies had an obvious and visible effect on the patient that was in keeping with the therapeutic concept—purging, emetics, stimulants, supressants, bleeding—in the expectation that these would affect the equilibrium of the nervous system and blood vessels.

To a great extent, belief about the cause of MS was related to the major scientific medical interest of the era in question. In the late 19th century, it centered around the possibility of a vascular, glial, or infective disease, and although these ideas did not disappear, later suspicion of an immunological cause, and the current interest in a genetic factor, essentially reflected the current major interest in medical science. Science often has an impact on the direction of disease therapy only when a cause of the disease is recognized. There are examples when therapy is discovered before the specific cause is known, such as diabetes, but there is usually some understanding of the mechanism of the disease. In multiple sclerosis, little was understood about the cause of the patches of demyelination, their recurrence, or why the process was ultimately a progressive one. Without some understanding of these fundamental processes, it was difficult to see what specific therapy might interrupt the process. Left with no specific therapy, the physician used any general measures available for a neurological disorder.

We will see that the developments in understanding of MS were not accompanied by corresponding developments in therapy; in the first hundred years after Charcot's 1868 lectures, therapy was surprisingly traditional and relatively unchanged. Some drugs and some physical techniques had a period of favor, but compounds of silver and arsenic, quinine, strychnine, potassium iodide, and all forms of antisyphilitic therapy were part of the therapeutic approach to MS for over a century.

THERAPY IN THE PRE-CHARCOT ERA

The physician to Lidwina of Schieden in the 15th century was confident and definitive when he announced that her progressive neurological disease was heaven sent, and attempts at therapy would be expensive and futile:

> *"Believe me there is no cure for this illness, it comes directly from God. Even Hippocrates and Gallenus would not be able to be of any help here. Let us admit this in all honesty rather than to bereave the poor father from his last means. The Lord's hand has touched this woman."*
>
> Godfreid de la Haye, c. 1405

A similar therapeutic nihilism was reflected in the late 17th century by the discussion between Margaret Davies of Myddle, and a surgeon in an apothecary's shop. He advised her not to purchase any more remedies, as her progressive lameness could last a long time, but would gradually progress and this slow progression would not be altered by any of the apothecary's medicines.

Although his physicians were puzzled by his nervous condition, Augustus d'Esté in the early decades of the 19th century was treated with a continuing array of therapies from many physicians; perhaps this reflected his social status as well as his constant search for relief. Sometimes he noted that his symptoms cleared without therapy, but as his disease progressed, he was subjected to leeches applied to his temples, purges, venesection, liniments, spa waters, and a long list of medications, which included prescriptions containing mercury, silver, arsenic, iron, antimony, and quinine, to mention just a few.[7,8]

Cruveilhier indicated that the 54-year-old embroiderer who resided bedridden at the Salpêtrière for 10 years, had been treated in the Necker hospital by Laennec with counter-irritation by moxibustion,* but she progressed, although there was little further change during the last three years of her life.

In the mid-19th century, diseases of the nervous system were treated in similar general ways, except that some were felt to need stimulant therapies and others sedative therapies. In 1852, Dr. John Neill and Dr. Francis Gurney Smith published a popular analytical compendium of medical science and discussed treatment for nervous diseases, using "nervous sedatives" such as foxglove, tobacco, Indian tobacco, aconite, hemlock, and hydrocyanic acid; and "alternatives" to bring the nutrition of the nervous system into balance, such as mercury, iodine, and arsenic.[9] Stimulants for the nervous system included musk, castor, asafoetida, valerian, garlic, oil of amber, skunk cabbage, coffee, and tea. Cerebral stimulants were alcohol, ether, Hoffman anodyne, chloroform, opium, camphor, hops, bittersweet,

---

*Moxibustion is a Chinese therapy performed by applying a cone of combustible material on the skin, usually over the back or chest, and then lighting it to produce a blister. The blister was thought to draw out noxious elements from the body.

henbane, thornapple, deadly nightshade, and extract of hemp. Treatment of paralysis, whether acute (apoplexy was treated separately) or chronic, was by restricting diet, reducing excitement, caring for the bowels and bladder, and administering strychnine. An incision would be made near the part affected, and a seton or foreign body inserted to produce drainage. Local treatment was vigorous rubbing of the paralyzed limbs using a stimulating liniment, applying blisters to the spine, or abrading along the course of the nerves and sprinkling the area with strychnine. Finally, the limbs would be stimulated by electricity or moxibustion.

THERAPY 1868–1899

Charcot was not impressed with any of the efforts to treat multiple sclerosis. At the end of his lecture, when he came to the point of discussing therapy he said:

> *"After what precedes need I detain you long … the time has not yet come when such a subject can be seriously considered."*[10]

But even the most therapeutically nihilistic physician struggles to find something that might help the patient, and even Charcot used the medicaments of the day for his MS patients. In addition, he subjected them to electrical therapy and to the suspension device he advocated for all forms of ataxia. In his translation of Charcot's lectures, Sigerson added a footnote to the therapeutic recommendations of Charcot indicating that other drugs were used, but with no better results. Such therapies were phosphorized oil, iodide of phosphetylamine, and calabar bean. One of Charcot's patients, Josphine C. Vauthier, was treated by his colleague Vulpian with calabar bean and belladonna.

Charcot's use of electricity was that advocated by the American neuropsychiatrist Hans Christian Orstead. In 1819, Orstead introduced a pattern of alternating current coupled with magnetism, or electromagnetism which was popular in the treatment of all forms of neurological diseases. He made electrical therapy well known on both sides of the Atlantic with his publication of a book on the subject, and he established a short-lived *Journal of Electrology and Neurology*.

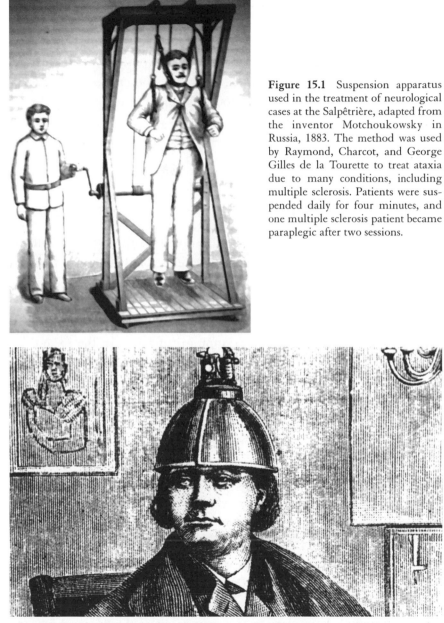

Figure 15.1 Suspension apparatus used in the treatment of neurological cases at the Salpêtrière, adapted from the inventor Motchoukowsky in Russia, 1883. The method was used by Raymond, Charcot, and George Gilles de la Tourette to treat ataxia due to many conditions, including multiple sclerosis. Patients were suspended daily for four minutes, and one multiple sclerosis patient became paraplegic after two sessions.

Figure 15.2 Vibrating helmet, part of the many types of apparatus devised to improve neurological disease at the Salpêtrière, and could be used with Charcot's vibrating chair, or separately as it was portable. These therapies were adapted for neurological disease at the Salpêtrière when it was noted the Parkinson patients seemed to improve after a period of vibration in a railway carriage. (*Scientific American*, 1892.)

In England, Moxon's therapy for his patients in the early 1870s included bleeding, cooling with sponges, Galvanic stimulation, Farradic stimulation, mist, effervescens, iron preparations, strychnine, belladonna, calumbae, potassium iodide, arsenic, nux vomica, silver nitrate, hyocyanide, atropine, ergot, quinine, and various other preparations, supplemented with a meat diet. Despite his many attempts to help his patients, he concluded:

> *"The results of treatment used in the foregoing cases will be seen from the reports to be most unsatisfactory; no approach to cure has been made."*

William Moxon, 1875[11]

Charcot's student Pierre Marie was much more positive about the future prospect of therapy in the 1880s; he felt strongly that infection was the cause of MS, and predicted that a vaccine like those of Pasteur or the lymph of Koch would soon be discovered for MS and would eliminate the disease.[12] However, there were limited approaches for treating an infection other than allaying the symptoms of fever. In the meantime, since MS was a sclerosis and due to an infection, he prescribed therapies he felt would benefit "sclerotics," such as iodide of potassium or sodium, and those that would benefit infections, such as mercury.

The late 19th century was an era of polypharmacy and enthusiastic therapies; empirical therapies were widely used for most serious illness, so it is not surprising that a wide variety of these treatments were aimed at improving people with neurological disease. In the 1890s, preparations of silver nitrate, arsenic, and mercury were the predominant medications applied to MS, but the list of medications sometimes used was very long. In 1885, A.B. Arnold recommended that large doses of narcotics, such as morphine, codeine, and opium, as well as cannabis, for the treatment of symptoms of MS, be coupled with sea bathing and electricity. He also recommended potassium iodide, strychnine, silver nitrate, and cod liver oil. The prominent American neurologist Charles Dana used all the approaches employed to treat any degenerative neurological disease, such as electricity, hydrotherapy, hygienic measures, and the usual list of medications offered by others.[13]

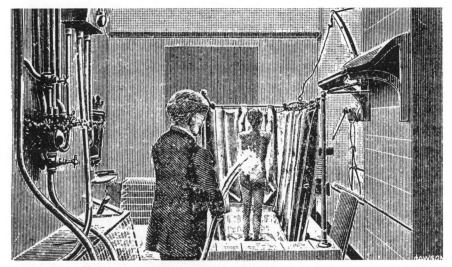

Figure 15.3 Hydrotherapy was used for all forms of neurological disease in the 19th century, with some variation in the kind of hydrotherapy if the person suffered from multiple sclerosis, locomotor ataxia, epilepsia, headaches, neurasthenia, impotence or hysteria. Some were as simple as a plunge in a cold tub of water or standing in a foot tub for three minutes, while dripping cold water from a sponge over the head and down the naked body. Others were the elaborate Scottish douche, hitting the body back and then front with a powerful jet of water, alternating with a shower of cold water from the above in the method of Fleury. (Dana, 1894.)

In 1893, Sir William Gowers said of MS that "even less can be done than for other degenerative diseases of the nervous system."[14] However, he recommended nerve tonics such as arsenic, nitrate of silver, quinine, and a number of other drugs. He also suggested benefit might come from hydrotherapy, electricity, maintenance of general health, putting aside all depressing influences, and avoidance of pregnancy.

In 1895, Arnold Edwards reviewed the therapy for MS and recommended silver nitrate, strychnine, ergot, barium chloride, and phosphorus. For tremor, he felt that the following were helpful, but only when in toxic doses: solanine, veratrum, intramuscular hyoscyamine or arsenic, or intramuscular curare. He felt the suspension apparatus used for ataxia by Charcot and Motschutkowsky was not of any value. Without further comment about benefit, he mentioned that electricity and magnetism were favored by the Germans.[15] In 1895, Sachs recommended a rest cure for MS and felt medication had no effect, but massage, hydrotherapy, and electrotherapy were useful to treat spasticity.[16]

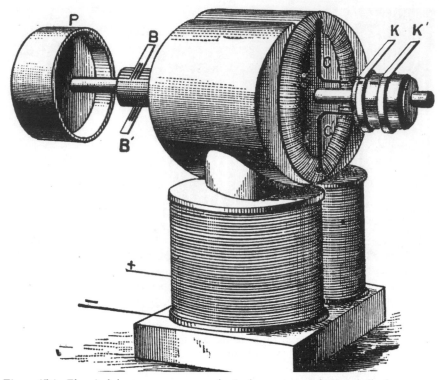

Figure 15.4 Electrical therapy was very popular in the treatment of MS and all other neurological diseases in the 19th and early 20th centuries. Therapies became very complex with high and low potential currents and sinusoidal currents. Greater currents were applied to spinal cord diseases, and the Dársonval battery was used to apply sinusoidal currents, with an electrode at the back of the neck and another over an affected part. "Voltaic alternatives" were said to be of value in optic atrophy according to Drs. Webster Fox and Eugene Riggs. (Dana, 1894.)

In 1898, C.E. Beevor believed that worry and overwork could cause MS, so his therapy included rest and avoidance of worry, mental and physical fatigue, and limitation of indulgence in wine and venery.[17] He was unsure what other therapies could work, but advocated nerve tonics, strichnine, quinine, iron, cod liver oil, and arsenic by increasing doses of liquor arsenacalis. He doubted that electrical therapy and baths were of any help.

Therapy 1900–1920

One of the continuing themes in the writings in the 19th century is the comparison of multiple sclerosis with syphilis. Even though Charcot,

Marie, Gowers, Beevor, Russell, and others stated clearly that MS was *not* a form of syphilis, any new therapy for syphilis was quickly applied to MS, since the two diseases produced major and sometimes similar changes in the nervous system. Many publications in the late 19th century were discussions of tabes doralis and MS together, to contrast and compare them. Arsenic, silver, and potassium iodide for syphilis were equally applied to the therapy of MS patients, as they were in other neurological diseases.

There was great interest in the development of therapies that might constitute a "magic bullet" and neutralize the specific abnormality of a disease. When a new therapy for syphilis was developed, such as Ehrlich's 606 (Salvarsan or arsphenamine) in 1910, it was recommended widely to MS patients within the year.* Even antisyphilitic therapies that could aggravate the symptoms of MS, such as the various fever therapies, were widely used. One can only imagine the distress of MS patients placed in the "fever box" or injected with typhoid vaccine or intramuscular milk to induce a fever. In 1911, Buzzard further encouraged the use of salvarsan in MS when he suggested that a spirochete might be the cause of MS.[18] Within a year, others were recommending it, referring to Buzzard's theory, recognizing that it might not be useful against the same spirochete as syphilis, but was still worth using just in case it was another spirochete that caused MS.[19] Interest in this approach was further sparked by announcements by Bullock (Gye), Steiner, and others over the next decade that they could isolate, transmit, and sometimes see the parasite of MS, which looked like a spirochete.[20,21]

At the National Hospital, Queen Square, intravenous typhoid vaccine was administered three times a week in MS cases. If there were severe reactions to the vaccine, intramuscular milk injections were substituted. In 1924, Henry MacBride and Arnold Carmichael wrote in *The Lancet* of their experience of treating 70 cases of MS with typhoid vaccine over the previous 15 months. The idea had originated in Vienna in the Wagner

---

*Paul Ehrlich's (1854–1915) "magic bullet" was originally a concept of natural chemicals to neutralize toxic substances and do so without side effects. Salvarsan was not a magic bullet in the sense that Ehrlich meant it; it was an external non-natural agent, and had side effects. Later, however, a magic bullet became thought of as a drug that had a specific, single, and dramatic curative effect on a disease.

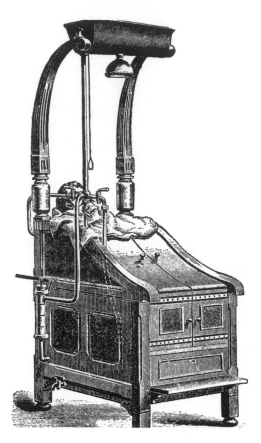

Figure 15.5 The hot box was probably the most distressing treatment of MS by many patients, as most are heat sensitive and become very weak and have their symptoms aggravated in hot environments. However, various methods of heating and fever therapies were in vogue as a treatment for MS up until the 1940s. Although a hot box like this would be found in a spa or hydrotherapy clinic, there were designs for a cheap hot box that patients could have in their home. (Dana, 1894.)

Jauregg Klinik, where doctors had postulated that MS was due to an intestinal infection. Various vaccines to kill intestinal bacteria were tried, and typhoid vaccine seemed to have the best effect. Eight to 12 intravenous injections were given one to three days apart, to increase patient's temperature to 100° F. The dose was increased from 25 million to 400 million units by the tenth or twelfth dose. Combining this with silver salvarsan was said to bring about a fairly good remission. Two cases were treated by subcutaneous doses with good results but no rise in temperature, which made doctors speculate that inducing an elevation in temperature might be unnecessary. Reflecting on his experience with this therapy during his early professional years at Queen Square, Dereck Denny-Brown said the results were poor and sometime disastrous.[22] However, typhoid injections and other forms of fever therapy were used up until the 1940s.

While interest in an infectious cause of MS gained ground after the writings of Pierre Marie and the spirochete enthusiasts, Oppenheim argued just as strongly that the cause of MS was a toxin such as lead, copper, or zinc coupled with some unknown factors.[23] Despite suggesting this specific cause, he offered no specific therapy to reduce or neutralize this theoretical toxin and his recommendations for treatment were similar to those of other physicians of his day—silver nitrate and potassium iodide, mild galvanic current to the back of the head, spa baths at Oeynhausen or Nauheim, and leeches. Even up to the present "detoxification methods" had periodic adherents, though they never gained widespread acceptance. Recognizing that there were no specific treatments, clinicians applied tried and true remedies, feeling that iodides could be beneficial, as were colloidal silver preparations either by inunction or intravenously, and fibrolysin given by intramuscular injections every five to seven days.[24]

An unusual therapy for MS used in 1910–1925 was roentgen ray therapy to the spine, again a reflection that X-ray therapy was a popular approach to many resistant diseases. In the mind of the public, it had the aura of modern science and powerful medicine, but it was one of the therapies the ARNMD committee warned against in 1921.[25]

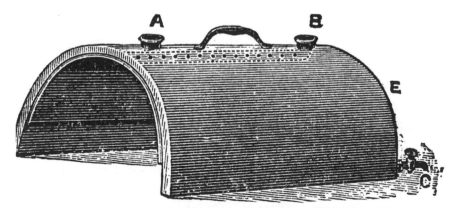

Figure 15.6   The vaporium designed by Dr. Percy Wilde was used to treat a limb afflicted with neurological symptoms. Boiling water poured in the double copper wall at B and drained out at C, until the metal was hot, and then both B and C were closed. The paralyzed limb was wrapped in hot flannel and placed in the vaporium. The whole apparatus was then covered with a blanket. (Dana, 1894.)

MS THERAPY 1920–1940

The ARNMD committee recommendations in 1921 rejected Oppenheim's toxic cause view and the detoxification therapies in MS, and expressed caution about therapies aimed at spirochetes.[26] Reviewing therapy of MS in 1921, Sachs and Friedman listed approaches they felt were helpful to MS patients. They recommended avoidance of extreme temperatures and dismissed treatments with iodides, silver, mercury, neoarsphenamine, and Farradic stimulation. MS patients were implored to avoid pregnancy, heavy exertion, and extremes of temperature. Tremor was treated with veronal and hyoscin. The most beneficial treatment was still thought to be arsenic given either by mouth or through injections of cacodylate of soda. Sodium nucleinate could also be helpful. Various spas were recommended, and warm baths, moderate and skillful message, and methodic exercises "are in order." Sachs and Friedman suggested that for spastic contractures, the Foerster surgical operation was useful even though Foerster himself was not enthusiastic about this procedure. Constipation should be as treated with enemas and incontinence with tincture of belladonna. Spasticity was treated with passive motion and warm baths, while ataxia was treated with Fraenkel exercises.

Douglas McAlpine reviewed the therapy for multiple sclerosis in *The Lancet* in 1925.[27] He was a leader in research on multiple sclerosis over the course of his career and wrote the classic book on multiple sclerosis three decades later, so it is worth reviewing his recommendations in detail to see the state of therapy in his era. He succinctly summarized current thinking about the disease. Onset was between ages 15 and 30 in most cases. The characteristic relapsing-remitting pattern, so useful in making the diagnosis, indicated to him that some organism or toxin was invading the nervous system from time to time and producing an inflammatory reaction that produced "patches" that blocked nerve transmission. He indicated that the classic pattern with Charcot's triad was present in only 14 percent of MS cases, and he divided other patterns into cerebral, retro-bulbar neuritis and spinal forms. His therapy was first general, dealing with any infection in the teeth, sinuses, or tonsils. The patient might need new teeth or tonsillectomy, but these approaches required caution, so that they did not precipitate an attack. Sinus infections were important, for there was only a thin plate separating the sinus from the optic nerve, and the infection might readily travel. General health must be maintained to avoid fatigue, manage constipation, and minimize alcohol and tobacco use. If there were a relapse, the patient should be put to bed on a light diet for a week or more.

McAlpine recommended that medical therapy should be arsenic, administered as *liquor arsenicalis*, two minims thrice daily, increasing to 20–30 minims daily, and given for four to five weeks. After that course, mercury and iodides were begun. Every so often over the next few years, a monthly course of arsenic should be given as a booster treatment. Tincture of belladonna was used for incontinence, and painful muscle spasms were treated with hot baths or radiant heat, and by sodium bromide at bedtime.

Special forms of therapy were again based on the suspicion that MS might be caused by a spirochete. Therapy began with six to eight injections of N.A.B. (neoarsphenamine) with concurrent oral mercury and potassium iodide. After this course, there was a pause for a few weeks and then the mercury and iodide were restarted. After another four weeks, the N.A.B. was begun again. McAlpine mentioned that in France, organic bismuth was being given intramuscularly into the buttocks and this could be used alternatively with N.A.B. or could replace it. His recommendation for typhoid vaccine, "allied to protein shock," was to induce a mild fever by injections intravenously of increasing doses, starting with 25 million units, given every second day for 10 injections.

If the disease had reached a very progressive stage, all therapies except the general ones and the arsenic were contraindicated. Some patients were noted to have emotional ("hysterical") overlay that should be reduced to improve their effort and function. Movement was encouraged, to delay the patient's becoming bed bound. Massage helped, but McAlpine felt electrical stimulation could be injurious. Deformities could be prevented by exercise and splints.

MANAGEMENT OF MS 1921–1942

A view of a prominent London clinician's care of a colleague with MS can be seen in the records of Dr. Frederick Parkes Weber, who managed a physician with MS over many years with various medications, electrical therapies, and referral to other physicians. Parkes Weber was an attentive physician, who consulted other physicians and established a long-term relationship with his patient through the years of attempted therapies, including discussion of those pursued and initiated by the patient himself.[28,29]

Frederick Parkes Weber, renowned physician and diagnostician, known for his extensive knowledge of rare diseases, was consulted in 1921 by AC, a surgeon from his hospital who had numbness in his legs and hands. Although he looked for an infection and treated AC for a urinary tract infection, Parkes Weber noted that there was clonus and a Babinski sign. Worried about a cord tumor, he referred AC to Sir Thomas Horder in Harley Street. The surgeon was convinced the illness was due to strain, especially that experienced in World War I. AC was given a course of IV novarsenobillon, "on the supposition that it might do good, if the disease was disseminated sclerosis." He was sent on a six-week rest to Cornwall. A year after onset, AC's walking was affected and he planned to give up surgery and consulting, but hoped to continue to teach. The unresolved question was whether the disorder was functional or organic, and if the latter, AC had to consider how he would make a living.

Parkes Weber had the habit of adding any relevant journal papers to a patient's file as he read them, and in 1921 and 1922 he added to the surgeon's file papers by Judson Bury and Anthon Feiling on symptoms in the nervous system.

A CSF examination was arranged, and AC was taken off work for three months and given regular massage. Parkes Weber discussed with Horder the recent Royal Society of Medicine meeting on the neurological complications of pernicious anemia (PA), but believed that AC's condition was likely disseminated sclerosis. Horder did not have the heart to do a gastric analysis for PA, as this would indicate they were looking for a serious condition. (PA was a fatal and "pernicious" disease in 1922.) In

the meantime, the surgeon was showing some improvement. A consultation with Professor Malaisé of Munich raised again the concern of a cord
tumor, but Hinds Howell was against surgery and suggested S.A.
Kinnier Wilson be called in. Wilson was definite—this was the spastic
form of disseminated sclerosis, and AC should be treated with colloidal
silver. Not yet content with the leading specialists of London (Horder still
was not sure this was MS), the patient was considering other specialists:
Nonn in Germany or Wagner in Vienna. The patient showed slow worsening over the next few years and Parkes Weber considered the possibility that a B. coli infection might be the cause of AC's disseminated
sclerosis; he raised this question at a meeting in 1927 where Worster
Drought was discussing MS.

Treatment of the surgeon by 1930 was a no-meat diet, injections of
sodium cacodylate, and a rest cure. His file was now accumulating more
papers on MS, and there was excited discussion about the work of Kathleen
Chevassut and James Purves-Stewart; AC was referred to Purves-Stewart
and may have received the new vaccine for MS. He was later treated with
Eulenmeyer's solution, atropine sulphate, and air douches. By 1940,
Kinnier Wilson felt AC had a mild nonprogressive form of MS, even
though he was having difficulty walking and used a brace.

Over the next two years, AC began to fail, fracturing his hip and
developing complications of bedrest. Parkes Weber added to his file the
work by Putnam on a vascular basis for MS. In the meantime, AC was
being treated with low-salt diet, sulfathiazole, thiazamide, and IM
cyclotropin (urotropin, salicylic acid, and caffeine). He died in 1942, and
his postmortem was performed by the famous forensic pathologist Sir
Bernard Spillsbury. The notes of this case are extremely informative on
how a patient with MS was managed over 21 years of his disease prior to
the current era of case management.*[30]

In 1926, Fisher in Canada pointed out some of the less-common early
signs of MS, advocating two main approaches to treatment: inspire con-

*I am grateful to Dr. Lesley A. Hall of the Wellcome Library for bringing this case from the
Parkes Weber files to my attention. She recently reviewed the papers of Frederick Parkes
Weber (1863–1962).

fidence in the patient, and keep the bladder clean with sodium phosphate and urotropin. He also attempted to relieve MS symptoms using the various remedies for other spinal cord disorders. He did not comment on his own experience, but mentioned that others had had excellent results with tryparsamide and mercuralized serum given intraspinally.[31]

Infection continued to be a primary concern in the aggravation, if not the causation, of MS, so tonsillectomy, adenoidectomy, and tooth extraction were commonly recommended to MS patients in the 1920s and 1930s.

Russell Brain reviewed MS therapies in 1930,[32] and the list seemed depressing in its length as well as in lack of results. There was a large array of possible treatments: malarial therapy, typhoid vaccine, milk injections, phlogitan, sulfosian, African relapsing fever spirochete inoculation, staphococcal vaccine, neoarsphenamine (salvarsan), Chevassaut vaccine, arsenic, sodium encodylate, neoarsenobillon, silver salvarsan, intravenous colloidal silver, antimony, Bayer 205, sodium salicylate, intramuscular urotropin, intramuscular quinine, intramuscular mercury, oral iodides, intramuscular sodium nucleinate, diathermy, and x-ray irradiation. However, Brain's sobering negative conclusion was:

"No mode of therapy is successful enough to achieve, at the most, a greater improvement than might have occurred spontaneously.... The multiplication of remedies is eloquent of their inefficacy."

Russell Brain, 1930[33]

Following the overview by Brain, the first systematic attempt to evaluate all the various remedies for MS was by R.M. Brickner in 1935–1936; he presented one of the first outlines of how a therapy might be evaluated in the future.[34] The list of therapies is 29 pages long; all the therapies applied to MS patients by physicians anxious to help their patients who are even more anxious for anything that might help. Brickner looked at 158 therapeutic reports and concluded that one could only evaluate the effect of a treatment if the investigator noted not only the number occurring while on the therapy, but the disease course before treatment, the progress of subjective and objective features during therapy, and the appearance of new symptoms and signs. He suggested it would be important to assess the patient by a careful check-up each year and follow each patient for five years. Brickner's favored therapy was quinine, and this was known widely as the "Brickner quinine treatment for MS." Although popular as a therapy, others asked for the controlled studies of this therapy that Brickner himself had suggested for therapies of MS.[35]

Tracy Putnam in New York agreed with Brickner's recommendations, but felt that the most important measure of therapeutic effect is the prevention of attacks, for that would encourage recovery. Putnam did a primitive statistical analysis on Brickner's list of 1,407 cases treated with the 158 therapies and calculated that half the patients had profited from the various therapies. In a few forms of treatment (salicylates, nuclein, liver extract, intrathecal lecithin, and sympathectomy) all the cases so treated had improved, but these were all in small series of 10 or fewer cases. Larger series also showed good results: 60 percent improvement with fever therapy; 58 percent with roentgen therapy; 49 percent with quinine; 48 percent with fibrolysin; 45 percent with arsphenamine (salvarsan); and 35 percent with the Purves-Stewart vaccine.

To his literature analysis, Putnam added results from patients he and his colleagues studied at the Boston City Hospital, but despite his optimistic view of the list of therapies in the Brickner review, here was another picture. Their results were dismal, with no improvement in MS patients treated with liver extracts, high vitamins, arsphenamine, suramin sodium, typhoid vaccine, quinine, or amphetamine. Twelve patients who had forced CSF drainage were no better (they might have felt substantially worse), and he noted that the 12 treated with fever therapy were all made worse. Thus, paradoxically, his review of therapies from the literature suggested great promise of benefit from the therapies applied in the 1930s, but the patients in his own practice showed little benefit.

In the 1930s, Putnam referred to observation of vascular change within the plaques and suggested microvascular thrombosis might be the cause of the scattered pathology. He had initially proposed psychotherapy as an approach to the treatment of MS, but later abandoned this and suggested the use of anticoagulants. Putnam became a strong advocate of the new anticoagulant dicoumerol (warfarin).* Even when others were giving up this therapy after a decade of poor results, he continued to use it with his patients.[36] Denny-Brown said that during that era, he was more impressed with the dangers of anticoagulants than with their benefits.[37]

The idea of a vascular lesion that caused the plaques of MS dates back to the writings of Rindfleisch in 1863. Initially, arguments centered around whether the primary lesion was in the vessels or whether the inflammatory process involved the vessels secondarily. Pierre Marie believed that infection was the primary cause, but that the vascular change was an important result, so his therapy was two-pronged, aimed at the infection, and also at the sclerosis associated with the vascular process. N.D. Royle in Australia did thoracic sympathetic trunk sections as early as possible on MS patients to increase blood flow to the spinal cord and brain before venous congestion caused the sclerosis.[38] Although the interest in a vascular cause of MS continued during the early decades of the 20th century, it was only with the development of anticoagulants in the 1940s that a specific therapy could now be brought to bear on this concept of MS.

MS THERAPY 1940–1950

Tracy Putnam suggested the possibility of venular thrombosis in the center of the plaque in 1931 and put forth the idea of anticoagulation in 1940.[39] There was a theoretical basis for Putnam's approach to this therapy along the following lines:

- Venous thrombosis seemed to be an essential factor in MS.
- The association between the vascular lesion and the plaque was assumed to be causal.
- Plaque-like change can be induced by experimental venous thrombosis in the spinal cord.

---

*When a hemorrhagic disease of cattle occurred in midwestern Canada and the United States in 1920, Ontario veterinarian Frank Schofield noted the cause was moldy clover. His observation was ignored until Karl Paul Link of Wisconsin isolated the toxic substance, dicoumerol from the clover. The Wisconsin university alumni for whom warfarin was named has received royalties from the sale of the anticoagulant ever since its discovery in 1940.

- Obstructive changes seen in the retinal vessels of MS patients may be thrombotic.
- The coagulation system in MS may be unstable in some cases.
- External factors such as allergens may be active in MS and these could cause vascular changes.

Although Thygesen says that each of these points could be argued, the decision to use anticoagulants seemed reasonable according to the understanding at the time. An even more flimsy theoretical basis for this therapy came from Lesny and Polacek in Czechoslovakia, who postulated that MS was rare in the yellow race; Mongolians do not get MS in Europe, but whites can get MS in China; coagulation of the blood is lower in Chinese, but prothrombin levels are increased in people with MS; therefore, anticoagulation was an appropriate approach to treatment. Again, each point could easily be argued, but it was as the framework on which to build a therapy that anticoagulation was an exciting new therapeutic adventure in medicine.

Reese treated 28 patients with dicoumerol, but found only subjective improvement and no objective change.[40] He did not feel justified in continuing the therapy, but Putnam argued that he used too low a dose and allowed fluctuations to occur in the prothrombin levels so that attacks would occur when the level was low. Later, Putnam and his group published a study of 43 patients; the relapsing cases showed a striking improvement, but the progressive cases remained unchanged or continued to progress. The researchers found there was an attack every two to three years in the time prior to therapy with dicoumerol. The extensive statistical study of 3,797 attacks in 810 patients over an average observation period of 9.7 years seemed to confirm the results with dicoumerol. However, we now know that attacks decrease over time, and Putnam was undoubtedly observing the natural history of the disease rather than an effect of therapy.

Müller found an MS attack occurred once every two years.[41] Two years later, Lesny and Polacek used Swedish heparin in 27 cases and a Czech preparation of dicoumerol in 40 patients for up to 14 months and reported that the good results were seen not only in the "fresh" cases, but also in those who had been paraplegic and now could walk again.

Putnam used anticoagulation drugs through the years of World War II, and as Talley indicates, believed in this therapy until his death.[42] He reported on anticoagulation therapy with dicoumerol in 43 patients and found striking improvement in the relapsing cases, but no change in the progressive cases, who remained static or progressed. Schumacher was critical of Putnam and his group; he noted that the average interval between attacks prior to treatment was longer than the average period of observation for each patient.[43] Also Putnam had a different system of including acute episodes in the pre- and post-treatment phases. Despite the theoretical basis for using this therapy, the number of negative reports and the experience of many clinicians made it likely that anticoagulation therapy would share the fading fate of so many others.

Putnam did not restrict himself to the use of anticoagulants, however; Talley reviewed his record and found 118 different drugs he prescribed for his MS patients. At the UCLA neurology clinic where Talley worked, 136 drugs were used on MS patients, mostly for the control of symptoms, and 45 of these were similar to Putnam's armamentarium.[44]

In 1949, Scheinker suggested another vascular theory with an accompanying therapeutic approach: the lesions of MS might be due to vasoparalysis. Therapies applied were caffeine, ephedrine, alcohol, and adrenal cortex extract, but the cases were poorly documented and interest in the therapy quickly waned.[45]

Though anticoagulants were still being widely used, there was increasing skepticism about their benefits and increasing recognition of their dangers and side effects. By 1953, a review of the course of 105 attacks of MS in 60 patients, 35 of whom were treated with anticoagulants, was carried out by Paul Thygesen in Denmark.[46] The patients were treated with dicoumerol (Synparin) for an average of 11 months. A parallel study was carried out by M. and T. Fog at the same time. Both groups found no effect from anticoagulant therapy. Thygesen's extensive study of his cases, and his review of other series, including some who used the same approach as Putnam, concluded that anticoagulation did not alter the number of attacks or the course of the disease.

Talley makes the interesting suggestion that the approach to a vascular cause and therapy for MS fed into an old and familiar concept of manipulation of the blood in the treatment of disease.

"Whether it was Putnam's blood thinning, or the increased blood flow from vasodilators, or the prevention of blood sludging through Swank's low-fat diet, these strategies made sense, not only in the then current theories of pathogenesis but also because of the powerful roots of these practices in the ancient traditional panoply of Western healing."

Colin Talley, 1999[46]

Around 1950, there was increasing enthusiasm for injecting materials directly into the intrathecal space, the theoretical benefit being delivery of the therapeutic agent more directly into the central nervous system.[47] Stern gave vitamins intrathecally to two patients and he said they "felt, ate, walked, and talked better" and one patient lost his diplopia.[48] He also reported similar improvements in a number of non-neurological conditions such as inoperable malignancy, heart failure, and Paget's disease. There was great public interest in vitamins as apparently miraculous substances. Newspapers reported of more and more discoveries of vitamins necessary for health. Because many vitamin deficiencies had neurological consequences, including demyelination, it seemed logical to use vitamins to treat a disease like MS, especially since the vitamins were easily available and inexpensive. Greater and greater oral doses were used in treating MS, but the intrathecal route was never widely used.

By the mid-1950s, McAlpine was recommending rest and rehabilitation in a sanitorium for three to six months for MS patients. Fever therapy was still being used and Compston mentioned Professor Clarke's unpublished Humphrey Davy Rolleston Lecture in 1947 to the Royal College of Physicians on the benefits of pyrexia therapy in MS, at a time its popularity as a treatment was fading rapidly.[49]

It is interesting to contemplate the various concepts that guided therapy for MS over the years. Therapy might be governed by the concept of etiology, the concept of pathology, the nature of the symptoms, or just the need to offer some kind of help. We also see intertwined enthusiasm for anything new, and the common and sometimes useful phenomenon of extrapolating from a beneficial therapy in another disease. When a new way of viewing disease was espoused by medical science, that view was directed at MS. When a new therapy was found for infection, rheumatological disease or cancer, it was soon applied to MS.

Up to 1960, there were few accepted criteria for the evaluation of MS cases undergoing a new therapy, even though clinicians well knew some of the confounders that might give the appearance of a dramatic response when none existed. Spontaneous remissions had been acknowledged as characteristic of the disease since the writings of Frerich, Türck, Vulpian, and Charcot. The tendency for the patient to want to get well and to please the doctor was also well-known. Putnam illustrated this tendency in the case report of a woman who came regularly for ultraviolet radiation while continuing to progress to a wheelchair and then becoming bedbound, each visit saying she was improving. Despite these well-known factors suggesting a benefit when it might not be there, over and over there was (and still is) the tendency to imply efficacy for an agent because of uncontrolled cases reports. Brickner was the first to suggest criteria for the evaluation of effective therapy in MS, primarily by comparing the response to the natural history and the course before therapy.[50] Putnam cautioned about the natural tendency of MS patients to recover and to have remissions, which could confound attempts to assess therapeutic effect of an administered agent. He noted that von Hoesslin in Munich showed that 17 percent of his series of 516 cases had remissions, some so complete that the person felt well again, with some remissions as long as 14–40 years. In Putnam's series of 133 cases, 69 percent had some improvement at some time in their disease course and 44 percent of those with a first symptom had this disappear, a tendency more common in ambulatory office patients than in those on the wards.

Just as the enthusiasm for anticoagulants was fading, another therapy captured the interest of physicians and patients. At the Mayo Clinic, Bayard T. Horton developed a histamine therapy that was enthusiastically used for many disorders from the cluster headaches once named after Horton, to arthritis and MS. Horton and his colleagues H.P. Waegener, John Aita, and H.W. Woltman treated 102 MS patients with daily intravenous histamine diphosphate.[51] The patients were followed for up to 15 months with improvement visible in 18 of the 24 acute cases, and 36 of the 78 chronic cases. Criteria for improvement were vague, but others began to use this therapy. Abramson administered the histamine by ion-tophoresis, with improvement in the 11 cases he treated.[52] Hinton Jonez at the Tacoma clinic in Washington offered massive doses of histamine for the treatment of MS, as a prevention rather than a treatment of acute attacks, and had a very large clientele seeking this help.[53] A country doc-tor in Tacoma, Jonez writes in his book, *My Fight to Conquer Multiple Sclerosis*, that he was attending a course on allergy at Jefferson Medical College in Philadelphia when he heard Foster Kennedy and Bayard Horton speak of MS and the possibility that it was an allergic disorder. Antihistamines were an exciting approach for allergists at that time, but Horton was using histamine as a form of desensitization, and in a private conversation, Horton told Jonez of his theory that MS was an allergic dis-ease. Jonez returned home and gave histamine to a Mrs. Johnson, who improved and "gave away her wheelchair." After that, he convinced the sisters at St. Francis Hospital to give space for his Tacoma MS Clinic, and for many years he continued his therapy with large doses of histamine.

POSTWAR THERAPEUTIC OPTIMISM

The postwar era of new therapies such as sulfas, penicillin, new surger-ies, vaccines, and sera fostered a hopeful attitude toward cures in the pop-ulace and a renewed therapeutic activism in physicians. The need to do something for the patient was always there, so the array of therapeutic options was always long, but now there was confidence that these new options would do more than ameliorate the symptoms—there was now a sense of the miraculous about medicine's potential. Even though many medical writers would say that a therapy was disappointing, in the next breath, they offered drugs that "were sometimes helpful." By the 1940s, there was a new sense that therapy might really alter MS. Patients were also becoming more active in their pursuit of answers and in the age of new research and promising "breakthroughs" touted by the media, offered themselves as "guinea pigs" for anything rumored to be in the off-ing. In the United States, the increased status of the neurologist, the direct-to-consultant and fee-for-service system, amid an atmosphere of buoyant confidence in the ability of medical science to find answers to cancer, heart disease, and diseases like multiple sclerosis, encouraged this hope. It also encouraged a system of offering some form of therapy, any form of therapy, for the seeker. Patients would beat a path to the door of anyone offering any new therapy for MS. In this atmosphere, patients would not accept that there was nothing that could be done, an attitude of many classical neurologists, and increasingly insisted they be given any new therapy or they would go elsewhere.

In the United States, the media encouraged the sense of hope by emphasizing the very American approach of recovery through personal strength and individual effort, overcoming all odds. *Reader's Digest*, the *Saturday Evening Post,* and other magazines of the day carried stories of individuals who found inner strength to defeat the crippling aspects of MS and get up and walk. Many of these were initiated by the National MS Society as part of efforts to increase public awareness and a sense of optimism about the future of the disease, especially through further research. Such stories occurred in the British, Australian, and Canadian media only decades later, perhaps because the MS Society activity in those countries was slower to develop.

It was appropriate that by the closing days of World War II, Reese could step back and ask, "What do we know of multiple sclerosis?"[54] First, he admitted the cause was unknown, or that it might be one disease or many, perhaps with many causes. He said that there were 108 years of negative results in the attempt to show that bacteria, viruses, spirochetes, and other agents were involved. It was uncertain that the cause was a myelin or lipid-destroying enzyme, or a constitutional altered humoral reaction, or faulty blood clotting, or a specific allergic reaction.

What was known was the appearance of the scattered white matter plaques, which were sometimes acute, subacute, or chronic; some were sharply delineated, and others faded. These were the end stage of tissue damage with myelin edema, fat-filled microglia, focal astrocyte prolifer-ation, and perivenular gitter cell infiltration. The myelin might be in var-ious stages of breakdown, leaving naked axons, and sometimes loss of axons. Lesions were very scattered and only severely damaged areas would mirror the clinical symptoms. He felt the age of the lesion, its "intensity," and its location were important; these lesions might coalesce into a larger plaque.

He was convinced that all the various theories of cause had led to no specific therapy of value and this included "an endless list of drugs": proteins, vaccines, sera (specifically the Laiguel-Vasastine-Karessios and the Stransky sera), lipoid and endocrine substances, and the heroic measures of fever therapy, forced spinal drainage, cervico-dorsal sympathectomy, and ganglionectomy, all of which "reflects our searches and our failures."

Reese was uncertain of Marburg's theory that the myelin breakdown was due to a primary axonal swelling, and favored the theory that the primary problem was in the myelin, perhaps due to a lypolytic enzyme or "ferment" as Brickner and others had argued. His evaluation of the various studies of the vascular basis of MS was vague, perhaps because it was an area of his own research. He offered no conclusion, but noted the enthusiastic endorsement of the vascular theory by Putnam, and its denouncement by the neuropathologist George Hassin. All of this argument about the role of the vascular system was being pushed aside about 1950 by the new interest in "neuroallergy" led by Ferraro and others, who believed the key to MS was in an antigen-antibody reaction that caused the breakdown of myelin.

Perhaps as a carryover from the earlier days of confusion of MS with the vitamin B12 deficiency syndrome of subacute degeneration of the cord, Reese felt that achlorhydria usually indicated the patient would not have remissions because of poor absorption of nutrients in the GI tract.* He also felt that MS patients did not tolerate well a spinal tap to obtain CSF or for forced drainage, not because they might have exacerbations of their MS, as some others believed, but because they had more headache and dizziness afterwards. Acute attacks were recognized to clear spontaneously, and more severe and persistent symptoms were unresponsive to therapies.

---

*Reading this comment by Reese made me understand why a senior neurologist in my training days would always do a Schilling test for pernicious anemia in every case of MS. I thought he was trying to avoid missing a case of subacute combined degeneration of the cord, a gratifyingly responsive disease to treat; he might have been assessing the prognosis for remissions.

So, how would a patient be managed in 1946? Try to prevent infections, regulate menstruation and pregnancy, and "combat vegetative-endocrine crises" by avoiding exposure to cold, emotional shocks, fad diets, and allergies, all of which would undermine the homeostatic equilibrium of the organism. Here the terminology of Reese reflects the kind of thinking of the humoral physicians of the 18th century and the alternative therapists of the 20th century. Reese became quite stern in his advice:

> "A warning may be issued: Never treat an early multiple sclerosis case too drastically, either medically, or physio- or hydro-therapeutically. Keep the patient in bed for four weeks and support him according to his needs, since our goal is to support the upset homeostasis, to arrest the disease process, and to protect especially against recurrences."[55]

Reese had assessed the white counts of MS patients, but observed only a slight increase in the eosinophil cells, suggestive of an allergic phenomenon; he noted there was no clinical evidence of allergy. He used Horton's histamine treatment with promising results in early and remittent cases. He could not confirm the evidence that MS patients had a hyperprothrombinemia, but he still treated his cases with dicoumerol, even though in 28 cases he treated, there was no objective improvement.

MS THERAPY 1950–1960

> "Strangely enough, one seldom reads about an attempted treatment which has not had a favorable, often 'dramatic,' effect on disseminated sclerosis. It is no less strange that all methods of treatment have been abandoned in the course of a short time."
>
> Paul Thygesen, 1953[56]

Thygesen was referring to the array of therapies over the century, including a hundred homeopathic remedies, nonspecific "Reiz-therapie," "specific" vaccines, radiotherapy; transfusions of various kinds, and several, often opposing, potent drugs and even psychotherapy and heroic surgery. His monograph in 1953 was an intensive review of MS features, and a careful assessment of the then popular therapy of MS with anticoagulation.

Up to the 1950s, MS therapies for the most part varied little from those of a century before, with some briefly popular agents and approaches, soon replaced by others. Physicians consistently recommended control over stress and activities, limits on pregnancy and physical exertion, and an array of medications that included potassium iodide, arsenic, strychnine, mercury, silver nitrate, quinine, cod liver oil, vitamins, and tonics; and physical measures that included hydrotherapy, massage, fever therapy, and horseback riding. Little changed during these many years, and the test for each particular therapy was the value the practitioner put on it. The experience of the physician was the bedrock value system for what worked and what did not. No matter what the latest article said, or what the city consultant believed, "in my experience" expressed by the patient's physician held sway.

Assessing the period of the 1947–1960, Talley reviewed 227 records from the private practice of Tracy Jackson Putnam, who had then moved to Beverly Hills, California.[57] He also reviewed 86 patient records from the UCLA Neurology Clinic, which demonstrated the very personal and

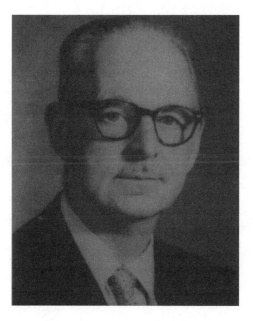

Figure 15.7   Tracy Putnam believed the basic lesion in MS was a vascular one and treated patients with anticoagulants. (Reprinted with permission from Elsevier, *Surgical Neurology*, 1988, 29:89–90.)

plaintive approaches of patients to the experts, seeking any therapy, and often coming with a lot of background information, asking for the latest treatment they had heard about. Telley convincingly argued that a look at the culture of 19th-century therapy, which carried over into the practicing community of the 20th century, revealed a lot about the approach of physicians toward the treatment of MS patients. How medical treatments "worked" and how care was provided by the neurologists was historically, culturally, and locally specific.

George Schumacher at Cornell University Medical College was asked by the new Advisory Board of the National Multiple Sclerosis Society to prepare a report on the current understanding and therapy of MS; this was published in a series of articles in the *Journal of the American Medical Association* in 1950.[58] Schumacher emphasized to the general medical community the importance of multiple sclerosis medically and socially, and added that it was not as gloomy a story in terms of prognosis or length of life as many had reported; most patients had almost normal life expectancy, though they were often disabled. He outlined the necessary disease features leading to the diagnosis, which would later be codified in what became known as the Schumacher criteria. He berated those who diagnosed only on the presence of certain signs ("cookbook medicine") or on symptoms alone, which he felt was worse, and inexcusable.

Schumacher felt there was no satisfactory therapy in 1950, but any future therapy that worked would have to limit the attacks and the progression. He dispensed with the therapies that had been used but were now discarded, some after long use and some after a brief period: these included arsenic, fever therapy, vaccines and sera, autohemotherapy, lecithin, X-ray therapy, sympathectomy, belladonna, endocrine therapies, and penicillin.

The therapies still under consideration at the half century were: 1) general measures, 2) drug therapies, and 3) psychotherapy. Under general approaches he listed good nutrition and vitamins (but not megavitamins), living in a warmer climate, and avoiding physical and emotional stress, and perhaps avoiding pregnancy. Avoiding infection was important, but the specific role of infection in disease was still unclear. Skin testing and elimination diets for allergies were not yet warranted despite some positive reports. A high-protein diet low in ash was recommended to avoid bladder stones. He recommended physical therapy, but not some of the enthusiastic programs that drove the patient to the point of exhaustion.

He compiled the literature on MS therapy since the review by Brickner in 1936.[59] Treatments aimed at the pathogenesis of the disease included anticoagulants, vasodilators (especially histamine and quaternary ammonium compounds), circulatory stimulants, vitamins (especially B vitamins and vitamin E), drugs to affect the immune state, and enzymes (cytochrome C). He listed a miscellaneous group of therapies used in MS including trypan red, cytochrome C, and ammonium chloride, which brought "no distinctive relief."

Schumacher's recommendations on drugs were in the two categories of those aimed at modifying the lesions in the nervous system, and those that were symptomatic therapies. He began by saying no drug had been shown to heal the primary lesion of MS. Histamine, given intravenously by Horton at the Mayo Clinic and by iontophoresis by Abramson, was an approach aimed at vasodilation, on the hypothesis that vasoconstriction was a primary factor in the cause of the lesions. Schumacher concluded that no patient had been cured by this method. Others gave papaverine and amyl nitrate on the same logic, but although retinal vasospasm and scotomas were said to improve in half the cases treated, these drugs had not been shown to be beneficial or practical in MS therapy. Other vasodilators that had been tried without effect, included aminophylline, belladonna, amprotropine phosphate, and alcohol. The vascular theory of MS causation led others to try a long list of sympatholytic and adrenolytic drugs to no avail, despite early "promising results." Schumacher criticized the anticoagulant trials as being too short, but thought them worthy of closer study, although he doubted the practicality of long-term therapy because of the inherent dangers.

Others theorized that there was vasoparalysis in the area of the plaque and used circulatory stimulants such as ephedrine, caffeine, alcohol, adrenal cortical extract, and desoxycorticosterone acetate, but Schumacher felt early promising reports were not based on sound scientific premises or on controlled studies.

Schumacher went on to review other forms of therapy such as transfusion therapies of Lehoczky (1944), Tschabitscher (1949), and Leo

Alexander (1950) and reached the same depressing conclusion. Hemolytic serum and vaccine therapies were of no value, and he concluded that the new reports on the use of ACTH should also be labeled as insufficiently substantiated. He was not convinced that the vitamin therapies, even in large doses, had any effect and he felt the new studies with vitamin B12, although underway, were unconvincing.

Schumacher concluded as negatively as Russell Brain had 20 years before:

> *"No case of unequivocal cure of established multiple sclerosis is on record. No case of complete relief of symptoms of significant duration has been proved to be due to a therapeutic measure. No study statistically summarized advances a sufficiently high percentage of good results in a significantly large number of patients to warrant general use of the method in question by practicing physicians.*
>
> *In summary of the drug treatment of multiple sclerosis it may be said that the outlook for cure of the disease by use of drugs is unpromising and that the outlook for symptomatic relief by drugs is less optimistic than would appear from the large number of reports which make claims of favorable effects."*

George Schumacher, 1950[60]

Despite the negative review by Schumacher, more and more therapies for MS were announced during the 1950s. Dr. Emanuel M. Abrahamson of New York stated that he had found a basic problem in MS patients, hypoglycemia due to hyperinsulinism; he devised a treatment to correct the hypoglycemia.[61] Dr. Hinton D. Jonas of Tacoma, Washington, adapted the enthusiasm and therapeutic method of Dr. Bayard T. Horton of the Mayo Clinic, who was treating many conditions with histamine desensitization. Jonas used massive doses of histamine in the treatment of MS by a regime of long-term self-injection and iontophoresis. He said he personally administered 150,000 doses, more than any other person, "without a single bad result." The Jonas method and Horton histamine therapy had a wave of popularity, which soon waned, as so many other "new breakthrough" therapies did, and continue to do.

Those who favored an allergic basis for the disease used a long list of other antihistaminic therapies as well, and in 1954, Drs. Milo G. Myer, Alan Johnston, and Arthur F. Coca announced that removing allergens would improve or even cure MS.[62]

In the 1950s, there was press attention to a new vaccine from Russia, but this turned out to be rabies vaccine, which caused adverse effects in MS patients.[63] However, about every five years for the next few decades, there was an announcement in the press of a "Russian vaccine" of interest in the MS community. During the cold war, everything Russian was under suspicion and open to scrutiny. In 1959, Dr. Richard Masland at the NINDB was contacted by two physicians at the CIA who said that they had serum from a Russian patient treated with a multiple sclerosis vaccine, and they wanted the serum tested.[64]

Those who theorized an emotional basis for MS favored psychotherapy, either as supportive or morale-building approach, or corrective psychotherapy. Psychotherapy was employed as a treatment, since many clinicians thought the vascular changes and plaques could be induced by stress and emotional factors. Smith Ely Jelliffe believed that repressed emotions caused plaques in the areas where the repression occurred in the nervous system. Employing psycho-dynamic approaches would have the advantage of reducing the cause of the lesions. A leading advocate of this approach was, again, Tracy Putnam, but within a few years Langworthy, Fuglsang-Frederiksen and Thygesen, and others concluded that this approach had no value in effecting a change in the course of MS (although it might have other benefits).

Since there were so many repeated disappointments about new therapies in MS, Thygesen asked why there was such continued optimism about new treatments for the disease.[65] He pondered that it was probably because clinicians who knew quite well that spontaneous remissions occurred, forgot this while treating their own patients. Also, there usually are fewer remissions and more attacks recorded in the pretreatment phase. Finally, Thygesen said most people with MS "are amiable people who hate to disappoint their doctor" and gave the responses the doctors wanted to hear.

THE ERA OF CLINICAL TRIALS

For centuries, therapy was based on empirical approaches to the concepts of disease in that era. If an imbalance of humors or influence of the wind direction or planet configuration was believed to influence the occurrence or healing of a disease, the therapy would be a logical approach to that cause. This is not so farfetched; we currently operate this way. If we believe MS is due to a vascular occlusion, we try anticoagulants; if we think it is an immune reaction, we apply every immunosuppressant known; if we think it is an infection, we use any vaccine or antibiotic that might reduce or eliminate an infectious process. In the last 50 years, we have gone through each of these phases. The results have been disappointing, but the theories persist.

Frustrating the efforts to find new therapies for patients is the lack of understanding of both the cause and the detailed pathophysiologic mechanisms involved. William Gowers a century ago said it would not be possible to find effective therapies until we knew more about causation.

In the 19th century, therapies were empirical, administered to patients if they seemed to help previous patients with similar problems. With experience, clinicians developed opinions on what was helpful and what was not. Although Pierre Louis in France and William Farr in England had developed ways to use statistical analysis in assessing outcomes in the late 18th and early 19th centuries, use of these methods only slowly entered the realm of clinical investigation and most papers through the 19th and early 20th centuries were case series of accumulated clinical experience, though some of these series were large. By the 1930s, clinicians began to complain that many reports of helpful treatments in MS were not sufficiently controlled and the American Neurological Association asked for improved standards for clinical studies.

For centuries, medical knowledge was based on authority and passed from generation to generation. Experience gave the physician an impression of what seemed to work. This empirical approach was the basis of medical practice until the scientific approach became a method of examining questions and testing hypotheses. The scientific method challenged ideas, theories, and accepted knowledge and became a way of approaching medical knowledge at the same time it propounded the idea that medical knowledge was there to be challenged, and the discarding of untenable beliefs was an exciting prospect.

One way that beliefs and theories were to be challenged was through experiment. Don't think—do the experiment, was the admonition of John Hunter in the 18th century. Thomas Jefferson chided physicians, even his prominent friend Dr. Benjamin Rush, for theorizing too much. Knowledgeable in science and medicine as well in the other philosophies, Jefferson said, "It is not to physic I object, but to physicians," as they did not observe enough and use common sense, when observation and experiment would give them valuable information. Experiment became the way to advance medical knowledge and Claude Bernard and Louis Pasteur were leaders of the approach.

During this time, knowledge of multiple sclerosis grew by the method of collection and analysis of case series. Charcot's list was not long, perhaps 39 cases of MS, but he examined many different neurological and psychological phenomena at the same time. Uhthoff, Bramwell, Müller, and others accumulated large series of cases and analyzed them in simple numerical ways. Use of statistical analysis in the assessment of these series was only slowly emerging.

Clinical trials did not enter the regular practice of MS work until the last half of the 20th century. There were early trials in medicine, and historians will often refer to the shipboard study of James Lind, who assigned a different treatment (vitriol, sea water, herbs and spices, cider, oranges, and limes) to each pair of sailors. The two on oranges and limes dramatically improved and were back to their duties within a week. It took him six years to publish his work, and the British Navy almost 50 years to adopt the treatment as policy (perhaps some things do not change). Another interesting experiment that may have a lesson for our future trials in MS is the story of William Withering and the discovery of the witch's potion that contained foxglove for dropsy. Many stories of discovery in medicine are told the way we like to hear them rather than according what happened. Withering had a long experience of the progress of dropsy and used the natural history of the disease to compare with a 10-year experience using digitalis before publishing his work. In the future, we may have to abandon placebo trials and use observational trials and compare the results to a knowledge of the natural history of MS, just as Withering did for dropsy.

Today, new agents are studied with a well-developed method of randomized clinical trials (RCT) first developed by Ronald Fisher in the 1920s and 1930s in agriculture and brought into medicine by Bradford Hill to study streptomycin and PAS in the treatment of tuberculosis in 1946. Clinical trials for MS were first used to study steroids, and then later for any new agent thought to be helpful. Such trials have been very useful in demonstrating effectiveness of drugs and in the future, will have to adapt to the challenges of ethical controls, high costs, limited measurement tools, and the need to use large groups of patients studied over a very long time.

The difficulties in assessing therapy in MS were recognized by the early writers, who noted that patients could have spontaneous remissions and periods without progression. Many drugs used in early studies of MS seemed to help because the number of attacks lessened, but it was later recognized that relapses decrease over the long-term in the disease even without therapy. Careful study of a control group was mandatory to assess results for any treatment. Indeed, the placebo group in almost every long-term study seemed to show some evidence of improvement, whether reduction in relapses or in symptoms.

In the 1970s, many MS trials began with agents borrowed from the development of drugs in cancer and rheumatologic research, with varying degrees of tightness in the design of the treated and controlled groups. By 1979, a committee under Joe Brown outlined suggestions for the design of a trial in MS[66] and this was followed by further refinements by Myers and Ellison[67] and Weiss and Stadlan.[68] Each well-designed trial in the past decade has taught investigators helpful lessons for the next trial.

In 1974, the National Advisory Commission on Multiple Sclerosis (USA) divided clinical trials into preliminary, pilot, and full studies. This classification was succeeded in 1977 by a system put forward by the U.S. Department of Health, Education, and Welfare (HEW) in 1977, dividing trial types into four phases. Trials were divided into phase 1 to study effects in normals, phase 2 to study MS to determine efficacy, and phase

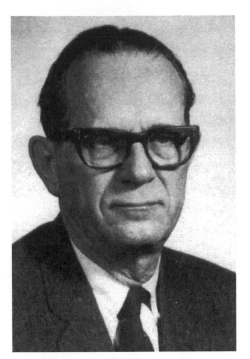

Figure 15.8 Joe Brown was professor of neurology at the Mayo Clinic. He led a group (Beebe, Kurtzke, Loewenso, Silberberg, Tourtelotte) to define a standard for the design of a trial of a new agent in MS (1979). (Courtesy of AAN and Dr. M. Cohen.)

3 on patients to determine subgroups and for definition of toxicity. Phase 4 is a postmarketing clinical trial.

Trials are difficult because large numbers of patients must be followed for a long time. Patients may drop out for various reasons, and this makes assessment of the trial results difficult, because the dropout group may not be random, but represent characteristics that change the remaining group. Many patients go into trials, not just to assist research, but to get "the new therapy," even though the agent has not yet been shown to be therapeutic.

Recruitment is also difficult because only a small proportion of an MS group will be appropriate for the trial and many of those may not be interested. Bornstein screened 932 volunteers to get 50 patients for a trial[69] and Ellison screened 1,118 patients to get 98 patients for a trial.[70]

The investigators and the patients must be blinded about who is on therapy and who is on placebo so that biases are reduced. Noseworthy noted in the Canadian cyclophosphamide trial that the unblinded neurologists saw a therapeutic effect while those who were blinded did not.[71]

Finally, when the results are compiled, there has to be an assessment of whether the statistical benefit constitutes a significant clinical benefit, whether the cost is worth the change seen, and how that is to be balanced against side effects and complications. Despite difficulties, the current trial methodologies allow us to get better answers to important questions. As this is written, there are many trials assessing new agents for MS so the outlook is very hopeful.*[72]

STEROID THERAPY

An early harbinger of steroid therapy was the suggestion by Judson Bury in 1912 that the administration of suprarenal extract had improved some cases of MS; he said that "two patients testified strongly to its beneficial effect."[73] As early as 1925, Hench theorized there was a "substance X" in the adrenal gland, and by 1949, he reported that he was able to "cure" rheumatoid arthritis; and this (unfulfilled) expectation garnered him a Nobel Prize.[†] "Compound E" was thought to be a miraculous cure for rheumatoid arthritis, and rheumatologists were excited to have a drug that finally could alter the course of the disease. The drug gave them a scientifically based therapy and a new place among medical specialties. Physical medicine was overtaking the field of musculoskeletal and rheumatic diseases after World War II, at a time when the rheumatologist's therapeutic armamentarium had a reputation for being on the fringe.[74]

The use of cortisone was limited by the small and costly supply, and it was said that the used syringes and bottles at the Mayo Clinic were returned to Edward C. Kendall, who first developed cortisone, so that any remaining drug could be salvaged. There was a rush to find ways to synthesize cortisone for a larger supply.[75] When more drug was available, cortisone was used on more diseases and it was not long before it was

---

*A full review of the modern trials for therapeutic agents in MS can be found in *Management of Multiple Sclerosis and Interpretation of Clinical Trials* by Donald W. Paty, Stanley A. Hashimoto, and George C. Ebers, Chap. 12 in *Multiple Sclerosis*, edited by Paty and Ebers.

† There was great excitement when cortisone "burst on the scene" in the late 1940s, although it was much like interferons in the early 1990s—much excitement and expectation, but for a very expensive drug that was in very short supply.

being tried on multiple sclerosis, but in doses we would now regard as extremely small.

Randt and Merritt treated MS patients with ACTH in 1950 in a small study that suggested slight improvement,[76] and Selye said that ACTH might give slight improvement in MS, but the effect lasted only a few days.[77] Henry Miller of Newcastle suggested that steroids be tried in MS because they appeared to have a positive effect on acute disseminated encephalomyelitis.[78] In 1951, Jonsson used cortisone on MS; others who tried it were Fog (1951), Glaser and Merritt et al. (1952), Merritt (1954), and Rucker (1956); they concluded that ACTH and cortisone were not suitable therapy for MS. Although the initial results were unconvincing, and many attempts were felt to be negative, that did not stop the drug's being widely used as a therapy.

During a three-year period (1958–1961), Henry Miller and his group carried out the first double-blind trial in MS using ACTH and saline injections in acute attacks of MS.[79] They matched their groups for age, sex, and duration of disease, as well for the proportion who had initial attacks, those who were having a repeat attack, and those who were having an exacerbation of an existing disability. The dose was 60 units of ACTH gel twice a day for one week, 40 units twice a day for one week, and 60, 40, and 20 units on the second, fourth, and sixth days of the third week. The control group had a similar pattern of saline injections. The investigators abandoned Alexander's complex scoring system, which they had planned to use in the trial.[80] It proved unworkable in patients as it was confusing in the area of disability prior to, and due to, the attack being treated; the investigators reverted to a more subjective evaluation by the blinded clinicians. They felt the ACTH was significantly better than saline, and this was especially impressive in optic neuritis.

The image of cortisone as a "wonder drug" kept it in the forefront of MS therapy in the 1960s–1970s even when most studies had negative results. Oral steroids have been studied in repeated trials since the 1960s without convincing results, including the negative trial by Miller in 1961.[81] Miller concluded that oral prednisone 15 mg daily for 8 months followed by 10 mg daily for 10 months was ineffective. In 1965, Tourtellote and Haerer also obtained negative results with methylprednisolone 8–12 mg daily for 18 months. In the meantime, because of the possibility of a greater effect by introducing steroids directly into the intrathecal space, the method was used extensively in the 1960s, though use waned in the 1970s when arachnoiditis was recognized as a complication in many who had repeated and long-term therapy by this route.

One of the early proponents of ACTH therapy was Leo Alexander (1905–1985) of New York.[82–84] The "Alexander Regime" was used widely over the next two decades, despite Cushingoid features and side effects, but was gradually replaced by briefer courses of ACTH for acute attacks and then IV methylprednisolone over a few days. In his 1961 book on MS, Alexander outlined his experience with a number of other therapies, including muscle adenylic acid (My-B-Den) and thiamine given to 209 cases but with disappointing results.[85] He used blood transfusions with minor improvement when they were given to previously stable patients who were having an attack.[86] His best results were still with ACTH

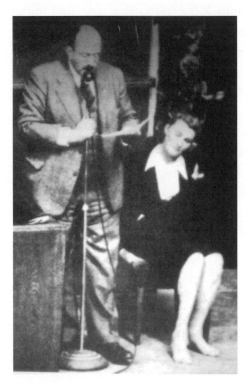

Figure 15.9 Dr. Leo Alexander was an advocate of ACTH therapy for MS in the short and longer term, called the "Alexander Regime." Alexander was a prominent New York neurologist who contributed to the literature on depression and many neurological disorders. His lasting contribution was drafting the Nuremberg Code following his investigation of Nazi medical experiments after World War II. This photograph shows Leo Alexander testifying at Nuremberg with a Polish survivor of a bone graft experiment. (Shevell MI. Neurology's witness to history: Part II. Leo Alexander's contributions to the Neremberg Code (1946–1947). *Neurology*, 1998, 50:274–278.)

given by the "Alexander Regime." He had negative results with oral cortisone, prednisone, and intrathecal hydrocortisone. His therapeutic regime with any MS patient was to provide explanation and encouragement if the patient was doing well, blood transfusion or ACTH in an acute attack, and ACTH if the MS was progressing.

Alexander wrote almost 300 papers on a variety of neurological and psychiatric conditions and published on MS for over 25 years. In 1947, he published a series of papers on MS with Tracy Putnam as a frequent co-author. It is of current interest that Alexander wrote on the loss of axons in plaques, the vascular changes in the plaques, as well as various treatments for MS and its symptoms, and methods of assessing outcome from clinical trials. He developed the first protocol for objectively assessing the features of MS patients in a clinical trial, but as we mentioned earlier, it

Dr. Leo Alexander and The Nuremberg Code

At the end of World War II, Leo Alexander, a distinguished American neuropsychiatrist with Austro-German background, was assigned by special orders to review the Nazi euthanasia program that focused on disabled adults and children. He was the first to describe the extent of this program, and also described the Dachau hypothermia and high-altitude experiments.[87,88] He was a medical expert for the prosecution at the "Nazi doctor trials." Perhaps his lasting legacy was related to his authorship of a later series of documents that would be the basis of the initial draft of the Nuremberg Code of Clinical Research Ethics.[89,90] It is ironic to note the involvement in Nazi medical experiments by two other prominent neurologists who contributed to MS research, Hallervorden and Shaltenbrandt, and also by neuroanatomist Pernkoff, whose great atlas is said to show anatomic dissection on German Jews. It has also been pointed out that the Nuremberg Code, which has been important in outlining ethical restrictions on clinical trials, a process led by the Americans, has never been signed by the United States, on the argument that it was meant for other countries such as Germany, and was not necessary for the United States.

did not find favor because it was complex, repetitive, and impractical for wide use.

Alexander served on the first medical advisory board for the nascent National MS Society but came into conflict with the Society when he was turned down for a grant. He enlisted the support of the Boston chapter of the Society, which broke with Society policy by giving him a research grant. The angry responses from Alexander and the patients and neurologists he contacted drove groups into various camps of support for Alexander or the National Society, culminating in a packed annual chapter meeting to vote on the issue. Sylvia Lawry and the National MS Society emerged bruised but victorious.

ACTH was used extensively for acute attacks of MS based on the reports from Alexander (1961), Henry Miller (1966), Rinne (1968), and Rose (1970). Although ACTH might be helpful in acute attacks, Miller felt it was ineffective in reducing relapses when used for longer periods. Rose carried out another early well-controlled MS trial with this agent in 1969, demonstrating a positive, but very modest improvement over placebo.[91] The study was one of the first major controlled double-blind trials in MS. Although ACTH had some effect on the timing of recovery, it was unclear if recovery was any better. Despite the marginal results, ACTH treatment became the standard for the next 15 years, replaced in the mid-1980s with high-dose intravenous methylprednisolone given over a few days, another therapy borrowed from the promising results with pulsed therapy in rheumatoid arthritis. This therapy had some effect on reducing immunological synthesis and oligoclonal banding patterns were minimally affected, but the effect might be primarily on inflammation.*

In the early 1980s, many neurologists began to replace ACTH treatment of acute MS attacks with high-dose intravenous methylprednisolone, a methodology used by rheumatologists in serious rheumatic disorders. There were a number of early trial series, but the first major trial was done by Compston's group at Cambridge.[92] Since then, this has been the preferred therapy for acute attacks, although a number of regimes are used.[93]

---

*A full review of the trials with ACTH and steroids was published by Lawrence W. Myers.

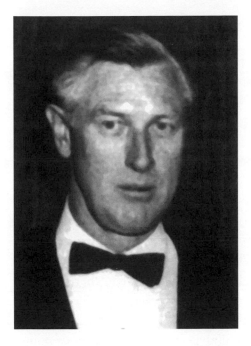

Figure 15.10   Augustus Rose, known to his colleagues as "Buck," was head of neurology at UCLA Medical Center. He led the major 10 center trial that demonstrated the benefit of ACTH in acute MS published in 1970. The trial was perhaps the most rigorous design and evaluation of any MS trial to that date. (Courtesy of AAN and Dr. M. Cohen.)

Nineteen trials on optic neuritis treated with oral steroids have been conducted over the last 50 years and at most have shown a modest effect on the speed of recovery, but no greater recovery than placebo and no difference in the eventual long-term outcome. An American Academy of Neurology Subcommittee produced a practice parameter on the treatment of optic neuritis by steroids in 2000, and concluded prednisone in doses of 1 mg per kg had no demonstrable effect. Higher doses might hasten recovery, but the eventual visual acuity was unaffected. As always, there are treatment proponents who argue the doses are still too small and there are studies underway to assess if very high-dose oral steroids in daily doses equivalent to the intravenous therapies may be more beneficial. Those who argue that the intravenous steroids achieve better results only because of dosage find support from recent evidence that oral methylprednisolone in very high dosage may be beneficial.

Steroids remain the standard management for serious acute attacks of MS. Their use is a safe outpatient procedure, but has annoying immediate side effects such as emotional change and insomnia, and there is a small but serious risk of avascular necrosis of the hip. This latter complication may be missed if symptoms and disability of hip disease are ascribed to the advancing MS.

After 50 years of using steroids in MS, the answers are not yet clear, or we are not hearing the answers that are there.

ATTEMPTS TO SUPPRESS THE IMMUNE SYSTEM

Although changes in the immune system are intricate and complex, and incompletely understood, for many years attempts have been made to alter the immune system in the hope of ameliorating the activity of multiple sclerosis. The observation of Glanzmann in 1935 that an immune disorder (EAE) could be produced in animals began a study of immune mechanisms in nervous system diseases like MS.[92] After Kabat noted the presence of increased gamma globulin in the CSF,[93] there was an increased interest in immunity in MS, and this interest grew during the 1960s and 1970s. Later, any agent that could suppress the immune system was applied to MS. Even steroids could be regarded as a means of reducing the activity of the immune system. However, it was evident that the understanding of the immune alterations in MS was incomplete; it was not clear how therapies should alter the immune system to effect a positive result. Also, a target antigen for the immune reaction has yet to be found. The EAE model has been used to test agents against an immune demyelination, but there are examples of quite different responses in animals and in later human MS experiments.

Plasma Exchange

Therapeutic plasma exchange (plasmapheresis; apheresis) has been attempted in MS since 1980, based on the hypothesis that the plasma may contain proteins or other substances that initiate inflammation and demyelination. A recent meta-analysis of six prospective, controlled studies suggested a modest, but significant benefit.[94] There was a modest reduction in the likelihood of progression at one year and a greater chance the patient would be improved. The therapy is complex, expensive, and has some complications; it is ill-suited for long-term therapy for a common chronic disease. Recent studies by Weinshenker suggested the need for more specific indicators of those most likely to benefit.[95] There is some indication that plasma exchange may be best for those in the throes of a severe attack that does not respond to steroids.

Immunosuppressant Therapy

It would seem logical in a disease that appears to be immunologically mediated to try to improve patients using drugs that have the capacity to suppress the immune system. Knowledge of the intricacies of the immune mechanisms in MS is imperfect, as is knowledge of the complexities of drug effects, so attempts are necessarily empirical. From the 1960s on, any immunosuppressant drug available was tried on MS. There have been repeated initial "promising results worthy of study in a larger trial" that ended in disappointment when such trials were done. Therapies that have been tried include azathioprine,[96] cyclophosphamide,[97] cyclosporine,[98] sulphinpyrazone,[99] total lymphoid irradiation,[100] and plasmapheresis.[101] Studies are now underway with autologous bone marrow transplantation. Although azathioprine is still widely used in Europe, most of the immunosuppressants have faded from the clinical scene because of lack of effect, or marginal effect in the face of serious side effects and long-term concerns. Others, such as cyclophosphamide and plasmapheresis, are reserved for a few rapidly progressing cases or severely involved patients.

Azathioprine (AZA)

In an uncontrolled and unblinded study of azathioprine (AZA) in MS, Frick and his colleagues found there was a reduction in relapse rate, but not in progression of the disease. Soon after this initial report, during a discussion at an MS symposium about whether azathioprine had any effect or not, J.H.D. Miller added a strong note of caution to the participants by reminding them that in Belfast, they had information on the onset and death dates of 471 patients, and the average length of life with the disease was 20 years:

> *"So that you must think twice before you submit patients to danger-ous therapy, because, on the whole, the majority of patients get along very well."*

At the same meeting, T.M. Bell warned that slow and latent virus infections seemed not to respond to natural interferons, which are involved in the mechanism for terminating most viral diseases; since there is little interferon production in these diseases and they are relatively unresponsive to interferon, it is possible that immunosuppressants might actually reactivate the disease. Since so little was known about the complexity of the immune system before, during, and after activity in MS, the empirical approach of using one immunosuppressant after another to assess its effect on MS bothered many during the 1970s and 1980s.

The major argument at the time, however, was whether AZA had any beneficial effect or not. Soon after the initial report, Cendrowski, Silberberg, Swinburne, Patzold, and others carried out separate studies that showed little benefit from AZA, although other later studies suggested some effect in early relapsing-remitting cases. When AZA was combined with steroids and compared with steroids alone, no difference was seen. The study of Ellison seemed to demonstrate that AZA was ineffective, but a large British-Dutch study soon after again raised the suggestion of a beneficial effect on MS elapses and progression, although even the study authors did not feel the results were convincing enough to recommend AZA as standard therapy for MS. A meta-analysis of all the many confusing studies, but limited to seven well-controlled studies on 793 patients suggested a minor benefit; but this minor effect had to be balanced against potential problems, such as gastric side effects, increased infections, increased risk of malignancy, and hepatic damage.[102]

Many things affect the use of a therapy; despite the various negative and positive studies of AZA use in MS, there was an interesting and marked difference in the use of this therapy in Europe and North America. Some European neurologists suggested AZA was a standard therapy, while their North American colleagues seldom used the drug. This might be partly related to the positive results that came mainly from European studies, or to a pattern of using more medications in continental Europe compared to an atmosphere of relative therapeutic nihilism in North America. AZA was available (not experimental), relatively easy to take by oral route, reasonably free of major immediate side effects, and could be used in patients who had few other options for therapy. North

American physicians were concerned about long-term effects on cancer risk and more reluctant to embark on long-term use; later European studies did not demonstrate a significant cancer risk. Some suggested that AZA had to be used in the long-term for its benefits to become obvious, but others argued the decrease in relapses was just the natural history of the disease, as attacks tended to decrease as the disease progresses.

Cyclophosphamide

Studies on EAE in the 1960s suggested that cyclophosphamide might be useful in MS, and many clinicians tried it on a few patients who had rapidly progressing disease. They were uncertain of the result, but convinced about the side effects that occurred to most patients, including hair loss and severe cystitis. Use of the therapy in uncontrolled studies of individual patients who were progressing rapidly grew. This led to the belief that some patients may have reached their disease plateau after the therapy. Cendrowski reported a negative trial in 1973[103] and Drachman found in 1975 that cyclophosphamide was not effective in treating acute attacks of MS.[104] There was some suggestion that this immunosuppressant could slow the progression of MS when the results were compared to historical controls. After years of anecdotal reports suggesting some benefit, Weiner reported beneficial results on the longer-term outcomes in the preliminary and later final results of a five-year multicenter trial.[105] Side effects were major and the study results were challenged by a group of Canadian investigators who found no benefit in a subsequent trial but again noted significant side effects.[106] The two groups debated their results in letters to editors, and the final report of the American trial again showed positive results. The arguments did not end, but the issue was resolved by the National MS Society, which said this therapy could not be recommended because of the serious side effects and the minimal, if any, benefits. Cyclophosphamide is still used in some severe and progressive cases that do not seem to respond to any other therapy.

Cyclosporine

Because cyclosporine, a very effective immunosuppressant, could inhibit EAE, and could suppress Il-2 production by T-cells and inhibit T-cell activation, it was tried by Ebers and Feasby in Canada in 1984, but continued progression occurred in all five patients treated. Rudge at Queen Square, London found a slight benefit to those treated with a high dose, but the side effects were potentially serious complications: kidney damage, hypertension, and encephalopathy and precluded this therapy's use as a treatment for MS. Later, Kappos demonstrated that the drug had no clinical benefit in MS and moreover had no visible MRI effect, something later studies would show with therapies that had a demonstrated effect.[107] A study in 1990 had a large dropout rate for the drug and the placebo group, usually a sign that the patients perceive no benefit; there was no measurable benefit, except for a subgroup that seemed to take longer to get to wheelchair status, and there was no MRI effect. This experience seemed to suggest that general immunosuppression is not an effective way to treat MS.

Methotrexate

Although available for over four decades, methotrexate has been in MS therapy only in the last few years, after Currier and his group in 1993 and Goodkin in 1995–1996 reported minor favorable results with weekly low doses. A report by Fischer et al. suggested some effect on cognitive function. There was no change in progression in the studies of methotrexate and no changes in T2-weighted total lesion area on MRI.

Mitoxanthrone

The most recent drug available for MS is mitoxanthrone (Novatrone®), which has clinical benefit in progressive cases that must be balanced against potential dose-related cardiac complications and the possibility of leukemia. It is given as an intravenous infusion every three months. It remains to be seen how this therapy will be used in a lifelong disease, as the side effects of the drug appear to be dose related, so the longer it is used, the greater the risk for serious myocardial damage.

Cladribine

Cladribine, developed at the Scripps Clinic in California, held some promise for MS therapy because it was capable of immunosuppression, with specific antilymphocyte and antimonocyte activity, and could reduce the burden of disease on the MRI scans of MS patients. After an initial promising trial in chronic progressive MS, the subsequent studies showed no clinical effect. This has been used to suggest that suppressing MRI activity may not translate into clinical effect, but it is worth noting that these trials with cladribine have been relatively short-term. It may be difficult to note clinical benefit in such short-term studies.

Other Therapies

Antilymphocytic sera and antithymocyte globulin have been tried with minimal or no measurable benefit and are not being used as MS therapy. Attempts to treat MS with IV Ig and IM Ig date back to 1982. The studies and strength of evidence have been reviewed in detail by Brill et al.,[108] and they place IV Ig therapy in a "second-resort" category. There is renewed interest in IV Ig, with some suggestion that it may have a beneficial effect, on evidence from a large Austrian study, even after a number of other small studies showed little or no benefit. Recent studies with Campath IH and pretreatment by steroids suggested a reduction in relapses but not progression, but with striking reduction in new MRI lesions during the trial. This therapy can also induce Grave's disease in one-third of subjects; some patients have relapses of previous symptoms if they are not pretreated with steroids.

In conclusion, the attempts to benefit MS patients who have an immune process as part of their disease by applying any agent that suppresses the immune system has been consistently unsuccessful. In reviewing all the studies with immunosuppressants, in 1986, Ellison put the problem for clinicians clearly: we don't know the right dose, duration, or pharmacologic interactions of the permutations and combinations of these treatments.[109]

IMMUNE MODULATION

Levamisole

Levamisole has been used in a number of small clinical trials over two decades, with results that suggest the agent may have no clinical benefit or may even worsen patients. Also troubling in the report that patients on this drug for other reasons developed adenocarcinoma of the colon and a CNS disease that looked like MS on MRI and in biopsy material.

Linomide

The immune-modulator linomide was promising as a drug that might provide benefit in relapsing-remitting and secondary progressive MS, with a striking reduction in MRI burden of disease, but a large clinical study had to be discontinued because of serious cardiac effects resembling pericarditis in 12 cases, with eight deaths.

Transfer Factor

In a series of studies between 1976 and 1989, agents that altered transfer factor were assessed as possible therapeutic agents, but the conclusion of these trials was negative, despite good theoretical grounds.

Myelin Basic Protein

In the search for a primary antigen in MS, myelin basic protein (MBP) has long been under suspicion. Early attempts to use either human or bovine MBP as a therapeutic agent were unconvincing or negative. Weiner et al. in Boston attempted a widely publicized trial with bovine MBP given orally to induce oral tolerance, but this was reported with negative results. In the meantime, many patients in the MS community were using oral myelin, which could be obtained from health food stores, even though the formulations and amounts were uncertain.

Vaccination

> "I have little doubt in fact, gentlemen, that in the employment of such a substance as the vaccine of Pasteur or lymph of Koch the evolution of insular sclerosis will someday be rendered absolutely impossible."
> Pierre Marie, 1895[110]

In 1895, Pierre Marie felt there would eventually be a vaccination for MS that could render the disease impossible. After a century, the attempts to find it continue. In the mid 1950s, there was interest in the vaccine therapies of William M. Crofton, a Dublin pathologist who moved to London and for years gave vaccine therapy for many illnesses including MS. BCG vaccination was attempted in the 1970s,[111] and there is a preliminary trial currently underway in France. Anti-T-cell vaccination studies are also in progress. The idea in the 1960s that the wide use of measles vaccine might reduce the incidence of MS in 30 years has not proved correct.

Stem Cell Transplantation

The discovery in the last decade that stem cells are present in the CNS has led to current experimental studies that show stem cells migrate when injected into experimental mice with a genetic myelin disorder. Research on direct transplantation of stem cells for oligodendrocytes into the brain and spinal cord is very promising.

Another approach is to use autologous stem cell transplantation to see if a "new" immune system can cure the disease; studies on this approach are underway in many centers.

Hematopoietic stem cell transplantation is one of the most important medical advances in recent decades and Joseph E. Murray and E. Donnall Thomas received the 1990 Nobel Prize for their discoveries in organ and cell transplantation.[112] About 30,000 transplantations take place each year and the number will continue to increase as the process becomes safer, more efficient, and convenient and as more conditions are found to be amenable to this approach. MS is one of the conditions under study and many centers are beginning early studies to assess the benefit of autologous stem cell transplantation. This is the first time MS investigators have seriously discussed a possible cure. Simplistically put, if the defect in MS is in the immune system, what if you could replace the immune system? It will not take long to know the answer, for MRI can be used as surrogate marker for activity after the transplantation; some of the preliminary results are promising.

Monoclonal Antibodies

Studies with monoclonal antibodies such as natalizumab (Antegren®) are continuing. Monoclonal therapy has a compelling theoretical basis as a therapy for MS. MRI studies show that it can reduce EAE and the burden of illness in MS patients. Further trials are underway to assess longer-term clinical effects in MS patients.

DIET

Diets have been a part of the therapy for MS, as for other diseases, as long as we have known of the disorder. Sometimes they have been part of a general strengthening of the patient's constitution, sometimes part of the disease treatment, and occasionally a specific therapy for the disease. Augustus d'Esté was treated with beefsteaks and Madeira wines. Most recommendations for MS patients have been for a generally balanced diet, with a light diet during a relapse, and minimal alcohol and tobacco.

During the discussion of etiological theories at the ARNMD meeting in New York in 1948, Richard Brickner suggested that there should be closer study of the things that precipitate acute attacks of MS. He gave an example of the "therapy" of grain desensitization, giving grain orally or by injection. He said this therapy actually made patients worse, relating the case of one patient who received grain desensitization and then "tobogganed straight downhill" to death. At the same meeting, another dietary approach was outlined by Foster Kennedy, who described a patient, a physician with MS, who was put on a series of elimination diets by Robert Loeb. He was "condemned to eat everything that flies, nothing that swims, and only lamb on land." He was instructed to avoid "multiple sources" of his foods, but when the physician lapsed and took a soup at a country inn which had "generic and multiple sources," he suffered dizziness and diplopia for two days.[113]

Roy Swank was the first systematically to study the relationship of diet and MS and suggest that a low animal fat diet was a specific therapy for MS.[114–116] He had assessed the incidence of MS from 1935–1948 in 18 counties in Norway and found considerable variation between different regions and between farming-dairying areas versus fishing districts and between inland and coastal areas. He assessed diet by a seven-day recording of food intake, compared these records to MS incidence rates, and suggested a strong association between the risk of MS and both butter fat consumption and fish consumption. Over a 50-year period (and Roy

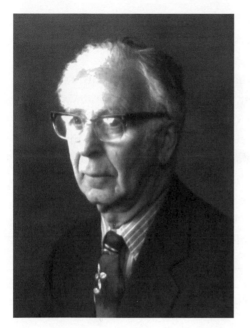

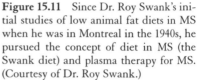

Figure 15.11   Since Dr. Roy Swank's initial studies of low animal fat diets in MS when he was in Montreal in the 1940s, he pursued the concept of diet in MS (the Swank diet) and plasma therapy for MS. (Courtesy of Dr. Roy Swank.)

Swank to this day continues to follow his patients who are faithful to the Swank diet), he reported less disease progression in his cases. However, the results in his patients were compared to published reports (historical controls) rather than to a randomized control group within his study, and such results were not convincing to the neurological community. Many other diets have appeared, some complex, and combining the features of gluten-free, low-fat, and antimigraine diets in many instances, usually accompanied by various supplements. Most of the diets have as their central theory the lowering of the amount of animal fat while increasing the amount of vegetable oils.*

B.W.A. Agranoff and D. Goldberg looked at MS deaths between 1949 and 1967 and compared them with food consumption data for the United States, concluding that there was a relationship to latitude, low temperature, and per-capita milk consumption.[117] All three variables

---

*Roy Swank was recruited to the MNI and McGill University by Wilder Penfield, who gave a young neurologist an offer he could not refuse: a clinical investigator position with rank of assistant professor, research funds for his work, and support for three months' travel each year. At age 92, Dr. Swank is writing a book in which he hopes to explain how the low-fat diet in MS works. (personal communication)

seemed to be independently related to MS risk. They also noted that fish and vegetable fat intake were inversely related. They also studied data on 20 countries belonging to the Organization for Economic Cooperation and Development (OECD) and again found correlation with fat intake, animal fat, butter fat and meat fat, and a negative association with vegetable and fish consumption. Knox found the same kind of relationship from WHO data and showed a correlation with intake of meat, eggs, butter, sugar, and milk. The correlation was particularly related to intake of total fat. Butcher emphasized the correlation between MS prevalence and milk consumption. He showed differences in the intensity of dairy cow breeding between Nordic and Celtic populations in Scotland: an MS gradient parallel to milk consumption in Norway, Australia, and South Africa as well as in Japan. Not all researchers believed the theory of the influence of animal fat on MS and in a reverse approach, in 1950 Crane suggested a treatment with fat-soluble vitamins, animal fat, and ammonium chloride.[118]

Alter et al. correlated the UN data on food consumption with MS prevalence in various countries and showed a correlation between MS and total fat and animal calories consumption, but a much smaller correlation with total protein and total calories consumption.[119] Alter discussed the harmful role of lipids in MS and the possible influence of early cow milk feeding on later development of MS. He pointed out that the distribution of MS followed a parabolic curve north and south of the equator and the distribution of animal fat in diets followed the same curve. Nangi and Narod looked at dietary factors in 23 countries and again found a correlation between incidence of MS and total fat, all meat and pork, but not beef consumption.[120] Most of these studies did not correct for a possible confounding affluence factor in many of these countries.

Englishman Roger MacDougall was a professor of theater arts at the University of Southern California when he developed symptoms of MS. His disease progressed so that he was "virtually helpless" and when he "could do little but lie and think," he read that diet might be involved in occurrence of the disease. He went on a strict diet and felt improved. Initially, he publically encouraged the diet he had used, which was that of Reginald Hawthorne, who had a health farm in Suffolk, but he later publicized his approach widely as the "MacDougall diet." He said he evolved this complex diet by trial and error, was returned to complete fitness, and able to bound up and down the stairs at age 62. The diet eliminated animal fats, refined sugar, and gluten, restricted carbohydrates and alcohol, and added multivitamins, magnesium, and calcium. Diets were being used widely by the MS community at that time; other popular diets were those of Shatin in Australia and Evers in Germany. Although MacDougall referred to his diet as empirical, he also accumulated a list of scientific publications he said supported the components of his diet (B12 deficiency could damage the nervous system; pellagra from B vitamin deficiency caused neurological features similar to MS, etc.). He wrote his story in 1970 in a book, *No Bed of Roses*. His dietary plan was adopted by many patients although most found it difficult, unpleasant, and expensive.

MacDougall arranged with a pharmaceutical company (Associated Preparations, Sutton, Surrey, England) to produce two preparations of multivitamins and minerals (Cantamac-MacDougall diet supplements) in the "correct proportions" that he had found beneficial. Cantamac-Vitamin Compound Formula was to be taken six times a day along with the MacDougall diet, or C-mac Vitamin B12 three times a day along with the diet. MacDougall stated that many thousands of people in 25 countries were using the diet, and he was receiving encouraging reports more or less daily—sometimes several on the same day (personal communication 1973). The literature he distributed indicated that the MacDougall diet was for degenerative disease, and this included "multiple sclerosis, rheumatism, arthritis, schizophrenia, gout, ulcers and many others." Despite its popularity in the MS community, MacDougall's diet was never widely advocated by neurologists. At the National Hospital, it would be "reluctantly passed to patients if they were anxious for a dietary approach."*

Malosse et al. studied dietary patterns in 29 countries and again suggested a correlation between MS incidence and milk consumption.[121] Similarly, Klaus Lauer studied data from 21 countries on three continents and found that of 76 commodities in diet, 16 passed their three-part steps

---

*Personal communication, Professor John Marshall, National Hospital, Queen Square, 1973.

for possible correlation with MS. These included animal fat, total fat, calcium, riboflavin, total meat, pork, margarine, coffee, and beer.[122–130] Lauer's review of studies in the United States, comparing dietary patterns with MS incidence, suggests a relationship between MS incidence and meat, dairy food, and low temperature.

In 1973, the preliminary results of a Belfast-London trial suggested that in a diet with low animal fat, a supplement of linoleic acid reduced the frequency, duration, and severity of attacks, but had no effect on disease progression. This was followed by a Newcastle study which also had positive results, and a Canadian study which showed no benefit. A 1976 report suggested that patients treated with evening primrose oil (naudicelle) might have more MS deterioration, but others argued that a coloring agent in the capsules used might have reduced the conversion of fatty acids to prostaglandins.

Professor E.J. Field, Director of the Demyelination Unit at Newcastle, was also a proponent of the restriction of animal fats in diets and diet supplementation with sunflower seed oil. He evolved a red cell blood test that he felt would diagnose MS susceptibility in children who could then be treated with diet. His test and the concept of treating susceptible children did not gain acceptance.

Analysis of three double-blind trials of linoleic acid (Dublin-London; Newcastle; London, Ontario) with a total of 87 treated and 85 controls over a 2 1/2 year period, found that patients with minimal or little disability on entry to the trial had a smaller increase in disability than the controls.[131] In addition, treatment reduced the severity and duration of relapses regardless of level of disability and duration, and this simple and healthy diet is widely used. There have been no further trials, primarily because dietary trials are hard to conduct over a long period, compliance is a major problem, and there are often confounding changes in the life and diet of the patients including use of medicines and alternative therapies.

Although linoleic and linolenic acid have been used to correct a hypothetical deficiency of unsaturated fatty acids in MS, they could also induce a minor immunosuppression. At McGill University, where Swank did his early work before moving to Oregon, David Horribin, a biochemist interested in demyelination, proposed evening primrose oil as a therapy, and established a company in Nova Scotia to produce the oil (Efamol®). He later developed a European pharmaceutical house to pursue research and development as well as marketing of Efamol® for MS, psoriasis, premenstrual syndrome, and many other conditions. Efamol® continues to be widely used by MS patients.

Specific diets are not currently widely prescribed by neurologists, but are widely used by patients. When pressed by patients, many neurologists will recommend a healthy, well-balanced low-animal fat diet in the form of a low-cholesterol diet, with or without a supplement such as evening primrose oil.[131]

OTHER THERAPIES

Vaccinations were first proposed by Pierre Marie in 1895; he believed MS was caused by an infection, and it would only be a matter of time before a vaccine such as Pasteur developed for other diseases would render MS "absolutely impossible." There have been individuals and clinics offering vaccines for MS throughout the 20th century, including William Mervyn Crofton, a Dublin pathologist, who developed vaccines for many diseases including MS, but his work was regarded as questionable. There are currently efforts to develop a vaccine for MS so the story is not yet complete.

Dr. P. Le Gac of France developed a therapy, known as the "Le Gac treatment" and popular in the 1960s, based on the theory that rickettsia organisms were responsible for the disease. The therapy combined antibiotics, physiotherapy, sea water, and seaweed baths.[132,133]

For a brief period in the 1970s, tolbutamide, an oral agent for diabetes, was widely used by MS patients. There were no major trials to support this use, but the drug was easily available from physicians, inexpensive, and relatively free of side effects. Parnate (tranylcypromine), a tranquilizer, had the same brief popularity.

Dumas and Foix first advocated blood transfusions for MS in 1924. Between 1924 and 1932, improvement and even prolonged remissions were reported in MS cases treated with blood transfusions. In 1932, a monograph by Laignel-Lavastine and Koressios at the University of Paris detailed positive results of blood serotherapy in 120 cases of MS, even though benefit might last only six months and the treatment had to be repeated.[134] Interest in this type of therapy waned in interest during World War II, even though the belief in the power of blood, plasma, and serum as a medicine grew in the public's mind during that period. Interest increased when Leo Alexander in Boston and Roy Swank in Montreal began to use blood transfusions and other blood products in MS. At the 1948 ARNMD meeting, Alexander presented a detailed analysis of 50 Bostonian patients treated with blood or plasma transfusions. He concluded that 46 percent showed improvement. A smaller group was treated with gamma globulin or saline with only two cases (11 percent) showing improvement. Allergic reactions occurred more often than in the general public, leading researchers to suspect some particular allergic phenomenon in MS cases.[135] The clinicians noted that the blood groups and Rh typing in the MS group corresponded to those in normal population. Alexander published his experience with blood transfusions in 76 patients and felt the only ones who benefited were those with mild cases, previously stable, who were now having an acute attack.[136]

Roy Swank, who had all his patients on the low-animal fat diet, began to use blood transfusions for their relapses in 1952; he gave transfusions to 12 percent of his MS population. In 1975, he switched to transfusions of fresh frozen plasma or plasma fractions. He gave a total of 1,336 infusions, 1,029 of fresh frozen plasma to 180 patients, and 307 of plasma fraction to 19 patients, with 58 receiving both. He used no controls, but felt the patients responded, and that the benefit was due to a missing factor in the plasma of MS patients. He also felt that whole plasma contained some substances toxic to MS patients and caused drowsiness and minor aggravation of symptoms in some patients, so the benefits were more rapid and freer of side effects if low molecular weight plasma fractions were used. This therapy was not accepted by the neurological community, but at this writing, Swank is still recommending it to patients.

Despite some attempts, and some heroic surgical interventions, no procedure for MS has found a place in the therapy for the disease. Although he felt it should be considered early in the disease, thoracic sympathectomy by Royle in Australia was a failure. Thymectomy was not effective unless azothioprine was added and the minor effect might have been due to the drug. Tonsillectomy, adenoidectomy, removal of teeth, and removal of dental amalgam were in vogue early in the century when infection was felt to play a major role in MS, but these have been discarded. Removal of dental amalgam returned as a procedure in recent years when scientifically tenuous concerns over mercury surfaced. Although the procedure is discouraged by most neurologists it has been widely sought by patients, who have always maintained a belief in a toxic theory for MS. In this, as in many other ways, they made their own decisions and ignored the advice of the MS "experts."

The list of unsuccessful therapies in MS is long and has included the various anticoagulants, antihistamines, antibiotics, antitubercular and antiviral agents, anti-inflammatory agents, snake venom, various diets and supplements, high colonic irrigation, metabolic inhibitors and stimulants, chelation, blood transfusions, hyperbaric oxygen, magnetism, and removal of dental amalgam.

PHYSICAL MEASURES

Patients with neurological disease were often treated with water therapy, spas, baths, and douching. Commonly used physical measures for MS were galvanic and faradic stimulation, used throughout the 19th century on most patients. At the Salpêtrière, patients were hung on the suspension apparatus to treat ataxia, including those with ataxia from MS. The patient was suspended in the air by straps under the chin and axillae. Exercise, first thought to be harmful, had become a treatment modality by the end of the 19th century, although neurologists cautioned against excess effort.

After World War I, physical therapy for war injury became highly developed and in peacetime, these therapies were extended to other neurological diseases. Methods developed from polio therapy were soon applied to MS. Like advances in surgery, the advances in rehabilitation were spurred on by war. Rehabilitation approaches at institutions after World War II were found to be applicable to MS, especially since the sufferers of the ravages of war and the sufferers with MS tended to be young adults.

Dorsal column stimulation was first introduced for the treatment of intractable neurological pain in 1970; it had a brief period of use after an MS patient being treated for pain was noted to have some improvement in MS symptoms. This was an example of an anecdote's being inflated by therapists and the media into a "breakthrough" therapy that was used on many patients world wide until it failed in virtually all and disappeared, with no mention of its early passing by the same media that trumpeted its birth.

Electromagnetic field stimulation (EMF) to the skull has been used in MS with the initial suggestion of improvement in all of the 16 cases treated, but without any controls.[137] In recent years, a return of public interest in magneto therapy and magnetism for many chronic conditions has seen an upsurge in a methodology that began with Mesmer in the 18th century. Mesmerism and magnetism were initially discredited by a committee of the Paris Academy and the addition of Benjamin Franklin, at the request of King Louis XVI. Their conclusion was that the alleged effect might not exist, and did not seem to be useful; if it did not exist, it certainly could not be useful. It is interesting that this committee with Franklin assessed mesmerism by methods that constitute multiple single-blind trials.

TREATMENT OF SYMPTOMS

Treatment of MS has long traveled in three directions: to reduce the impact of an attack, to treat symptoms, and to affect the underlying disease; if not to cure it, at least to reduce its progression. Treating symptoms was the center of most therapeutic regimes in the first century after Charcot, since all the writers on the disease recognized that no therapy was curative.

> *"One should be clear in differentiating the disease process (in MS) per se from the causes of symptoms since it may at times be quite independent."*
>
> Namerow and Thompson, 1969

Much of the therapy applied to Augustus d'Esté was directed at improving his vision, reducing his muscle spasms and weakness, and improving his bladder and his impotence.

Many agents aimed at reducing the effects of spasticity have been tried over the last century, for this is one of the most debilitating features of MS. Physical therapies, exercise, warming the limbs, and electrical stimulation had some minor benefit, but the advent of agents such as diazapine, dantrolene sodium, and more recently baclofen and tizanidine, gave physicians better tools to reduce spasticity and the symptoms of increased muscle tone. While neurologists struggled to find better drugs for spasticity, increasing numbers of patients were quietly using

Botulinum Toxin for Spasticity

An interesting new twist on an old observation is the use of botulinum toxin for spasticity. It was first used in MS by Joseph Tsui at the University of British Columbia. Justinus Kerner (1786–1862) noted that sausage poisoning was due to a toxin, and after experiments on himself, he suggested the toxin could be useful as a therapy. Warned against such dangerous behavior, Kerner tasted extracts of the poisoned sausage and noted they tasted sour and caused mild symptoms of botulism such as dryness of the mouth and pharynx. In the last chapter of his monograph, he suggested the toxin could be used to block the conduction in nerves. His publication made him well-known and he earned the nickname Wurst-Kerner because of his association with sausage poisoning. Incidentally, botulus is the Latin for sausage and was used by Müller to name the disease botulism in 1870. The final step was the discovery by Emile-Pierre van Ermengem that the toxin that produced botulism was produced by a bacterium, *Clostridium botulinum*, a discovery made after an outbreak of poisoning after a funeral in the village of Elzelles. Alan B. Scott showed the correctness of Kerner's prediction in experiments in animals in 1973 and in humans in 1980, and the therapy is now used for a variety of movement disorders, spasticity, and as Kerner predicted, hyperhydrosis and hypersalivation. Its use in spasticity is limited because the doses have to be large, over wide areas of muscles, and may need to be repeated after several months.[138]

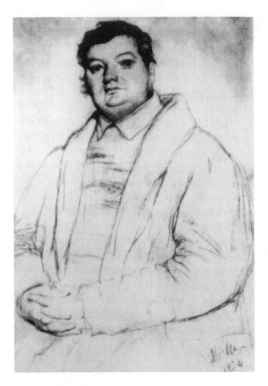

Figure 15.12 Justinius Kerner (1786-1862) first suggested that the poison of botulism be used in diluted amounts as a treatment, and in recent years, this has been used to treat many movement disorders, muscle spasms, and the spasticity of multiple sclerosis. (Crayon painting by O. Müller, 1834.)

cannabis, which gave them better relief from pain and spasms, even if it impaired their alertness and balance. Destructive surgery such as Bishoff's myelotomy, or phenol injection, were irreversible approaches to destroy the reflex arc and made nursing easier. It is a measure of the sense of hope of MS patients that even those who were bedridden would reject a therapy because it was irreversible. There might be a new therapy in the future that could offer relief, but not if they took this irreversible step. Baclofen administered into the subarachnoid space by an implanted pump has been a complicated means of therapy, but allows a large dose of the drug to be administered. Botulinum toxin has been found to be useful in many movement disorders, and can also reduce spasticity when injected directly into muscles. It has limited practicality currently, since large doses must be administered at great expense and the treatment may have to be repeated after some months. There are current trials with marijuana to assess if this is an effective way to reduce spasticity, as many patients claim, and large amounts of research funds have been set aside for this purpose by the British and Canadian medical research councils. Such trials are difficult to design and control so the number of applications for research funding has been small.

Tremor was the MS symptom that first attracted the attention of Charcot, and his initial presentations were to differentiate MS from Parkinson's disease. In 1895, Edwards thought it was the most characteristic symptom of MS.[139] Many agents to combat it have been tried, but it is still one of the most resistant symptoms in MS. Isoniazid in high doses, beta-blockers, anti-Parkinson drugs, primidone, carbamazepine, clonazepam, glutethimide, weights applied to the limbs, stereotactic lesions in the thalamus, and chronic thalamic stimulation have been tried with limited success. Caution must be used with thalamic stimulation on lesions, however, as Reginald Kelly reported demyelination along the track of stereotactic probes some decades ago. Ondansetron is being studied currently, but cerebellar tremor is one of the most disabling symptoms of MS to date.

Nineteenth-century reports of MS noted the involvement of speech, but usually in a late stage of the disease. Landon Carter Gray said in 1893 that speech was one way to differentiate MS from Parkinson's disease—the speech in MS is jerky or scanning and staccato, hesitant, with irregular jerky muscle movements of the mouth and tongue, and the teeth are uncovered when speaking. In Parkinson's disease it is just the opposite, and the speech is "slow, deliberate, and seemingly wise."[140] No successful therapies have been developed for speech difficulties in MS.

Heat sensitivity was noted early as a symptom in MS. In the first medical report of a case by Ollivier d'Angers in 1824, the patient was noted to become weak in a hot spa. Heinrich Heine noted that his vision was worse in hot weather. Lyman talked about his case of MS developing an acute attack when sitting in the sun and Dercum had a patient who developed MS after sunstroke. In 1887, Oppenheim noted that hot baths worsened symptoms in MS. Gowers and Russell said that the pyrexia associated with infection could aggravate MS.* The obvious recommendation was removal from hot environments.

---

*In the popular TV program *West Wing*, the President of the United States had an acute exacerbation of MS, a condition diagnosed seven years before, when he developed an infection and the treatment was to treat the infection and reduce the fever.

When fever therapy became prominent in the treatment of syphilis, it was applied to MS patients. There were many techniques used to cause fever, including typhoid or milk injections, inducing fever by pyrogens from other infections, and using a hot box.[141] Patients must have been much worse after such therapy.

In 1959, Edmund and Fog noted that fever therapy brought out transient new signs in MS patients in 75 percent of the 41 patients they studied.[142] Although not specific to MS, it was much more frequent an observation in MS patients. Floyd Davis of Chicago showed that in a person suspected of having a meningioma but who had MS, a hot bath at 102°F caused visual blurring.[143] At 104° F, there was weakness of the right arm and leg, numbness of the right hand, a central scotoma, and a Babinski sign. He then suggested the "Hot Bath Test for MS," which was useful in the decades before MRI, as one of the methods of increasing the evidence for a diagnosis of MS. Davis went on to show that altering calcium ions in nerves changed conduction; he began a series of experiments to try to improve conduction with chemicals.[144]

Many of the earliest descriptions of MS noted that there could be deterioration of vision, either acutely or slowly over years. Optic neuritis was noted by Charcot. What became known as Devic's disease was probably first noted by Allbutt, who recorded optic neuritis associated with acute spinal cord disease.[145] MacLaurin in Australia described the features of retrobulbar neuritis,[146] and William Gowers painted beautiful pictures of vision changes with optic neuritis.[147] Uhthoff found abnormal fundi in 52 of 100 cases of MS.[148] Five of his patients had apparently normal vision and no signs of changes in their fundi. Retrobulbar neuritis later turned out to be MS in many. In 1909, Gordon said it was the first symptom of MS in five of 56 cases, and Fleischer found in 1908 that in cases of retrobulbar neuritis, 21 of 30 patients developed MS. Marburg found this in 14 of 24 cases, but a few reports found a much smaller percentage of cases led to MS, suggesting some variability in diagnosis.

The first efforts to treat the visual effects of MS were by local eye soaks and eye cups. Patients were kept in dim rooms and asked to avoid eyestrain. Specific therapy was applied first by the use of steroids, but arguments about their effectiveness in optic neuritis continue despite a half century of trials.[149,150]

An interesting combination of the visual blurring and heat sensitivity of MS is the phenomenon described by Uhthoff and now named after him.*[151] He reported on 100 cases of optic neuritis with the neurologist Gnauck, and noted that three of these had desaturation of color vision with exercise and fatigue.[152,153] The phenomenon bearing his name was exemplified in a fourth patient (XVIII) whose visual acuity after walking around Uhthoff's examining room dropped from 6/200 and 1/6 in the right and left eyes, to 4/200 and 14/200. Little attention was paid to this phenomenon for many years even though the transient effects of fever therapy and of hot baths was well known. Although other cases of visual blurring with exercise or hot baths were noted and recorded by Selhorst,[154] the association of the symptom to Uhthoff occurred in the report of Ricklefs.[155] The symptom is usually associated with mild bilateral optic atrophy in MS patients and comes on about 30 seconds after exercise commences, and stops a few minutes after exercise ceases. It may be present in up to a quarter of MS patients on history, and if detailed studies such as evoked potential studies, visual contrast sensitivity, and other tests are done, about half the patients will show a change.[156] Patients have often noted improvement in their vision after drinking ice water or cold beer or after getting into a cool swimming pool or lake.

Brickner was a proponent of the vasoconstriction or vasospasm theory of MS and felt the theory was supported by the heat sensitivity noted in MS patients. In 1948, he outlined his evidence for this, which included precipitants such as hot baths, sitting under a hair dryer, hot drinks, and hot food. Other precipitants that could worsen symptoms or cause an attack and suggest a brief period of vasospasm included bright lights, violent exercise, eating, and smoking. This led to the suggestion that patients

---

* Like Marcus Gunns, Jackson, Gowers, and others at the National Hospital, Queen Square, and Henri Parinaud with Charcot and his contemporaries at the Salpêtrière, Uhthoff developed an interest in assessing the ophthalmological aspects of the neurological patients with Westphal's neurology clinic in Berlin. Wilhelm Uhthoff (1853–1927) was a prolific writer on neuro-ophthalmological conditions; unlike Charcot, he was noted for his warm and kindly manner with patients and associates. Although such designations always engender argument, Bielschowsky referred to Uhthoff as the "true originator" of clinical neuro-ophthalmology.

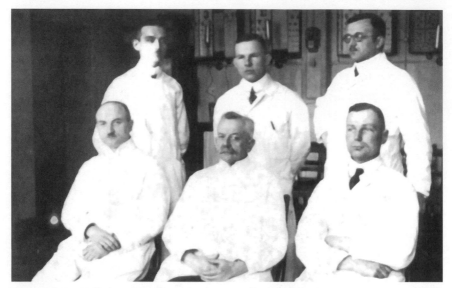

Figure 15.13 Wilhelm Uhthoff with his house staff. He collected one hundred cases of multiple sclerosis when many felt it was a rare disease. He detailed the ocular and visual changes in the disease. He is remembered for the observation that exercise can cause the vision to transiently decrease. (Courtesy of Hans K. Uhthoff, Ottawa.)

should be treated by the method that had become known as the Brickner treatment, using histamine by iontophoresis. Selhorst raised questions about the pathophysiology of heat sensitivity in MS patients and questioned whether the effect is just a thermal one, as central temperature changes only minimally, but the symptom's onset is very rapid in some patients.[157] Some patients with visual blurring do not complain of Uhthoff's symptom with exercise or heating. It is more likely that a circulating product of metabolism affects the demyelinated or thinly remyelinated areas.[158]

It is interesting that although sensory symptoms were mentioned by the early writers, other clinicians, including Osler and Marie, believed a relative absence of sensory symptoms was characteristic of MS.

In 1887, Oppenheim was the first to emphasize that sensory symptoms were not only common, but even characteristic of the disease. Attempts to reduce sensory symptoms were by rubbing, massage, warm flannel wrapping, and soaks in cold tubs. In recent years, a tricyclic antidepressant or carbamazepine is often used, with very limited success. A recent study compared MS patients with controls, an important approach since sensory symptoms are common "normal" symptoms. Sensory symptoms were more common in the MS patients and differed in severity and quality.[159]

In Rae-Grant's study, pain was present in 67 percent of the MS patients at some time in their disease course; although this was the same in controls, twice as many MS patients had active pain problems at the time of the study, and the pain was more often neuropathic in type, with burning, itching, electric, and formicatory pain. Lhermitte's phenomenon was present at some time in the course in two-thirds of the MS patients.* Respiratory symptoms of shortness of breath, difficult deep breathing, frequent hiccups, coughing, and sighing were present in 20 percent compared to 7.5 percent in the controls.[160]

The specific phenomenon described by Lhermitte, Bollak, and Nicholas in 1924 relates to sudden electric shock-like sensations spreading down the body or limbs associated with flexion of the neck or trunk (Lhermitte's sign or phenomenon),[161] a sign of posterior column involvement. This occurs in cases of MS, tumors, arachnoiditis, subacute combined degeneration of the spinal cord, and Pott's disease. Although it is now regarded as a sign associated with neck flexion, it occasionally occurs with trunk flexion, as Lhermitte reported, and indicates thoracic pathology in those cases.[162]

Jean Lhermitte and his colleagues described the phenomenon in a 24-year-old cashier:

> *"In August 1923 the patient first noticed a phenomenon that she described thus: When I try to lower my head, I feel a violent shock in the nape of my neck, and a pain like an electric shock runs through my whole body, from my neck to my feet, down my vertebral column."*[163]

---

*Jean L. Lhermitte (1877–1959), the son of an artist, and student of Pierre Marie, made a number of contributions to neurology, including the treatment of war neurosis, the description of anterior internuclear ophthalmoplegia (Lhermitte's syndrome), and recognition of the importance of the inferior olivary nucleus in myoclonus. As pointed out by Pearce, the phenomenon in MS for which he is remembered is the Lhermitte "sign," which is really a symptom, rather than a sign.

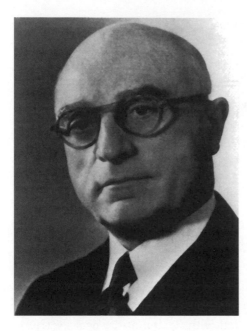

Figure 15.14 Jean Lhermitte was director of the Dejerine Laboratory for Brain Research at the Salpêtrière, and students including Douglas MacAlpine from London, came to study with him. Walter Reise of Virginia, also a student with Lhermitte, described him as a man reflecting with equal force the continuity and unity of life, and work. (Critchley, 1953.)

He went on to add that the patient had to keep her body straight and move cautiously so as not to invoke the electric shock. He said this had not been noted before in the symptoms of MS, but had been mentioned by Babinski in 1918 in a case of concussion to the spine. Lhermitte himself had published it as a symptom of neck injury.* Although Tinel had noted such an electric sensation when demyelinated peripheral nerves were percussed, Lhermitte correctly deduced that the fibers causing the symptom in MS and in cervical injury were in the spinal cord.

Fatigue is one of the most common and distressing symptoms of MS, but surprisingly was not often commented on as a symptom of MS until the 1980s.[164] Murray published the serendipitous observation that amantadine therapy was useful in about half the MS patients he studied. One of his patients, a physician, was bothered primarily by overwhelming fatigue, which made it difficult to get through his long office day seeing patients. When he took amantadine (Symmetrel®), an antiviral agent, to

---

*This was reported in 1917 by Marie and Chatelin after head injury. It was first mentioned as a symptom in MS by Bureil and Devic in 1918. It became identified with Lhermitte in the neurological literature after 1930.

prevent the influenza that was occurring in his practice at that time, he noted the MS fatigue was reduced. After a period on and off the drug with corresponding improvement and worsening of his fatigue, Murray carried out a small open trial with some improvement in the symptoms in two-thirds of his patients and then carried out a double-blind controlled study with similar results. He then organized a Canadian Cooperative Trial showing benefit in about half the cases.[165] Longer experience indicated fewer patients got long-term benefit, but for many years amantadine was the only agent that modified MS fatigue. The stimulant pemoline (Cylert®) was popular in the United States to treat MS fatigue, but did not show greater benefit than a placebo in trials, and was later removed from the market because of a hepatotoxicity side effect. Recently, there have been small studies suggesting that modafinil and also high doses of enteric coated aspirin (1250 mg daily) may be helpful.

It had been noted since 1925 that some patients with MS might have seizures. Early reports of MS record "comas" and "seizures" and other paroxysmal symptoms without clear descriptions of the episodes.[166] The opinion was that seizure occurred in five percent of MS cases and it remained for Ebers and the Canadian Network of MS Clinics to show in a large multicenter national study that incidence was indeed six percent.

Harris reported that 64 of 1,622 patients with MS (four percent) had trigeminal neuralgia. Conversely, White and Sweet in a 1969 review of literature on 10,220 patients with trigeminal neuralgia found 172 cases (1.7 percent) with MS. Further studies have repeatedly found the incidence of trigeminal neuralgia in MS in the 7–8 percent range.[167] Trigeminal neuralgia in MS occurs in younger patients, though it is usually a disorder of the elderly; and in a few patients it can be bilateral, which is very unusual in the late-onset type. Therapy has been with carbamazepine (Tegretol®) since the late 1960s; other agents (baclofen, gabapentin, mexilitine) have also been used. If these fail, then surgical procedures often bring relief.

It is not common for MS patients to show evidence of respiratory failure, but this can happen in the late stages due to weakness of the chest wall muscles and accessory muscles of respiration. On a historic note, it is interesting that John Kurtzke, who contributed so much to the understanding of MS, published his first paper on MS as a fourth-year medical student on four cases of respiratory failure in MS.

COGNITIVE CHANGE IN MS

Cognitive and emotional change has been noted in MS patients through the known history of the disease. There has been controversy about how common this symptom is, and whether it is a reaction to the emotional stress of the disease, due to the demyelinating lesions in the nervous system, or a combination of these.[168,169] Despite repeated observations and comment in the medical literature, physicians tended to tell patients that mental change was not part of the disease, and the apparent emotional changes were just what one would expect in such a serious and disabling disease. It would be expected for young adults to be disturbed and upset about having a disabling disease with the possibility of greater disability in the future. One emotional change that seemed to stand out was euphoria, an unexpected cheerfulness, jocularity, and tendency to make light of everything.

A change in attitude toward the issue of cognitive change in MS seems apparent in the work of 19th century writers who noted this was a common feature of MS, perhaps because they tended to see and diagnose patients later in their disease course. In the mid 20th century, many argued that cognitive changes did not occur in MS. This attitude was fostered in some part by the MS societies, and accepted by many neurologists, who stated that patients remained mentally alert throughout their disease course.

Even the most knowledgeable neurologist may miss clinical observations that do not fit the accepted pattern or theory used in framing a disease or are not useful in diagnosing or managing patients. As we have seen, neurologists repeatedly ignored the experience of seeing more than one patient with MS in the same family, saying they had seen it, but it was unusual. They paid little attention to common symptoms in their MS patients such as sensory symptoms, pain, and fatigue. These were not accepted as characteristic symptoms of the disease, even when each of these symptoms was seen in over half of the cases. (Until recent decades, pain was said to be absent in MS and fatigue was not mentioned often as a characteristic symptom until the 1980s).

Donald Paty noted negative reaction to his suggestions in the 1970s that cognitive dysfunction should be a focus of study by the National MS Society in the United States, and some scientists expressed concern about opening up such a discussion. Efforts were made and slowly research and systematic studies revealed the nature and the extent of cognitive changes. Recent research has shown that these may begin very early in the course of the disease.

That cognitive and emotional changes could occur in the disease was noted in many of the earliest cases described. The cook Darges, briefly described by Cruveilhier in 1841, was said to have normal intelligence but demonstrated outbursts of unexpected laughing and crying.[170–172] He said, "She became seized with an emotion difficult to describe. She blushed, laughed, and cried." Mental changes were also noted in the cases of Vulpian,[173] Frerichs,[174] Valentiner,[175] Morris,[176] Moxon,[177] Seguin,[178] Wilks,[179] and Osler.[180] In his second lecture on MS, Charcot described mental changes, memory difficulty, slow learning, blunting of emotions, indifference, pathological laughing and crying, and occasional transition into classical forms of mental illness. He commented:

> *"There is marked enfeeblement of the memory; conceptions are formed slowly; the intellectual and emotional faculties are blunted in their totality. The dominant feeling in the patients appears to be a sort of almost stupid indifference in reference to all things. It is not rare to see them give way to foolish laughter for no cause, and sometimes, on the contrary, to melt into tears for no reason. Nor is it rare, amid this state of mental depression, to find psychic disorders arise which assume one or other of the classic forms of mental alienation."*
>
> Jean-Martin Charcot[181]

In *A Manual of Diseases of the Nervous System* (1893), Gowers said slight mental change was common and characteristic in MS and might include memory failure, alternating complacency and contentment, demonstrating a happy personality in spite of grave disability, and, rarely, a form of mental disturbance bordering on chronic insanity.[182] In 1895,

Edwards on the other hand felt that intelligence was almost always affected and described patients' facial appearance as "air de béatitude."[183] Charles Dana also felt mental change was not only common, but characteristic of MS.[184]

In 1904, Eduard Müller reviewed the literature on MS in Germany and noted that euphoria was more common than depression, and that lack of insight was common.[185] He commented that pathological crying and laughing was an organic change, not a psychological one, but the cause of the other emotional changes and the euphoria was uncertain. The impact of such changes in the patient was well described by W.N.P. Barbellion (B.F. Cummings), in his account of his MS in *The Journal of a Disappointed Man*.[186] He noted "kaleidoscopic changes" in his emotions at periods of his disease and described well the roller coaster of his emotions from deep depression to pleasure and exultation.

In the 1920s, Sachs and Freedman indicated that mental changes occurred in 15.6 percent of MS cases.[187] Sanger Brown and Thomas Davis argued that the mental and emotional changes in MS were due to the organic cerebral changes in the disease.[188] They published an expanded version of their 1921 ARNMD paper a year later, dividing their discussion into sections on euphoria, depression, mental deterioration, hallucinations, schizophrenia-like states, personality change, and the course of the mental symptoms of MS.[189] They suggested that mental changes were organic; patients were not abnormal before getting the disease; they allowed that stress and personality factors could alter reactions to the disease. Jelliffe put forward the alternative view that these mental changes were due to emotional and psychodynamic factors, and even suggested that psychological factors could be involved in the development of some forms of MS.[190] The ARNMD committee was noncommittal and stated that there was no specific psychic disorder characteristic of the disease.[191]

A further "stocktaking" ARNMD meeting occurred in Paris in 1924. Henri Claude, a young psychiatrist, did not agree that mental changes were common in MS, and felt that many of the suggested cases were misdiagnoses, even though he allowed that some minor symptoms could occur, such as puerilism, attention difficulties, depression, and apathy, but usually only in advanced cases of MS.[192] In fact, he felt that the serious mental changes reported were in *formes frustes* or in different, but related diseases.

In 1926, S.A. Kinnear Wilson and S.S. Cottrell were the first to systematically evaluate the mental and emotional changes in MS. The clinicians felt they were more specific features of MS than the classical Charcot triad, which tended to be seen only late in the disease course.[193] Cottrel was a young American psychiatrist working with the more senior and prominent Wilson at the National Hospital for Nervous Disease, Queen Square, London. Their work was important for another reason— it was one of the first studies to address a specific methodology of work, using representative samples, successive cases, operational definitions, reliable data collection techniques such as semistructured interviews, and data analysis. They did not specifically measure cognitive change, although they discussed these features in their patients. They discussed "spes sclerotica," "eutonia sclerotica," "euphoria sclerotica," and emotional liability as characteristic of MS. They felt that 70 percent of their MS patients had some degree of euphoria, due to organic changes, but cognitive change was rare.

In his influential overview of MS in 1930, Russell Brain[194] indicated that the mental changes in MS had received too little attention, so the review by Wilson and Cottrell was important in bringing such symptoms to the notice of neurologists. Brain felt there was not enough attention paid to the common "hysterical manifestations" of MS patients. When Bramwell in Edinburgh, and Buzzard in London, at the turn of the 20th century and Brain in the 1930s referred to "hysterical MS," they did not mean that these cases were psychologically induced, hysterical, or what became known as conversion reactions, but were cases of MS who had mental changes with strong emotional overtones, resembling the behavior of patients with hysteria.

Kinnear Wilson wrote an essay on pathological laughing and crying in MS in 1928,[195] and used as an example a 32-year-old man with typical signs of MS who began to have exaggerated emotional responses, so that he would weep when reading of a stranger's death or burst into long uncontrollable, but almost silent laughter at mere trifles.

"In the course of my examination I asked the routine question whether he had any difficulty with the bladder, and replying in the affirmative, he added he had already 'ruined four pairs of trousers' and went off into an apparently interminable series of peculiar hollow laughs, which convulsed the whole ward as well as himself. So facile became the mechanism that he would laugh whenever he began to speak, as though the stimuli of contracting muscles were sufficient to set it off."[196]

In 1929, André Ombredane attempted a systematic assessment of MS patients in Paris hospitals.[197] His MD thesis, later published as a book, focused on 50 cases studied by a systematic psychometric evaluation, plus 10 from the literature. He separated mental changes into a sclerotic mental state, which included mood (74 percent), and cognitive change (72 percent), and a second category of dementia and psychosis. He concluded that affective disorders and euphoria were associated with intellectual deterioration. A further puzzling conclusion was that intellectual deterioration was related more to a diffuse toxic state than to plaques. Although widely quoted and influential, his report is hard to evaluate: he rated fatigue as cognitive impairment and fatalism as a form of depression. His work, the only MS research of his career, was thoroughly reviewed by Berrios and Quemada,[198] who analyzed the data by the statistical techniques of 1990 and concluded that there were too many hidden factors in his data to make possible any definite conclusions on the correlation of emotional change and intellectual change. These limitations did not prevent Ombredane's report from being influential for many years. Berrios and Quemada suggest the direction of neuropsychiatry of MS would have been different if this flawed study had not been published before.

In 1938, David Arbuse reviewed the literature on psychiatric aspects of MS and concluded that mild euphoria was present in most MS cases and inappropriate laughter and crying was not infrequent.[199] Sugar and Nadell[200] agreed with Wilson and Cotrell, and Arbuse, but could not decide if the changes were psychologic or due to organic changes. Borberg and Zahle[201] agreed that in their series of 330 patients, "light euphoria" was the most common psychological symptom. Pratt compared mental symptoms in MS and muscular dystrophy and confirmed that the MS patients were more cheerful, with more mood swings and euphoria.[202]

There have been a number of reviews of euphoria in MS, all suggesting it is a reflection of organic change. Rabins used pre-MRI studies to show that euphoria was associated with greater brain involvement in MS, particularly in the periventricular areas, but occurred in less than 10 percent of patients.[203] Current MRI correlations indicate that the cognitive and emotional changes have specific neuroanatomical correlations.

Once better neuropsychometric techniques were developed in the postwar period, cognitive and psychological changes were separated; they were difficult to compare since they reflected different approaches and different schools of thought and often were not based on a solid epidemiological approach. Stenager argued that in the 150 years since Charcot's descriptions, the observations about cognitive and emotional change in MS have moved from broad case-based generalizations about the MS patient to detailed, specific studies of emotional trauma, depression, and memory.[204,205] Even more recently, MRI has allowed speculation that localization of specific mental changes and measures of whole-brain N-acetylaspartate (WBNAA) may be useful in assessing progressive neuronal cell loss in specific brain areas.[206]

Only in the last three decades have psychometric techniques clarified definitions, approaches, and results in MS studies.[207] In addition, there have been approaches that recognized that subtle changes required specific tools, that changes needed to be isolated from other phenomena such as depression and fatigue, and to be correlated with them. Paradoxically, as we are learning to separate and more effectively measure cognitive and affective changes, the separation has made it possible to learn how these changes are so often linked.[208–210]

PROGNOSIS IN MS

Many early observers of multiple sclerosis thought patients lived only a few years after diagnosis, mostly because observers only saw and made the diagnosis of MS in the end stages of the disease. The wide use of the

Charcot triad ensured that physicians could only be confident about the diagnosis when it was well established and late, and would be reluctant to make the diagnosis in the absence of late disease features. But by 1942, Kolb in Baltimore noted there was only a slight reduction in life expectancy in MS cases.[211] Foster Kennedy expressed the feelings of many neurologists of his day:

> *"The diagnosis of multiple sclerosis is not just a diagnosis. It is also a prognosis, a prognosis of utter disaster to any human to whom it is given."*
>
> Foster Kennedy, 1950[212]

By 1948, it was thought the average life of an MS patient from onset to death was 27 years. It is now recognized that the life expectancy of MS patients is not much shorter than that of the normal population, but there may be many years of disability, and some individuals and some forms of MS progress more rapidly.

THE MODERN AGE OF MS THERAPY BEGINS

In previous decades, MS societies in many countries were influential in developing research, not only because of their grants, but because of peer review research committees and other activities that brought researchers together. In the 1980s, investigators organized to take research, clinical trials, and clinical measurements to a new level.

In his address on being awarded the Dystel Prize, given by the Dystel family in memory of their talented son who had his career cut short by MS, Dr. Kenneth P. Johnson of the University of Maryland considered when the modern age of MS therapeutics began.[213] He indicated two events that in his personal experience as a career MS researcher marked a change in the approaches to MS therapy. One was in 1978 when Byron Waksman, Director of Research Programs at the NMSS, indicated his wish to test the theory that human interferons might have a therapeutic effect on MS as antiviral agents.

The second milestone was the meeting on Grand Island outside Buffalo on the Niagara River in the winter of 1982, sponsored by the

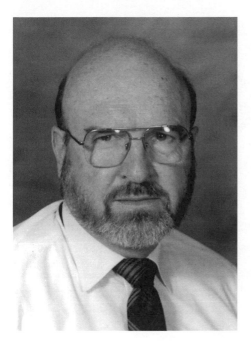

Figure 15.15 Dr. Robert Herndon. (Courtesy of Dr. Robert Herndon.)

United States and Canadian MS Societies, and cochaired by Robert Herndon and Jock Murray.[214] At that meeting, a discussion of treatment trials led to the formation of a committee to foster clinical trials in MS. The European participants at the meeting decided to form a European Committee for Treatment and Research in MS (ECTRIMS), which has become a very influential organization. With some United States and Canadian colleagues, Johnson initiated the Americas Committee for Treatment and Research in MS (ACTRIMS). These organizations have been influential in the development of clinical research and clinical trials in MS on both sides of the Atlantic.

Discussion at the Grand Island meeting centered around the potential for new agents, the need for more specific measurements and outcomes, and statistical methods to be applied. A recommendation for a group to assist in planning and design of new trials resulted in the formation of the Advisory Committee on Clinical Trials of New Agents in Multiple Sclerosis of the National MS Society.[215] There was optimism, caution, and skepticism at the meeting and it led to activities that preceded the flurry of trials in the next decades. Kenneth Johnson referred

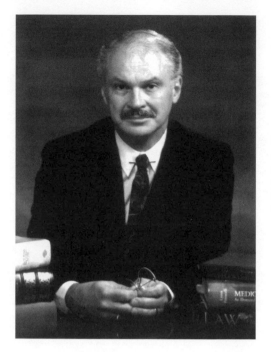

Figure 15.16 Dr. Jack Conomy initiated the Consortium of MS Centers to
encourage interchange between all
professionals involved in MS care and
research. (Courtesy of Dr. Jack
Conomy.)

to the meeting as a turning point in current MS research and Rudick and
Cookfair referred to it as "a watershed event in the recent history of MS
therapy, representing activism and optimism in the context of widespread
therapeutic nihilism and skepticism about the feasibility of clinical trials
in MS."[216] Another important meeting was held in Charleston, South
Carolina on outcome assessment in multiple sclerosis clinical trials.

In 1985, Dr. Jack Conomy of the Cleveland Clinic brought a small
number of clinical investigators, Barry Arnason, Don Paty, Howard
Weiner, and Jock Murray, together to discuss a collaboration of MS
research clinics. The collaboration began slowly, but the membership of
comprehensive MS treatment and research clinics increased from 5 to 85 by
2000. Annual meetings now bring together up to 800 healthcare professionals from all fields; these participants focus on people with MS and
investigations of this disease. In Europe, another organization,
Rehabilitation in MS (RIMS) also began, and in recent years, these organizations have held meetings together to further encourage collaboration.
MS research at the beginning of the 21st century is clearly an international

endeavor. As an example of this effective collaborative spirit, in the fall of 1999, ECTRIMS, ACTRIMS, RIMS, and the CMSC met together in Basel, Switzerland, for a joint meeting; they had another meeting in Baltimore in 2002. Other important MS meetings are the Charcot Symposium, and the MS meetings held annually in conjunction with meetings of the American Academy of Neurology, the American Neurological Association, the European Neurological Society, and other organizations.

INTERFERONS

"The fact that patients have been willing to participate in placebo-trials for as long as 5 years testifies to their dedication and courage."
Kenneth Johnson, 1997[217]

In the 1950s, it was noted that during a viral infection in tissue culture, a soluble substance was released into the surrounding milieu; this tissue culture fluid could be harvested and used to protect other cells. The substance was protein capable of "interfering" with viral infection in cells and was named interferon.

Interferons were independently discovered by two groups in the 1950s, Issacs and Lindenmann (1957),[218] and Negano and Kojima,[219] although work on viral interference had been going on since 1935.[220] In 1964, Wheelock and Sibley noted the appearance of interferon in the serum after viral infections.[221] Soon other biological effects were noted, such as the antiproliferative and immunomodulatory properties of interferons. Three types of interferons were recognized and named for the primary cells of their origin: leukocyte interferon, fibroblast interferon, and immune interferon. The first two shared many properties and were later classified as type 1, and the distinctive immune interferon was classified as type 2. Later, type 1 was renamed alpha and beta interferon and type 2 was named gamma interferon. A number of other interferons have subsequently been identified. They were involved in diverse biological actions of cytokines, including inhibition of the proliferation of normal and transformed cells, regulation of differentiation, host responses to various pathogens, and modulation of the immune system, including activation of natural killer cells and macrophages. Although initially studied in multiple sclerosis because of its antiviral properties, the benefits of interferons demonstrated later were likely due to their immuno-modulatory function.[222]

The antiproliferative property of interferon led to interest in it as a potential anticancer agent, and there were efforts to produce interferon variations by cloning and development of recombinant forms of interferons in the 1970s and early 1980s. The initial promise of interferon as an anticancer agent did not materialize, and Cantell notes that there were periods when interest in the interferon work lessened. Glaxo and Imperial Chemical Industries dropped out of collaboration with the Wellcome Foundation and the Medical Research Council in Britain. The Wellcome group produced Wellferon. There was much publicity in the popular press about interferon as a "wonder drug" in the early 1970s, so pressure and support for research continued from other directions. Production of small amounts of interferon was increased when Cantell, who supplied much of the interferon from the Finnish Blood Center, began to use Namalwa cells in 1974.* In the meantime, the use of interferon in other diseases, such as MS, began in parallel. After initial promising results, further trials were possible when recombinant techniques for producing interferon became available. In 1980, Charles Wessman took out a patent on coliform-produced interferon in the name of Biogen, a company on the verge of bankruptcy that saved itself by assigning these rights to Schering-Plough for $8 million.[223] Now greater amounts of interferon were being produced. The original interferon beta-1b was made by Cetus Corporation and Chiron Company manufactured the material used by Berlex in their early clinical trials. Other companies such as Berlex developed their own methods of producing interferon, and surprisingly, even the government of Cuba geared up to produce interferon on a large scale. Enough interferon was available for trials on a number of diseases, including MS. During the 1970s–1980s, Thomas Merigan at Stanford and Michael Oldstone at the Scripps Clinic studied the effects of

---

*Namalwa was a young Ugandan girl who died of Burkett's lymphoma, and like Helen Lane (HeLa cells), lives on in the cell cultures of labs around the world.

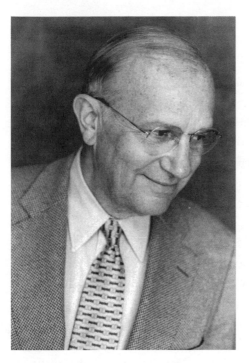

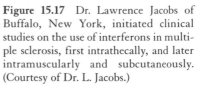

Figure 15.17 Dr. Lawrence Jacobs of Buffalo, New York, initiated clinical studies on the use of interferons in multiple sclerosis, first intrathecally, and later intramuscularly and subcutaneously. (Courtesy of Dr. L. Jacobs.)

interferon in mice and were interested in the possibility of a trial of interferon in relapsing-remitting MS. There have been several reviews of the early trials of these drugs.[224–226]

In 1977, Lawrence Jacobs of Buffalo began to use interferon that had been produced for some years at Roswell Park Cancer Institute by a tedious process called the "roller bottle" technique, using the tissue from the foreskins of recently circumcised infants. Because a purchaser returned a supply of interferon, it was offered to Jacobs, who was interested in the possibility of using it in research on amyotrophic lateral sclerosis (ALS) or multiple sclerosis. ALS seemed the appropriate disorder to study because of its rapid and fatal course, but MS was selected because there were so many patients available for study.*

A series of patients was given intrathecal injections of interferon-beta. Even with as few as 10 patients receiving interferon and 10 receiving placebo, there was a statistically significant reduction in exacerbations

---

*Theodore Munsat later showed that interferon did not benefit the ALS patients.

and disease severity in the treated group. Jacobs decided to use intrathecal natural interferon-beta because the interferon did not appear to cross the blood–brain barrier in appreciable concentrations. He carried out weekly intrathecal injections for four weeks and then monthly intrathecal injections for five months. The attack rate reduced from 1.79 to 0.76 per year in the treated patients, compared to a drop of 1.98 to 1.48 per year in the placebo group over a two-year period. There were major practical disadvantages to the regimen: patients developed serious flu-like side effects associated with intrathecal injections. Also, a mild chemical meningitis appeared to occur with an elevation of white cells and protein in the CSF.

Jacobs presented the results of an open trial in 20 patients showing a significant reduction in relapses with interferon, using the patients as their own controls.[227,228] Despite criticisms of the small study and of differences between the number of lumbar punctures in the treated and placebo group, the study raised interest in the use of interferons in the long-term treatment of MS.

At that time, Kenneth Johnson of San Francisco was in the midst of a trial with Thomas Merrigan at Stanford University and Michael

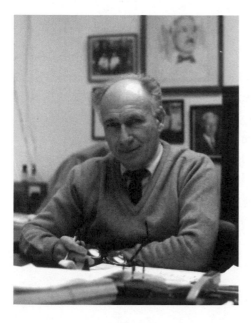

Figure 15.18 Dr. Byron Waksman was one of the early workers on the immunology of MS and when he became medical director of the National MS Society, fostered the career of many young investigators who are still actively contributing to the field. Waksman recognized early the potential of interferons in MS and encouraged the research and trials in this area. (Courtesy of Dr. Byron Waksman; photo by P. Shaw.)

Oldstone of the Scripps Clinic using alpha interferon. Johnson relates that Byron Waksman stimulated interest in the possibility of interferon in MS therapy, and the group met in an airport hotel in San Francisco to plan the trial.[229,230] With no guidelines or experience, they made reasoned decisions about how the agent would be used. They decided on continuous therapy rather than intermittent doses at the time of relapses; administration by the subcutaneous route; and using the largest amount that patients could accept and tolerate. The results were not statistically significant, but showed a trend toward benefit. When Johnson moved to Baltimore, he was approached by Schering-Plough Corporation about using recombinant alpha interferon, which he administered in a dose of 2 million international units (MIU) subcutaneously three times a week, but this treatment also showed only a trend toward benefit.

The popular press began to talk about a "breakthrough" in reference to the MS treatment trial studies at the Scripps Clinic in La Jolla, California, and the University of California, San Francisco, even thought the initial results were disappointing; there was no statistical significance, but some patients felt better. In the meantime, Torben Fog treated patients by administering 2.5–5 MIU of interferon beta-1a intramuscularly, but without effect. In retrospect, the dose was small and the patients had chronic progressive disease, both factors which might cause the trial to fail. Ververken and his colleagues tried interferon-beta on three patients without effect, but again these were chronic progressive patients.[231] The attempts continued and interest was supported by the observation by Abreu in 1982 that interferon beta would inhibit EAE.[232,233] In 1983, Biogen asked Kenneth Johnson and Hill Panitch to test gamma interferon, but 7 of the 18 patients recruited experienced new relapses on the drug, indicating this form of interferon stimulated disease activity.[234] This showed that cytokines were important in the pathogenesis of MS and led to the idea that if natural gamma interferon could be inhibited, it might lead to an effective therapy. It also pointed out that response in EAE might not predict clinical response in MS patients.

In 1984, Knobler reported the reduction of exacerbations in MS patients given intramuscular alpha-interferon in a double-blind crossover

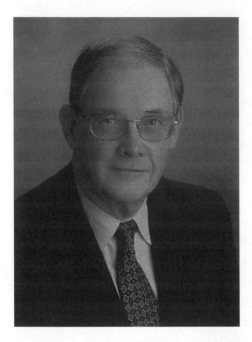

Figure 15.19 Dr. Kenneth Johnson was involved in the development of the initial trials of interferons in MS; and he continues to study long-term results of glateramir acetate. He was the founder of ACTRIMS. (Courtesy of Dr. K. Johnson.)

trial, with six months on each arm of the study.[235] There was a reduction of exacerbation in both groups, but the effect on the placebo group was after a period on interferon, so this may have been a carryover effect of the drug; the severity of the episodes in the interferon-treated group was less. Nine trials of alpha-interferon over the next 12 years led to the conclusion that alpha-interferon was not effective clinically and perhaps not on MRI either.

Despite much criticism and skepticism about the first trial of intrathecal interferon, Jacobs and his team persisted and designed a double-blind study of intrathecal interferon on 69 patients, showing a reduction in exacerbations of MS in the treated group, but noting something that has been seen in other studies—a reduction in the number of attacks in the placebo group.[236–238] Interest increased as there was evidence that a drug might finally be altering the course of MS, but the intrathecal route seemed impractical for most patients and for long-term use. Michel Revel at the Weitzman Institute in Israel had developed beta-1a in CHO cells in the late 1970s. Jacobs collaborated with the German biotechnology firm Bioferon, which was making a recombinant as well as a human

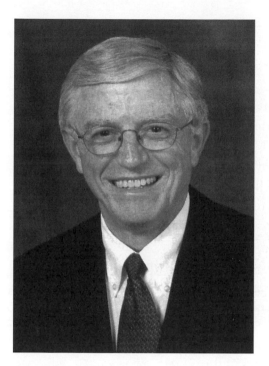

Figure 15.20 Dr. John Whitaker (1941–2001), Chairman of Neurology at the University of Alabama, died as this book was being completed. He contributed to MS care and research throughout his career and was involved in many of the pivotal trials on the new agents for the treatment of MS.

fibroblast interferon. The recombinant type was made from Chinese hamster ovary cells and replicated the human fibroblast interferon made from foreskin.

Richard Smith of the Scripps Clinic showed that the C-56 inducible protein response to systemic administered interferon in monkeys was similar to the response to intrathecal administration, suggesting interferon could be administered systematically and still have an effect in the brain. It would be of great benefit to patients to be able to take interferon by systemic injection rather than through repeated lumbar punctures. Studies suggested that six million units injected once weekly was a dose that achieved the desired effect with a minimum of side effects.

When sufficient supplies of beta-interferons became available, a multiple sclerosis collaborative research group (MSCRG) was formed by Lawrence Jacobs, Andres Salazer, and Robert Herndon to study its effect in MS patients. Were the positive results due to a suppression of a virus involved in the etiology of MS, or to a suppression of other viral infections that might aggravate or exacerbate MS, or did they indicate an independent action on the immune system because of the immunomodulatory effects of beta-interferon?

Triton Biosciences, a small company in California, approached Kenneth Johnson about doing a trial with recombinant beta-interferon, nonglycosolated, made by Chiron from E. coli. Cautious after the disturbing trial with gamma-interferon, the company first arranged a pilot, dose-finding and safety trial. The six-month trial showed there was a dose response, but 16 MIU was not well tolerated, so all patients were put on 8 MIU. The subsequent trial began in 1988 using 8 MIU, 1.6 MIU, and placebo. Two of the Triton scientists, Joy Wallenberg and Steve Marcus, were given credit by Johnston in his Dystel Prize address for having shaped the nature of this and subsequent trials by deciding to use the very expensive MRI imaging as part of the trial design.[239] In the meantime, Triton was purchased by Shering AG and renamed Berlex Laboratories. A trial was begun in 1988 with interferon beta-1b (Betaseron®) and Jacobs organized one with interferon beta-1a (Avonex®).

To study the effects of interferon beta-1b, 30 patients enrolled in 1986 received doses varying from 0.8 to 16 MIU of betaseron beta-1b

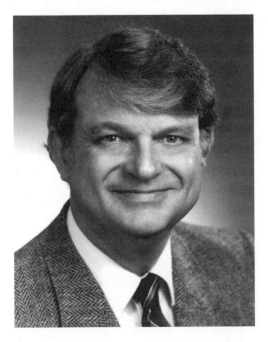

Figure 15.21 Dr. Donald Paty of Vancouver has been a pioneer of modern approaches to MS, contributing to the concept of multidisciplinary research clinics, MRI use in clinical trials, epidemiology, classification of MS, and design of clinical trials. (Courtesy of Dr. Donald Paty, Photo by Campbell, Vancouver.)

(Betaseron®). The study results showed a dose-related trend for reduction of acute attacks and for the number of patients free of attacks. Side effects, particularly flu-like symptoms and injection-site reactions, were significant but manageable. The results were positive enough to warrant developing a large, multicenter trial, using seven centers in the United States and four in Canada from the summer of 1988 to early 1993. This pivotal trial showed that Betaseron® in a dose of 8 MIU every second day injected subcutaneously led to a 30 percent reduction in the frequency of acute MS attacks, and a 50 percent reduction in moderate and severe attacks, throughout a period of almost five years. The study was not adequately powered to demonstrate measures of disability, but the placebo group trended toward clinical worsening, an important observation. Placebo groups in trials usually do better than expected, for a number of factors: selection, care, improvement of attitudes and expectations, and a tendency for the number of attacks to reduce over time. Aside from the important clinical information, perhaps the most persuasive data came from the MRI information on these patients, which Donald Paty had suggested should be an outcome measure in this trial, as he had used it in two previous trials. There was a dramatic reduction both in new lesions and in the accumulated lesion burden, as confirmed by the frequent MRI subset analysis of 52 patients at the University of British Columbia under Paty's direction. A not-unexpected but puzzling feature was the development of neutralizing IgG antibody against the interferon beta-1b. Although the titers were quite high in some patients, it did not clearly correlate with exacerbation rates, side effects, or other measures. To add to the confusion, in later years, antibody titers often fell as treatment continued. Subsequent observations indicated that the presence of antibody has not been consistently related to outcome, that antibodies can disappear in the midst of treatment, and that occasionally antibodies are found in placebo groups, so that the assays can be problematic.

William Sibley says that the most exciting day in his career, after almost 50 years in MS research, was that day in January 1993 when researchers broke the codes and found the remarkable effect of Betaseron®. He chaired the committee that wrote the paper published in *Neurology*.[240]

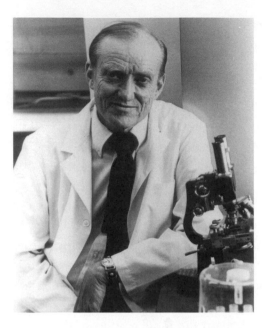

Figure 15.22 Dr. William Sibley as a resident in neurology was asked by Dr. Houston Merritt to survey the status of MS therapy for the Advisory Board of the National MS Society, which initiated a career in MS research, centered on virology, clinical trials, and the role of stress in the disease. (Courtesy of Dr. William Sibley.)

A major event in the treatment of MS occurred on March 11, 1993 when the hearing at the FDA met to review the Betaseron® trial for approval for marketing the drug in the treatment of MS. Even though the clinical data were impressive, demonstrating for the first time a significant alteration of the underlying disease in MS, it was the MRI data that were most persuasive. Betaseron® was approved in the summer of 1993 by a very rapid process.[241]

The excitement was understandable, but the expectations in the MS community were out of proportion to the objective results of the trial. It is always difficult to extrapolate from a focused controlled trial to the realities of individual patients, but appropriate expectations would be that patients would experience two-thirds of their usual number of attacks on this drug, but the attacks would be less severe, and their MRIs would show improvement, especially when assessed for the appearance of new lesions over time. MRI improvement was out of proportion with the clinical improvement. Publicity was worldwide and the demands for the drug led to concerns about its supply and availability. Although the criteria for approval of the drug for use in individual patients tended to comply with the criteria for the clinical trial, not always a very realistic or rational approach, patients with more progressive or more severe disease than allowed in a trial also wanted the drug.

Berlex, the company producing Betaseron®, decided to use a lottery to distribute drug to those who wanted the new therapy since it did not feel it could meet the demand. Eight hundred phone lines were set up. This created a public relations disaster, even though it did focus the therapy toward those who were expected to benefit from it. If patients had insurance to cover the high cost, or could afford it, and were selected by the lottery to receive it, treatment was initiated. Before this could be more of an issue, enough drug, and other drug options such as interferon-beta 1a and copolymer 1 came on to the market.

In the meantime, the work on interferon-beta 1a was finishing a multi-center, double-blind, placebo-controlled phase III trial with intramuscular recombinant human fibroblast interferon (Avonex®) in 301 patients with relapsing MS. This study also had positive results, and was stopped early, in August 1994. The interferon used was approved by the FDA in 1996.[242,243] The study showed important aspects of data analysis using the Kaplan-Meier survival curves. It was the first trial to show slowing of progression of MS, although there was a trend in that direction with Betaseron®. It also provided information that increasing cerebral atrophy was developing in MS patients over time and showed that Avonex® could slow the atrophic change. The measurements of burden of illness on the MRI was also reduced by the treatment.[244,245]

By January 2000, 84,000 patients world wide were taking Avonex®. Most recently, Jacobs has reported the results of the CHAMPS trial on patients at risk for clinically definite MS who have had one attack (two are required for the classification of clinically definite MS) and have positive MRIs suggestive of MS.[246] This shows that Avonex® can delay the progression of MS as measured by when patients might have the second attack, which classifies them as clinically definite MS (CDMS). Similar results have come from the ETOMS trial with Rebif®. Also underway is the IMPACT trial in patients in secondary-progressive MS.

As Knobler points out, a number of important lessons were learned from these three pioneering studies.[247,248] The interferons were not practical for treating acute attacks, but seemed to be helpful in patients with relapsing-remitting disease in the longer term. Also, the natural interferon produced many side effects, which might be reduced by more purified recombinant variations. Finally, the drug could be administered by subcutaneous injection and this was an acceptable form of long-term therapy.

As so often occurs in the development of a pharmacological agent, the release of a drug for use occurs only after a series of painstaking laboratory and then clinical steps taken over many decades. This was demonstrated in the arrival of the three interferon drugs now on the market for the treatment of MS (Betaseron®, Avonex®, and Rebif®).*

Clinical trials continue to refine and define the appropriate timing, dose, route, and indications for these drugs, combination therapy with these drugs, and combinations with other drugs. Although the effect of these new drugs has been modest, it has been a major first step in altering the outcome of MS, and the next few years will undoubtedly bring us further in the struggle to conquer this disease, which Gowers indicated a century ago was one of the most difficult of the neurological diseases to treat.

> "For the practicing neurologist, knowing the mechanism of action of IFN8k (beta interferon) does not yet affect clinical decisions. However, in the future this knowledge may result in more effective treatment of MS, through recognition of which patients will benefit optimally from IFN8k therapy. Tests that detect disease progression before clinical worsening are needed ... the trail ahead is likely to be long and tortuous."
>
> H. Moses and S. Sriram, 1999[249]

COPAXONE® (COP-I)

> "The 14th of June 1995 was a milestone for me—as on this day the file on Copolymer 1 (Cop 1) was submitted, under the name Copaxone®,

---

*Because of protection of Avonex® under the Orphan Drug Act in the United States, Rebif® was not initially permitted approval for marketing there. Both are interferon beta-1a and the Act does not allow competitors, to encourage drug companies to develop drugs for uncommon diseases. One could argue that MS is common, and there are differences in dose and route of administration. These arguments were accepted when the EVIDENCE trial of 2001 showed some benefit of Rebif® over Avonex® in a short-term trial. Rebif® was approved in early 2002.

by the Teva Pharmaceutical Company to the FDA (Federal Drug Administration) for approval as a New Drug Application for the treatment of multiple sclerosis ... after over 27 years of persistent research effort, perseverance and tenacity of purpose."

Ruth Arnon, 1996[250]

The development of another important agent in the treatment of MS can be traced to three individuals, Dr. Michael Sela, Dr. Ruth Arnon, and Dr. Devora Tietelbaum, who worked in the 1960s on synthetic copolymers that would stimulate EAE. To their surprise, many of these agents inhibited rather than stimulated EAE.

Ruth Arnon recently related the 27-year saga to bring copolymer I, (Cop 1), later named Copaxone®, to the market.[251] It is the very personal story of the day-to-day efforts, typical of those involved in research, to relentlessly follow faint leads, larger hypotheses, and walks through the forests of complex basic research knowledge and techniques to pursue a question. In a book like this, I can only lightly touch on the achievements of many whose struggle ended with a large step forward, while recognizing that there are many others who struggled as valiantly and as long, pursuing an important possibility, which might add new knowledge, but not an advance that would be noticed except by those who used that experience to pursue a new course. Fortunately, Arnon and her colleagues made a significant recognizable advance, but so many make an equal struggle, which comes to an equally accurate conclusion, but with no major clinical advance results. Those tireless workers also provide an important contribution to the body of knowledge that lets the next person take a further step forward.

Following the production of random copolymers that resembled myelin basic protein in the laboratory of Professor Ephraim Katchalski at the Weitzman Institute in Israel, the team expected these agents to produce encephalitogenic activity. Surprisingly, the copolymers had the opposite effect: the capacity to protect against experimental allergic encephalomyelopathy. Dr. Oded Abramsky carried out the first clinical trial in MS patients, and Dr. Helmut Bauer and Murray Bornstein planned others. Bornstein carried out three trials that showed the copoly-

---

*Four hundred volumes and 60,000 pages of data.

mer called Copolymer I reduced the number of exacerbations of MS with remarkably few side effects.[252] Problems in the production of a consistent product delayed the development of further trials, as did the interruption of the Gulf War, but the drug was available for further large trials in 1991.[253] The multicenter trial was positive and in September 1996, the FDA Expert Panel recommended approval of copolymer-1, by then well known by that name and the abbreviated Cop-1. Its new awkward name became glatiramer acetate; later the commercial name became Copaxone®. MRI was not used in the multicenter trial, but a subsequent European—Canadian study showed Copaxone® reduced the MRI lesion burden. The "designer drug" for MS patients was released in the United States in the spring of 1997, 25 years after the drug was first produced.

As with the interferons, further studies are being conducted with expected refinement in the routes, doses, and indications for this interesting drug. A trial of oral Copaxone® (the CORAL study) was completed in 2001 and did not show significant benefit for the oral preparation over a placebo. Combination trials using Copaxone® with other drugs are underway, combining with azathioprine, Avonex®, and other agents. Fortunately, the original group of patients in the multicenter trial has been regularly followed into the 11th year in 2002, the longest therapeutic study of a monitored MS population on one of the four immune modulating drugs, with patients assessed every six months.

As clinical trials are completed and experience grows, the guidelines for use of the new agents in MS will be modified. There is a current guideline from the NMSS in the United States, a Canadian guideline from the Canadian MS Clinic Network, and a European guideline. These are being updated; other agencies such as the MS Council in the USA are drafting new guidelines. It is too much to expect one international guideline, but the free communication and collaboration of the players in each group assure some unanimity in the results of these efforts.

FUTURE THERAPIES

Almost 40 trials of new agents and procedures, or other approaches with current therapies, are underway as this is written. A later history will show whether autologous stem cell transplantation, monoclonal antibodies, plasmapheresis, IV Ig, donepezil, mitroxanthrone plus interferon, mycophenolate, fampridine, variations on current therapies, and many other approaches will find a place in the treatment of MS patients.

THE FUTURE OF PLACEBO TRIALS IN MS

The modern randomized clinical trial (RCT) developed from the work of Ronald Fisher in agriculture experiments and was applied to medicine by Bradford Hill in 1946 with the first trials on streptomycin on TB. Within a few years, the first trials were being done with the RCT methodology by Henry Miller and others studying steroids in MS. The methods of selection, blinding, randomization, crossover techniques, intention-to-treat analysis, statistical methods, and complex ethical issues related to trials have developed to a high degree just as the RCT has been challenged by the results of its own success. Once a therapy has been accepted by clinical trials as beneficial, the gold standard of a placebo-controlled RCT may be ethically questionable except in certain clearly defined circumstances. When therapies such as the interferons, gluterimer acetate, and mitroxanthrone became accepted therapies, it was no longer reasonable to assign patients to a long-term placebo group. This will call for new strategies such as the use of MS patient groups who have not been shown to benefit from therapy, or who elect not to use these therapies, or by the use of natural history comparisons. The Sylvia Lawry program will look at the possibility of using placebo groups from clinical trials as a comparison, and others are exploring the large national history databases accumulated by many MS clinics such as the London, Ontario data. These issues have been explored by the Task Force on Placebo-Controlled Clinical Trials in MS (March 6–7, 2000) and are reviewed by Lublin et al.[254]

ALTERNATIVE THERAPIES: THE PARALLEL SYSTEM

"Clinical charisma and the exploitation of frightened vulnerable patients and their relatives litter the historical highways and byways

of therapeutic endeavor in multiple sclerosis. It has not been a golden road."

Alistair Compston, 1998[255]

Physicians, who represent the "conventional" or professional medicine recognized by the state and society, often use specific legislation, controls, responsibilities, protections, and rewards to classify other forms of therapy and their practitioners as alternative. This was so even before medicine acquired recognition through Royal Colleges or through state laws, and there has long been a sense of who was the recognized healer and which were the recognized healing arts before the profession of medicine was organized. In fact, much of the activity of organizing medicine and the formation of medical associations, particularly in the 19th century, was specifically about keeping other practitioners out, even before medicine had therapies that were any more efficacious than those of the "quacks" being excluded. It is sobering to note that the therapies practiced by the physicians in the past would be frowned upon as quackery by the profession today.

Alternative medicine has always been with us and has waves of acceptance. The boundaries between what has been called peripheral, unconventional, complementary, alternative, or more derogatory terms such as quackery, has never been clear. Therapies once in the forefront of medical approaches to symptoms and diseases are now in the list of alternative or complementary therapies, and alternative therapies eventually shown to be beneficial enter the realm of medical therapy. To understand the difference between the two approaches, it is important to recognize that they represent two different philosophies. Just to compare specific therapies, or whether one therapy is more beneficial than another, is missing a central point. Alternative medicine is a different system, based on belief and sometimes longstanding historical and cultural practices rather than science. Physicians often forget that science is a relative newcomer to the philosophy of medicine; for thousands of years, medical practice looked very much like current-day alternative medicine. One need only look at the therapies administered to Augustus d'Esté or B.F. Cummings (aka W.N.P. Barbellion) to note the similarity of physician therapies in the

19th and early 20th centuries to the alternative therapies of today. These patients were treated with arsenic, strychnine, potassium iodide, mercury, and belladonna, and with herbs, minerals, baths, massage, various electrotherapies, and complex diets.

Any chronic disease for which there is not effective treatment tends beget many alternative approaches to treatment; MS is a good example of this. One need only consult the frequently updated *Multiple Sclerosis: A Guide to Treatment and Management* (formerly called *Therapeutic Claims in MS*) to see the long, but necessarily incomplete list of the most frequently used medical and alternative approaches to MS.[256,257] But physicians had (and undoubtedly currently have) a similar long list of questionable therapies. Speaking in 1930 about the wide range of medical therapies, Russell Brain concluded, "The multiplication of remedies is eloquent of their inefficacy."[258]

Many alternative therapies have a long history of use in medicine as well as for MS. For instance, spa therapy, herbal preparations, stimulants, minerals, detoxification, and rest therapies have been used for over 150 years in MS, and wax and wane in popularity. Other therapies change as medical theories change, as with antisyphilitic therapy, antimicrobials and antibiotics, anticoagulants, immunosuppressants, and antioxidants, formerly medical therapies that are now regarded, if used, as unconventional or alternative.

Electric therapy has a very long history, and anything electric continues to impress. There are a vast number of ways that electricity is used to measure, stimulate, and rejuvenate the disturbed system. Magnetism was a fad of the 18th century that never really disappeared, resurfacing in popularity at the end of the 19th century and revived in the late 20th century with various stimulators and magnetotherapies. There has been recent interest in expensive magnetic pads for MS patients that go in their chairs, beds, or shoes to magnetically rebalance the system or provide a vital force to the body of an MS patient.

Alternative and complementary medicines in MS are not a small or peripheral issue. More MS patients use alternative therapies and go to alternative therapists than take prescribed medicines or attend physicians. Some will see their neurologist once every 6–12 months, but see an alternative therapist many times a month or even many times a week. Studies in Canada, the United States, and Europe have all shown a high use of alternative therapies by MS patients, with many using three to six different therapies at the same time, periodically dropping one and picking up another. About one-third do not tell their physicians what they are doing, mostly because they think the doctors will be judgmental or critical.

Richard Thomas wrote a holistic guide for MS therapy that suggests a long list of forms of natural therapies. This included acupuncture, cupping, acupressure, healing or faith healing, therapeutic touch, homeopathy, reflexology, crystal and gem therapy, aura-soma oils, aromatherapy, and flower remedies (olive for exhaustion, crab apple for shame about the disease, mustard for depression—and a "rescue therapy" that combines five of these flowers).[259] A more recent monograph by a physician is the review by Allan C. Bowling.[260] In the 1970s, Paty carried out a trial of acupuncture in MS, but there are few well-designed trials in the vast array of agents and therapies used in MS.

MS therapy with hyperbaric oxygen was suggested after a one-year study of this therapy in Dundee, Scotland, which followed two reports of benefit in EAE, and a preliminary report in MS patients by Neubauer in 1980.[261] Following this, in 1983, Fischer and his colleagues published a randomized double-blind control study in the *New England Journal of Medicine* suggesting benefit with this treatment.[262] The first ARMS center for hyperbaric oxygen was formed in Dundee in 1982 and many centers then appeared around the country as patient enthusiasm increased, despite unimpressive follow-up results by Barnes and others.[263] The treatment then became controversial. ARMS representatives discounted negative reports, releasing another report on 147 cases treated in Glasgow, and concluding that the treatment was beneficial and safe.[264] After each well-controlled study reported negative results, interest waned generally, but this therapy is still offered by groups that own hyperbaric chambers on both sides of the Atlantic.

In 1983, Jane Clarke published a book suggesting a new theory for the cause of MS—that overheating caused the disease, and lack of repair, of myelin was caused by a deficiency of copper/molybdenum in patients' diet; therapy based on this concept was developed.[265] Most recently, interest has been sparked in the media about bee venom therapy, the Cari Loder diet, and Procarin, but such alternative approaches arise frequently, fading slowly as the next one comes to the fore.[266,267]

Lourdes

Bernadette Soubirous was a 14-year-old French girl who saw a vision of a young Virgin Mary in a grotto at Lourdes in 1858. Soon after, stories of cures circulated from the crowds who came to the site. From the earliest years, people with MS joined the pilgrims to Lourdes. Charcot said that anyone who could be cured in such a fashion was hysterical, but in terms of the power of suggestion in people who were suffering from hysterical or emotional disorders, religious faith was a stronger force than medical authority. Organized groups of MS patients went to Lourdes in the late 19th century, assisted by Catholic societies. In 1897, Henry Head requested permission from the St. Luke, St. Cosmas, and St. Damian Society to examine the people with neurological disease returning from Lourdes. The MS Society of Great Britain and Ireland organized groups of MS patients to Lourdes in the 1960s. The Catholic Church has no cases of MS among those who are accepted as cures at Lourdes.[268]

MS patients have sought miracles as well as medical cures. There is a long history of MS patients visiting Lourdes, and in the 1960s the MS Society in Britain made arrangements for MS patients to join excursions of pilgrim-sufferers to Lourdes. It goes even further back to correspondence of Henry Head requesting permission to examine the neurological cases going to Lourdes in 1895; although he was allowed to do so, there was concern from the physician members of the Society of St. Luke, St. Cosmas and St. Damian who normally examined the pilgrims, that Head was not a Catholic. Examination of the records of a 25-year period of cases accepted by the Catholic Church as cures at Lourdes reveals no cases of MS.[269]

It is important to point out that there are good reasons why someone might believe he had found an important therapy for MS. It might appear that a therapy produced a reversal of severe MS when this in fact had occurred spontaneously. If 100 people each year tried the new therapy and 20 felt they were better (the placebo rate in MS is higher than this) and continued the therapy, even though the improvement occurred spontaneously or by the placebo effect, after five years, there would be 100 people who claimed they were helped by the treatment and indicated how they had benefited. Those who worsened after a time would fall by the wayside, going on to other forms of therapy, and therapists would continue to accumulate only the good responders. It is common for therapists to deceive themselves by noting that after some years, they have hundreds of people who seem to have benefited, some even dramatically.

> *"Multiple sclerosis soon acquired a regrettable reputation for maverick medicine based on shameless exploitation of its capricious natural history which favored the uncritical and those devoted to extrapolation from anecdotal experience."*
>
> Alistair Compston, 1998[270]

THE ORGANIZATION OF TREATMENT CLINICS

In the 19th century and the first half of the 20th century, MS case series and studies came prematurely from general neurology clinics. In the postwar period, a further development in clinics devoted to multiple sclerosis began. Prior to World War II, there were clinics in Europe and the United States usually related to the personal interests of specific neurologists, and organized around those interests in therapy and assessment. Very few were exclusively organized for MS patients, and most were large general neurology clinics that assessed MS cases, as they did other groups seen in large numbers, such as epilepsy, neuropathies, and muscle diseases. After World War II, clinics were set up to accumulate larger populations of MS patients for organized programs of documentation, assessment, and research. The first of these was started by Leo Alexander in Boston, the second by Melvin Thomas at the University of Pennsylvania in 1956. A few notable early clinics included the Atlanta MS clinic under Dr. Robert Kibler, the Newcastle Demyelinating

Diseases Research Unit at Newcastle-upon-Tyne under Dr. Henry Miller, and the MS Clinic at the Montreal Neurological Institute (MNI) under Dr. Bert Cosgrove and Dr. Roy Swank. Cosgrove began the first Canadian clinic in the 1940s. Donald Paty of Vancouver, formerly of Atlanta, who spent some time in the Newcastle unit, became a leader in the concept of a comprehensive organization of MS services, research, and education.[271] He said that he was first impressed with the advantages of a well-organized clinic for MS care and research in Kibler's unit in Atlanta. Paty organized the large and active unit at the University of Western Ontario in 1972. The system of MS clinics across Canada was strongly influenced by Paty's model and he later moved to Vancouver, where the comprehensive clinic model was combined with major research efforts in neuroimaging, genetics, epidemiology, and systems approaches to the study of MS patients. The clinics are now linked in a Canadian network of MS clinics.

To encourage the development of comprehensive clinics in North America, Dr. Jack Conomy of the Cleveland Clinic called together a small number of physicians to plan how such an organization could foster collaboration and education of health professionals involved in the care of MS patients. After years of struggle, the Consortium of MS Centers has grown to a membership of 85 clinics and has played an important role in the multidisciplinary communication about issues related to MS care and research. Collaboration of MS researchers and clinicians has also developed in Europe with ECTRIMS and RIMS, in North America with ACTRIMS, and South America with LACTIMS.

Jack Antel of Montreal pointed out to me a subtle change that occurred in the 1960s and 1970s—the advent of the clinical neurologist with special training in the "basic sciences" of neurology addressing the basic questions of MS. In the previous century, we saw advances made by clinicians often very skilled at neuropathology. In the 1950s, clinical neurologists recognized that other skills were necessary and there were individuals who trained in epidemiology, immunology, neurochemistry, infectious diseases, and more recently, neuroimaging, genetics, and the skills of clinical trial design. In MS research today, there is a cadre of international experts with a vast array of skills being brought to bear on

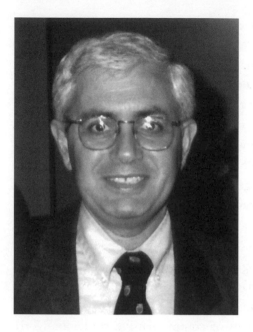

Figure 15.23 Dr. Jack Antel, as head of the Montreal Neurological Institute (MNI), leads a large group committed to research in MS. (Courtesy of Dr. Jack Antel.)

the underlying questions in MS. In recent years, there has been a shift from the clinician to the clinician-scientist to the basic scientist, whose training and skills are even more finely honed for the difficult questions we need to answer.

An example of all this is the group addressing multiple sclerosis questions at the Montreal Neurological Institute (MNI). This was one of the early dedicated MS clinics in the 1940s with the clinicians Bert Cosgrove, Roy Swank, and Colin Russell seeing a large number of patients and looking at clinical questions. Two decades later, the MS group was mostly clinical neurologists with special training in laboratory science. Today, the group is mostly basic scientists.

DATABASES

Attempts have been made since early in this century to collect population studies of MS, and this approach was accelerated by epidemiological studies to characterize the geographical patterns of MS, which were in full swing in the 1950s and 1960s. Local databases were developed in British Columbia and in some European countries, but these always suffered from incomplete ascertainment and the concern that the MS diagnosis was not always confirmed. Many researchers developed their information from wide advertising, and from MS society rolls, approaches which had many deficiencies and limitations. An effort was made to establish a nationwide database in Canada in 1974, but the focus shifted to the need for a nationwide organization of MS clinics at each university setting. MS CoStar was adapted as a computerized database system for MS by Studney and Paty in 1980, but did not find wide use, despite numerous attempts to have it adopted in North America and Europe. At this writing, a uniform database has not been adopted but there are many discussions underway.

The major European database for multiple sclerosis (EDMUS) continues to grow and expand. The NARCOMS Registry database was initiated in 1996 by The Consortium of MS Centers under the leadership of Timothy L. Vollmer to collect data from a large number of MS patients (now over 20,000) and to aid in recruitment of patients for studies and trials. It has the advantage of large numbers, but the disadvantage of unregulated enrollment methodologies, so how close this population of patients is to the cross-section of MS patients is uncertain. A similar European database is being developed. There are important natural history studies under way, a long-standing series from the London, Ontario and Halifax, NS clinics, as well as other clinics in France, Germany, Sweden, and elsewhere. There are also prospective databases being developed at the National MS Society and at the Brigham and Women's Hospital in Boston. The Sonya Slifka Longitudinal Multiple Sclerosis Society of the National MS Society will follow 2000 people with MS long-term. Its study group came from various areas of the United States and the study sample is representative of a cross-section of Americans with MS. The study was initiated in 1999 and named in honor of the mother of the Chair of the National Board of Directors of the NMSS, Mr. Richard Slifka. The Society contracted with Dr. Sarah Minden and Abt Associates, Inc. of Cambridge, Massachusetts to do the study long-term. A database on Devic's disease has been initiated at the Mayo Clinic by Brian Weinshenker.

A novel database suggested by John Noseworthy and Henry McFarlane is the placebo population from all clinical trials, as this could constitute a well-studied and documented group to establish the natural history of MS (at least in the short-term of studies) for comparison in future trials when it may be unethical in many instances to use a placebo. This database is being established by Professor W. Ian McDonald under the auspices of the MS International Federation in Munich. It has been named the Sylvia Lawry Center for MS Research in honor of the founder of the Federation and the National MS Society. The database will be directed by Professor Albrecht Neiss.

Therapy in MS usually develops and progresses in small steps. Dramatic discoveries like insulin and penicillin are the exception, and even these had long histories of growing knowledge that led to discovery. In MS, an important step has been taken in the past decade with the development of drugs that alter the course of the underlying disease.

When the next book on the history of MS is written, I hope and expect that many more dramatic steps will be described. Such was the hope of Barbellion:

"It would be nice if a physician from London, one of these days, were to gallop up hotspur, tether his horse to the gait post and dash in waving a reprieve—the discovery of a cure!"

W.N.P. Barbellion (B.F. Cummings), 1919[272]

REFERENCES

1. Charcot JM. Oeuvres complètes. *Leçons sur les maladies du système nerveux*. Vol. 1. Paris; 1894:269.
2. Gray LC. *A Treatise on Nervous and Mental Diseases*. London: HK Lewis; 1893:373-378.
3. Marie P. *Lectures on Diseases of the Spinal Cord*, trans. Lubbock M. London: New Sydenham Society; 1895;153:134-136.
4. Gowers WR. *A Manual of Diseases of the Nervous System*, 2nd ed. Vol 2. London: J&A Churchill; 1893:544, 557-558.
5. Putnam TJ. The Centenary of Multiple Sclerosis. *Arch Neurol Psych*. 1938;40(4):806-813.
6. Wilson SAK. *Neurology*. Bruce AN, ed. London: Edward Arnold; 1940:148-178.
7. Firth D. The Case of Augustus d'Este (1794–1848). The first account of disseminated sclerosis. *Proc Royal Soc Med*. 1940-41;34:499-52.
8. Firth D. *The Case of Augustus d'Esté*. Cambridge: Cambridge University Press; 1948.
9. Neill J, Smith FG. *Analytical Compendium of Medical Science*. Philadelphia: Blanchard and Lea; 1852.
10. Charcot JM. *Lectures on the diseases of the nervous system delivered at la Salpêtrière*. Sigerson G, ed. and trans. London: New Sydenham Society; 1877.

11. Moxon W. Eight cases of insular sclerosis of the brain and spinal cord. *Guy Hospital Reports*; 1875;20:437-478.
12. Marie P. *Lectures on Diseases of the Spinal Cord*, trans. Lubbock M London: New Sydenham Society; 1895;153:134-136.
13. Dana CL. *Textbook of Nervous Diseases*. 3rd ed. New York: William Wood; 1894.
14. Gowers WR. A Manual of Diseases of the Nervous System, 2nd ed. Vol. 2 London: J.&A. Churchill; 1893:544, 557-558.
15. Edwards A. *Disseminated Sclerosis*. Manchester: John Heywood; 1895.
16. Sachs B. A Treatise on the Nervous Diseases of Children. New York: William Wood; 1895:345-356.
17. Beevor CE. *Diseases of the Nervous System*. London: H. K. Lewis; 1898:272-278.
18. Buzzard EF. The treatment of disseminated sclerosis: A Suggestion. *Lancet*. 1911;1:98.
19. Bury, Judson. *Diseases of the Nervous System*. Manchester: Manchester University Press; 1912.
20. Bullock WE. The experimental transmission of disseminated sclerosis to rabbits. *Lancet*. 1913; Oct.25:1185-1186.
21. Gye NE. The experimental study of disseminated sclerosis. *Brain*. 1921;44:213-222.
22. Denny-Brown D. Multiple sclerosis: The clinical problem. *Am J Med*. 1952;12:501-509.
23. Oppenheim H. *Text-book of Nervous Diseases for Physicians and Students*, trans. A Bruce. Edinburgh: Otto Schulze; 1911.
24. Marburg O. Sie Sogenannte akute multiple sklerose (encephalomyelitis periaxialis scleroticans) *Jahrb Psychiat Neurol*. 1906;27:1.
25. Association for Research in Nervous and Mental Disease. *Multiple Sclerosis (Disseminated sclerosis)*. New York: Paul B. Hoeber; 1922.
26. Ibid.
27. McAlpine D. The treatment of disseminated sclerosis. *Lancet*. 1925;2:82-83.
28. Weber FP. Documents at the Wellcome Library, London. PP/FPW/B226/3; PP/FPW/B226/4; PP/FPW/322 and PP/FPW/B/332.
29. Hall LA. A "Remarkable Collection:" The papers of Frederick Parkes Weber, FRCP (1863–1962). *Medical History*. 2001;45:523-532.
30. Ibid, p. 523-532.
31. Fisher A. On some of the less common early signs of disseminated sclerosis with a report of some cases. *Can Med Assoc J*. 1926;15:1483-1486.
32. Brain WR. Critical review: disseminated sclerosis. *Quart J Med*. 1930;23:343-391.
33. Ibid.
34. Brickner RM. A critique of therapy in multiple sclerosis. *Bull Neurol Inst NY*. 1935-1936;4:665-698.
35. Talley C. *A History of Multiple Sclerosis and Medicine in the United States, 1870-1960*. PhD dissertation. San Francisco: University of California; 1998.
36. Putnam TJ, Chiavacci LV, Hoff H, et al. Results of treatment of multiple sclerosis with dicoumarin. *Arch Neurol*. 1947;57:1-13.
37. Denny-Brown D. Multiple Sclerosis: The clinical problem. *Am J Med*. 1952;12:501-509.
38. Frith JA. History of multiple sclerosis: an Australian perspective. *Clin and Exp Neurol*. 1988;25:7-16.
39. Talley C. *A History of Multiple Sclerosis and Medicine in the United States. 1870-1960*. PhD Thesis. San Francisco: University of California. 1998.
40. Reese HH. Disseminated sclerosis and dicoumerol therapy. *Tran Am Neurol Assoc*. 1944;70:78.
41. Müller R. Studies on disseminated sclerosis. *Acta med Scand*. 1949;133(suppl 222):1-214.
42. Talley C. *A History of Multiple Sclerosis and Medicine in the United States, 1870-1960*. PhD Thesis. San Francisco: University of California. 1998.

43. Schumacher GA. Multiple sclerosis and its treatment. *JAMA*. 1950;143:1059-1065, 1146-1154, 1241-1250.
44. Talley C. *A History of Multiple Sclerosis and Medicine in the United States, 1870-1960*. PhD Thesis. San Francisco: University of California. 1998.
45. Scheinker IM. Recent advances in research and treatment of multiple sclerosis. *Ohio State Med J*. 1949;45:27.
46. Thygesen P. *The Course of Disseminated Sclerosis: A Close-up of 105 Attacks*. Copenhagen: Rosenkilde and Bagger; 1953.
46. Talley C. *A History of Multiple Sclerosis and Medicine in the United States, 1870-1960*. PhD Thesis. San Francisco: University of California. 1998.
47. Stern EL. The intraspinal (subarachnoid) injection of vitamin B1 for the relief of intractable pain and for degenerative diseases of the central nervous system. *Am J Surg*. 1938;39:495.
48. Ibid, p. 495.
49. Compston A. The Story of Multiple Sclerosis. Chapter 1 in *McAlpine's Multiple Sclerosis*. London: Churchill Livingstone; 1998: 3-11.
50. Brickner RM: A critique of therapy in multiple sclerosis. *Bull Neurol Inst NY*. 1935-1936;4:665-698.
51. Horton BT, Waegener HP, Aita JA, Woltman HW. Treatment of multiple sclerosis by the intravenous administration of histamine. *JAMA*. 1944;124:800-812.
52. Abramson HA. Histamine iontophoresis in the therapy of multiple sclerosis. *NY State Med J*. 1949;49:1151.
53. Jonez HD. *My Fight to Conquer Multiple Sclerosis*. New York: Julian Messner; 1952.
54. Reese HH. Multiple Sclerosis and the Demyelinating Diseases. Critique of theories concerning multiple sclerosis. *JAMA*. 1950;143:1470-1473.
55. Ibid. p. 1470-1473.
56. Thygesen P. *The Course of Disseminated Sclerosis: A Close-up of 105 Attacks*. Copenhagen: Rosenkilde and Bagger; 1953.
57. Talley, Colin. *A History of Multiple Sclerosis and Medicine in the United States, 1870-1960*. PhD dissertation. San Francisco: University of California; 1998.
58. Schumacher GA. Multiple sclerosis and its treatment. *JAMA*. 1950;143:1059-1065, 1146-1154, 1241-1250.
59. Brickner RM. A critique of therapy in multiple sclerosis. *Bull Neurol Inst NY*. 1935-1936;4:665-698.
60. Schumacher GA. Multiple sclerosis and its treatment. *JAMA*. 1950; 143:1059-1065, 1146-1154, 1241-1250.
61. Abramson HA. Histamine iontophoresis in the therapy of multiple sclerosis. *NY State Med J*. 1949;49:1151.
62. Talley C. A *History of Multiple Sclerosis and Medicine in the United States, 1870-1960*. PhD Thesis. San Francisco: University of California. 1998.
63. Dick GWA, McKeown F, Wilson DC. Virus of acute encephalomyelitis of man and multiple sclerosis. *Brit Med J*. 1958;1:7-9.
64. Richard Masland; personal communication.
65. Thygesen P. *The Course of Disseminated Sclerosis: A Close-up of 105 Attacks*. Copenhagen: Rosenkilde and Bagger; 1953.
66. Brown JR, Beebe GW, Kurtzke JF, Loewenso RB, Silberberg DH, Tourtellotte WW. The design of clinical studies to assess therapeutic efficacy in multiple sclerosis. *Neurology*. 1979;29:3-23.
67. Myers LW, Ellison GW. The peculiar difficulties of therapeutic trials for multiple sclerosis. *Neurol Clinics*. 1990;8:119-141.
68. Weiss W, Stadlan EM. Design and statistical issues related to testing experimental therapy in multiple sclerosis. In: Rudick RA, Goodkin DE, eds. *Treatment of Multiple*

Sclerosis: Trial Design, Results and Future Perspectives. New York: Springer-Verlag; 1992:91-122.

69. Bornstein MB, Miller A, Slagle S, et al. A pilot trial of COP 1 in exacerbating-remitting multiple sclerosis. *N Engl J Med.* 1987;317:408-414.

70. Ellison GW, Myers LW, Mickey MR, et al. Multiple sclerosis: patient accural problems in a therapeutic trial. *Neurology.* 1983;33(suppl 2):71.

71. Noseworthy JH, Ebers GC, Gent M. The Canadian cooperative trial of cyclophosphamide and plasma-exchange in progressive multiple sclerosis. *Lancet.* 1991;337:441-446.

72. Paty DW, Ebers GC, eds. *Multiple Sclerosis.* Philadelphia: FA Davis; 1998: 192-228.

73. Bury, Judson. *Diseases of the Nervous System.* Manchester: Manchester University Press; 1912.

74. Canton D. Cortisone and the politics of empire, imperialism and British medicine 1918-1955. *Bull Hist Med.* 1993;67:463-493.

75. Marks HM. Cortisone 1949: A year in the political life of a drug. *Bull Hist Med.* 1992;66:419-439.

76. Randt CT, Trager CH, Merritt HH. A clinical study of the effect of ACTH on chronic neurological disorders in seven patients. *Proc 1st Clin ACTH Conf,* ed JR Mohr. Philadelphia: Blakiston; 1950:595.

77. Selye H. *The Physiology and Pathology of Exposure to Stress: a Treatise on the Concepts of the General-Adaptation-Syndrome and the Diseases of Adaptation.* Montreal: Acta Inc.; 1950.

78. Miller HG, Gibbons JL. Acute disseminated encephalomyelitis and acute disseminated sclerosis: Results of treatment with ACTH. *BMJ.* 1953;2:1345-1349.

79. Miller HG, Newell DJ, Ridley A. Multiple sclerosis: trials of maintenance treatment with prednisolone and soluble aspirin. *Lancet.* 1961;1:127-129.

80. Alexander L. New concept of critical steps in the course of chronic debilitating neurologic disease in evaluation of therapeutic response. *Arch Neurol Psychiat.* 1951;66:253-258.

81. Miller HG, Newell DJ, Ridley A. Multiple sclerosis: trials of maintenance treatment with prednisolone and soluble aspirin. *Lancet.* 1961;1:127-129.

82. Alexander L. Minutes of the Medical Advisory Board, National Multiple Sclerosis Society; 1949.

83. Alexander L, Berkeley A, Alexander AM. *Multiple Sclerosis: Prognosis and Treatment.* Springfield, IL: Charles C. Thomas; 1961.

84. Alexander L, Cass LJ. The present status of ACTH therapy in multiple sclerosis. *Ann Intern Med.* 1963;58:454-471.

85. Alexander L, Berkeley A, Alexander AM. *Multiple Sclerosis: Prognosis and Treatment.* 1961.

86. Alexander L, Loman J, Lesses MF, Green I. Blood and plasma transfusions in multiple sclerosis. In: *Multiple Sclerosis and the Demyelinating Disease.* Proceedings of the Association for Research in Nervous and Mental Disease (Dec. 10–11, 1948). Vol 28. Baltimore: Williams and Wilkins; 1950:178-202.

87. Shevell MI. Racial Hygiene, active euthanasia and Julius Hallervorden. *Neurology.* 1992;42:2214-2219.

88. Shevell M, Evans BK. The "Schaltenbrand experiment." Würzburg, 1940: Scientific, historical and ethical perspectives. *Neurology.* 1994;44:350-356.

89. Shevell MI. Neurology's witness to history: the combined intelligence operative subcommittee reports of Leo Alexander. *Neurology.* 1996;47:1096-1103.

90. Shevell MI. Neurology's witness to history: Part II. Leo Alexander's contributions to the Neremberg Code (1946-1947). *Neurology.* 1998;50:274-278.

91. Rose AS, Kuzma JW, Kurtzke JF, Namerow NS, Sibley WA, Tourtellotte WW. Cooperative study in the evaluation of therapy in multiple sclerosis: ACTH vs placebo—final report. *Neurology.* 1970;20:1-59.

92. Milligan NM, Newcombe R, Compston DAS. High dose methylprednisolone in the treatment of multiple sclerosis: Clinical effects. *J Neuro Neurosurg Psych*. 1987;50:511-516.

93. Myers LW. Treatment of multiple sclerosis with ACTH and Corticosteroids. Chapter 6, In: *Treatment of Multiple Sclerosis: Trial, Design, Results, and Future Perspectives*, eds Rudick RA, Goodkin DE. London: Springer Verlag; 1992:135-156.

94. Vanuakes EC, Pineda AA, Weinshenker BG. Meta-analysis of clinical studies of the efficacy of plasma exchange in the treatment of chronic progressive multiple sclerosis. *J Clin Apheresis*. 1995;10:163-170.

95. Weinshenker BG. Therapeutic plasma exchange. In: Rudick RA, Goodkin DG, eds. *Multiple Sclerosis Therapeutics*. London: Martin Dunitz. 1999:323-333.

96. Yudkin PL, Ellison GW, Ghezzi A, et al. Overview of azathioprine treatment in multiple sclerosis. *Lancet*. 1991;338:1051-1055.

97. Hauser SL, Dawson DM, Lehrich JR, et al. Intensive immunosuppression in progressive multiple sclerosis. *N Engl J Med*. 1983;308:173-180.

98. Kappos L, Patzold U, Dommasch D, et al. Cyclosporine versus azathioprine in the long term treatment of multiple sclerosis: results of the German multi-centre study. *Ann Neurol*. 1988;23:56-63.

99. Noseworthy JH, Ebers GC, Vandervoort MK, et al. The impact of blinding on the results of a randomized, placebo-controlled multiple sclerosis clinical trial. *Neurology*. 1994;44:16-20.

100. Devereux C, Troiano R, Zito G, et al. Effect of total lymphoid irradiation on functional status in chronic multiple sclerosis: importance of lymphopenia early after treatment—the pros. *Neurology*. 1988,38(2):32-37.

101. Noseworthy JH, Ebers GC, Gent M. The Canadian cooperative trial of cyclophosphamide and plasma-exchange in progressive multiple sclerosis. *Lancet*. 1991;337:441-446.

102. Paty DW, Ebers GC, eds. *Multiple Sclerosis*. Philadelphia: F.A. Davis; 1998: 475-477.

103. Cendrowski W. Combined therapeutic trial in multiple sclerosis: hydrocortisone hemi succinate with cyclophosphamide or cytosine arabinoside. *Acta Belg Neurolog*. 1973;73:209-219.

104. Drachman DA, Paterson PY, Schmidt RT, Spehlman RF. Cyclophosphamide in exacerbations of multiple sclerosis: therapeutic trial and a strategy for pilot drug studies. *J Neurol*. 1975;38:592-597.

105. Weiner HL, Mackin GA, Orav EJ, et al. Intermittent cyclophosphamide pulse therapy in progressive multiple sclerosis: Final report of the Northeast Cooperative Multiple Sclerosis Treatment Group. *Neurology*. 1993;43:910-918.

106. Noseworthy JH, Ebers GC, Gent M. The Canadian cooperative trial of cyclophosphamide and plasma-exchange in progressive multiple sclerosis. *Lancet*. 1991;337:441-446.

107. Kappos L, Patzold U, Dommasch D, et al. Cyclosporine versus azathioprine in the long term treatment of multiple sclerosis: results of the German multi-centre study. *Ann Neurol*. 1988;23:56-63.

108. Brill V, Allenby K, Midroni G, et al. IGIV in Neurology: Evidence and Recommendations. *Can J Neuro Sci*. 1999;26:139-152.

109. Ellison G. Treatment aimed at modifying the course of multiple sclerosis. In: *Multiple Sclerosis*, McDonald WI, Silberberg DH, eds. London: Butterworths; 1986:153-165.

110. Marie P. *Lectures on Diseases of the Spinal Cord*, trans. Lubbock M. London: New Sydenham Society; 1895;153:134-136.

111. Adams JM. *Multiple Sclerosis: Scars of Childhood: New Horizons and Hope*. Springfield: Charles C. Thomas; 1977.

112. Ho AD, Haas R, Champlin RE, eds. *Hematopoietic Stem Cell Transplantation*. New York: Marcel Dekker; 2000.

113. Kennedy F. On the diagnosis of multiple sclerosis. In: *Multiple Sclerosis and the Demyelinating Diseases*. Proceedings of association for research in nervous and mental disease; 1950;28:524-531.

114. Swank RL. Multiple sclerosis: a correlation of its incidence with dietary fat. *Am J M Sc*. 1950;220:421-430.

115. Swank RL, Lerstad O, Ström A, Backer J. Multiple sclerosis in rural Norway: its geographic and occupational incidence in relation to nutrition. *N Engl J Med*. 1952;246:721-728.

116. Swank RL. Plasma and multiple sclerosis—past and present. In: *Multiple Sclerosis: Immunological, diagnostic and therapeutic aspects*. Rose FC, Jones R, eds. London: John Libbey Eurotext.

117. Agranoff BWA, Goldberg D. Diet and the geographical distribution of multiple sclerosis. *Lancet*. 1974;2:1061-1066.

118. Crane JE. Treatment of multiple sclerosis with fat-soluble vitamins, animal fat and ammonium chloride. *Conn State Med J*. 1950:14:40.

119. Alter M, Yamoor M, Harshe M. Multiple sclerosis and nutrition. *Arch Neurol*. 1974;31:267-272.

120. Nanji AA, Narod S. Multiple sclerosis, latitude and dietary fat: is pork the missing link? *Med Hypoth*. 1986;20:279-282.

121. Malosse D, Perron H, Sasco A, Seigneurin JM. Correlation between milk and dairy product consumption and multiple sclerosis prevalence: a worldwide study. *Neuroepidemiology*. 1992;11:304-312.

122. Lauer K. Dietary changes in temporal relation to multiple sclerosis in the Faeroe Islands: an evaluation of literary sources. *Neuroepidemiology*. 1989;8:200-206.

123. Lauer K. Multiple sclerosis in relation to meat preservation in France and Switzerland. *Neuroepidemiology*. 1989;8:308-315.

124. Lauer K. The food pattern in geographical relation to the risk of multiple sclerosis in the Mediterranean and Near East region. *J Epidemiol Comm Health*. 1991;45:251-252.

125. Lauer K. A possible paradox in the immunology of multiple sclerosis: its apparent lack of "specificity" might provide clues to the etiology. *Med Hypoth*. 1993;40:368-374.

126. Lauer K. A factor-analytical study of the multiple-sclerosis mortality in Hesse and Baden-Wuerttemberg, Germany. *J Public Health*. 1993;1:319-327.

127. Lauer K. The risk of multiple sclerosis in the USA in relation to sociogeographic features: a factor-analytical study. *J Clin Epidemiol*. 1994;47:43-48.

128. Lauer K. Multiple sclerosis in the Old World: the new old map. In: *Multiple Sclerosis in Europe: An Epidemiological Update*. Firnhaber W, Lauer K, eds. Alsbach/Bergstrasse: LTV Press; 1994:14-27.

129. Lauer K. The Fennoscandian focus of multiple sclerosis and dietary factors: an ecological comparison. *L'Arcispedale S. Anna*. 1996;46(suppl):17-18.

130. Lauer K. Diet and multiple sclerosis. *Neurology*. 1997;49:(suppl2):S55-S61.

131. Dworkin RH, Bates D, Miller JHD, Paty DW. Linoleic acid and multiple sclerosis: a reanalysis of three double-blind trials. *Neurology*. 1984;34:1441-1445.

132. Bates D. Dietary supplements in multiple sclerosis: a review. In: *Multiple Sclerosis: Immunological, Diagnostic and Therapeutic Aspects*. London: John Libbey; 1987;179-188.

133. Le Gac P. Nouvelles données sur la sclérose en plaques. *J Méd Bourdeaux*. 1960;137:346.

134. Laignel-Lavastine M, Koressios N-Th. *Sérotherapie hemolytique de la sclérose en plaques*. Paris: Librairie M. Lac; 1932.

135. Alexander L, Loman J, Lesses MF, Green I. Blood and Plasma Transfusions in multiple sclerosis. In: *Multiple Sclerosis and the Demyelinating Disease*. Proceedings of the Association for Research in Nervous and Mental Disease (Dec. 10–11, 1948). Vol 28. Baltimore: Williams and Wilkins; 1950;178-202.

136. Alexander L, Berkeley A, Alexander AM. *Multiple Sclerosis: Prognosis and Treatment*. Springfield, IL: Charles C. Thomas; 1961.

137. Sandyk R. II. Therapeutic effects of alternating current pulsed electromagnetic fields in multiple sclerosis. *J Alt and Comp Med.* 1997;3:(4):365-386.
138. Erbguth FJ, Naumann M. Historical aspects of botulinum toxin: Justinus Kerner (1786-1862) and the "sausage poison." *Neurology.* 1999;53:1850-1853.
139. Edwards A. *Disseminated Sclerosis.* Manchester. John Heywood; 1895.
140. Gray LC. *A Treatise on Nervous and Mental Diseases.* London: HK Lewis; 1893:373-378.
141. Brain WR. Critical review: disseminated sclerosis. *Quart J Med.* 1930;23:343-391.
142. Edmund J, Fog T. Multiple sclerosis—visual and motor instability. *Arch Neurol Psychiat.* 1955;73:316-323.
143. Davis FA. The hot bath test in the diagnosis of multiple sclerosis. *J Mount Sinai Hosp NY.* 1966;33:280-282.
144. Davis FA, Stefoski D, Rush J. Orally administered 4-aminopyridine improves clinical signs in multiple sclerosis. *Ann Neurol.* 1990,27:186-192.
145. Allbutt T. Clifford. On the ophthalmoscopic signs of spinal cord disease. *Lancet.* 1870;1:76-78.
146. MacLaurin H. Case of amblyopia from partial neuritis, treated with subcutaneous injection of strychnia. *NSW Med Gaz.* 1873;3:214.
147. Gowers WR. *A Manual of Medical Ophthalmology.* London: J & A Churchill; 1979.
148. Uhthoff W. Untersuchen über die bei multiplen Herdsclerose vorkommenden Augerstörungen. *Arch Psychiat.* 1890;21:303-410.
149. Glaser G, Merritt HH, Traeger CH. ACTH and cortisone in multiple sclerosis. *Minutes of the Meeting of the Medical Advisory Board.* National Multiple Sclerosis Society; June 1951.
150. Miller HG, Newell DJ, Ridley A. Treatment of multiple sclerosis with corticotrophin (ACTH). *Lancet.* 1961;2:1361-1362.
151. Selhorst JB, Saul RF. Uhthoff and his Syndrome (1800-1895). Editorial. *J Neuroophthalmol.* 1995;15:63-69.
152. Uhthoff, W. Untersuchen über die bei multiplen Herdsclerose vorkommenden Augerstörungen. *Arch Psychiat.* 1890;21:303-410.
153. Selhorst JB, Saul RF. *Uhthoff and his Syndrome (1800–1895).* p. 63-69.
154. Ibid, p. 63-69.
155. Ricklefs G. Uber das Uhthoffsche Symptom bei multipler Sklerose. *Klin Monatsbl Augenheilkd.* 1961;139:385-390.
156. Regan D, Murray TJ, Silver R. Visual acuity and contrast sensitivity in MS: Hidden visual loss. *Brain.* 1977;100:563-579.
157. Selhorst JB, Saul RF. *Uhthoff and his Syndrome:* p. 63-69.
158. Selhorst JB, Saul RF. *Uhthoff and his Syndrome:* p. 63-69.
159. Rae-Grant AD, Eckert NJ, Bartz S, Reed JF. Sensory symptoms of multiple sclerosis: a hidden reservoir of morbidity. *Multiple Sclerosis.* 1999;5:179-183.
160. Ibid. p. 179-183.
161. Lhermitte J, Bollack A, Nicholas M. Les douleurs à type de décharge électrique dans la sclérose en plaques: un cas de forme sensitive de la sclérose multiple. *Rev Neurol. (Paris)* 1924:56-62.
162. Liveson JA, Zimmer AE. A localizing symptom in thoracic myelopathy: a variation of Lhermitte sign. *Ann Intern Med.* 1972;76:769-771.
163. Lhermitte J, Bollack A, Nicholas M. *Les douleurs à type de décharge électrique:* p. 56-62.
164. Murray TJ. Amantadine Therapy for Fatigue in Multiple Sclerosis. *Can J Neuro Sci.* 1985;12(3):251-254.
165. Canadian MS Research Group. A randomized controlled trial of amantadine in fatigue associated with multiple sclerosis. *Can J Neuro Sci.* 1987;14(3):273-278.
166. Matthews WB. Tonic seizures in multiple sclerosis. *Brain.* 1958;81:193-206.
167. Zakrzewska JM. *Trigeminal Neuralgia.* London: Saunders; 1995:7-8.

168. Stenager E, Knudsen L, Jensen K. Historical notes on mental aspects of multiple sclerosis. In: *Mental Disorders and Cognitive Deficits in Multiple Sclerosis*. Jensen K, Knudsen L, Stenager E, Grant I, eds. London: John Libbey; 1989:1-7.

169. Richardson JTE, Robinson A, Robinson I. Cognition and multiple sclerosis: A historical analysis of medical perceptions. *J Hist Neurosci*. 1997;6:302-319.

170. Cruveilhier J. *Medical Tracts*. 1828. Wellcome Library. 621.4.

171. Cruveilhier J. *Anatomie pathologique du corps humain, ou descriptions avc figures lithographiees et coloriees, des diverses alterations morbides dout le corps humain est suceptibles*. Vol 2. Paris: J. B. Baillière; 1835-1842.

172. Cruveilhier J. *Anatomie Descriptive*. 4 Vols on the nervous system with illustrations. Paris: Béchet; 1836-1841.

173. Vulpian EFA. Note sur la sclérose en plaques de la moelle épinière. *Union Méd*. 1866;30:459-465, 475-482, 541-548.

174. Frerich FT. Ueber Hirnsklerose. *Arch für die Gesamte Medizin*. 1849;10:334-350.

175. Valentiner W. Ueber die Sklerose des Gehirns und Rückenmarks. *Deutsche Klin*. 1856147-151, 158-162, 167-169.

176. Morris JC. Case of the late Dr. CW Pennock. *Am J Med Sci*. 1868;56:138-144.

177. MoxonW. Eight cases of insular sclerosis of the brain and spinal cord. *Guy Hosp Rep*. 1875;20:437-478.

178. Seguin EC, Shaw JC, Van Derveer A. A contribution to the pathological anatomy of disseminated cerebro-spinal sclerosis. *J Nerv Ment Dis*. 1878;5:281-293.

179. Wilks S. *Lectures on Diseases of the Nervous System*, delivered at Guy's Hospital. London: J&A Churchill; 1878:282-284.

180. Osler W. Cases of insular sclerosis. *Can Med Surg*. 1880:1-11.

181. Charcot JM. Lectures on the diseases of the nervous system. *Delivered at la Salpêtrière*. Vol. 2. Sigerson G, ed. and trans. London: New Sydenham Society; 1881.

182. Gowers WR. *A Manual of Diseases of the Nervous System*, 2nd ed. Vol. 2. London, J & A Churchill; 1893:544, 557-558.

183. Edwards A. *Disseminated Sclerosis*. Manchester. John Heywood; 1895.

184. Dana CL. *Textbook of Nervous Diseases*. 3rd ed. New York: William Wood; 1894.

185. Müller E. *Die multiple Sklerose des Gehirns and Rückenmarks*. Ihre Pathologie und Behandlung. Jena: Gustav Fischer; 1904.

186. Barbellion WNP (pseudonym for BF Cummings). *The Journal of a Disappointed Man*. London: Chatto and Windus; 1919.

187. Sachs B, Friedman ED. General symptomatology and differential diagnosis of disseminated sclerosis. *Arch Neurol Psychiat*. 1922;7:551-560.

188. Association for Research in Nervous and Mental Disease. *Multiple Sclerosis (Disseminated sclerosis)*. New York: Paul B. Hoeber; 1922.

189. Brown S, Davis TK. The mental symptoms of multiple sclerosis. *Arch Neurol Psychiat*. 1922;7:629-634.

190. Jelliffe SE. Emotional and psychological factors in multiple sclerosis. In: *Multiple Sclerosis: An investigation by the Association for Research in Nervous and Mental Disease*. New York: Paul B. Hoeber; 1921:82-90.

191. Association for Research in Nervous and Mental Disease. *Multiple Sclerosis (Disseminated sclerosis)*. New York: Paul B. Hoeber; 1922: 129-130.

192. Claude H. Quelques remarques sur le diagnostic de la sclérose en plaques. *Rev Neurol*. 1924;31:727-730.

193. Cottrell SS, Wilson SAK. The affective symptomatology of disseminated sclerosis. *J Neurol Psychopath*. 1926;7:1-30.

194. Brain WR. Critical review: disseminated sclerosis. *Quart J Med*. 1930;23:343-391.

195. Wilson SAK. Some problems in neurology. II. Pathological laughing and crying. *J Neurol Psychopath*. 1924;4:299-333.

196. Wilson SAK. Some problems in neurology. II. Pathological laughing and crying. *J Neurol Psychopath*. 1924;4:299-333.

197. Ombredane A. *Sue les troubles mentaux de la sclérose en plaques*. Thesis. Paris: Presses Universitaires de France; 1929.

198. Berrios GE, Quemada JI, Andre G. Ombredane and the psychiatry of multiple sclerosis: a conceptual and statistical history. *Comp Psychiat*. 1990;31(5):438-446.

199. Arbuse DI. Psychotic manifestations in disseminated sclerosis. *J Mount Sinai Hos*. 1938; Nov/Dec: 403-410.

200. Sugar C, Nadell R. Mental symptoms in multiple sclerosis. *J Nerv Ment Dis*. 1943;98: 267-280.

201. Borberg NC, Zahle V. On the psychopathology of disseminated sclerosis. *Acta Psychol et Neuro*. 1946;21:75-89.

202. Pratt RTC. An investigation of the psychiatric aspects of disseminated sclerosis. *J Neurol Neurosurg Psychiat*. 1951;14:326-335.

203. Rabins PV. Euphoria in Multiple sclerosis. In: *Mental Disorders and Cognitive Deficits in Multiple Sclerosis*. Jensen K, Knudsen L, Stenager LE, Grant I, eds. London: John Libbey;1989:119-120.

204. Stenager E, Knudsen L, Jensen K. Historical notes on mental aspects of multiple sclerosis. In: *Mental disorders and cognitive deficits in multiple sclerosis*. Jensen K, Knudsen L, Stenager E, Grant I, eds. London: John Libbey; 1989:1-7.

205. Stenager E. Historical and psychiatric aspects of multiple sclerosis. *Acta Psychiat Scand*. 1991;84:398.

206. Rao SM, Leo GJ, Ellington I, et al. Cognitive dysfunction in MS. *Neurology*. 1991;41(I): 692-696, (II):685-691.

207. Archibald CJ, Fisk JD. Information processing efficiency in patients with multiple sclerosis. *J Clin Exp Neuropsych*. 2000;22:686-701.

208. Stenager E, Knudsen L, Jensen K. Historical notes on mental aspects of multiple sclerosis. In: *Mental disorders and cognitive deficits in multiple sclerosis*. Jensen K, Knudsen L, Stenager E, Grant I, eds. London: John Libbey; 1989:1-7.

209. Richardson JTE. Cognition in MS. International Society for the History of Medicine. 1st annual meeting; May 8, 1996. Buffalo, NY.

210. Rao SM, Leo GJ, Ellington I, et al. Cognitive dysfunction in MS. *Neurology*. 1991;41(I):692-696, (II):685-691.

211. Kolb LC. Multiple sclerosis in the American negro. *Arch Neurol*. 1942;47:413-416.

212. Kennedy F. On the diagnosis of multiple sclerosis. In: *Multiple Sclerosis and the Demyelinating Diseases*. Proceedings of Association for Research in Nervous and Mental Disease. (Dec. 10–11, 1948). Vol. 28. Baltimore: Williams and Wilkins; 1950;524-531.

213. Johnson KP. *The John Jay Dystel Lecture*. San Diego, CA: American Academy of Neurology; May 2000.

214. Herndon RM, Murray TJ. Proceedings of the International Conference on Therapeutic Trials in Multiple Sclerosis. *Arch Neurol*. 1983;40:663-710.

215. Herndon RM, Murray TJ. Proceedings of the International Conference on Therapeutic Trials in Multiple Sclerosis. *Arch Neurol*. 1983;40:663-710.

216. Rudick RA, Cookfair DL. Conduct of a clinical trial in multiple sclerosis. In: *Multiple Sclerosis: Clinical and Pathogenic Basis*. Cedric S, Raine HF, McFarlane WW, eds. Tourtellotte. London: Chapman and Hall; 1997:341-353.

217. Johnson KP. The historical development of interferons as multiple sclerosis therapies. *J Mol Med*. 1997;75(2):89-94.

218. Issacs A, Lindenmann J. Virus interference I: the interferon. *Proc Roy Soc Lond*. 1957;147:258-267.

219. Nagano Y, Kojima Y. Inhibition de l'infection vaccinale par un facteur liquide dans le tissu infect par le virus homologue. *C R Soc Biol*. 1958;152:1627-1627.

220. Cantell K. *The Story of Interferon: the Ups and Downs in the Life of Scientist.* Singapore: World Scientific; 1998.
221. Wheelock EF, Sibley WA. Circulating virus, interferon and antibody after vaccination with the 17-D strain of yellow fever virus. *New Engl J Med.* 1965;173:194-198.
222. Moses H, Sriram S. Interferon beta and the cytokine trail: where are we going? *Neurology.* 1999;52:1729-1730.
223. Cantell K. *The Story of Interferon: the Ups and Downs in the Life of Scientist.* Singapore: World Scientific; 1998.
224. Jacobs L, Johnson KP. A brief history of the use of interferons as treatment of multiple sclerosis. *Arch Neurol.* 1994;51:1245-1252.
225. Johnson KP. The historical development of interferons as multiple sclerosis therapies. *J Mol Med.* 1997;75 (2):89-94.
226. Paty DW, Ebers GC, eds. *Multiple Sclerosis.* Philadelphia: F.A. Davis; 1998.
227. Jacobs L, O'Malley J, Freedman A, Ekes R. Intrathecal interferon reduces exacerbations of multiple sclerosis. *Science.* 1981;214:1026-1028.
228. Jacobs L, O'Malley J, Freedman A, Ekes R. Intrathecal interferon in multiple sclerosis. *Arch Neurol.* 1982;39:609-615.
229. Johnson KP. The historical development of interferons as multiple sclerosis therapies. *J Mol Med.* 1997;75(2):89-94.
230. Johnson KP. *The John Jay Dystel Lecture.* San Diego, CA: American Academy of Neurology; 2000.
231. Ververken D, Carton H, Billiau A. Intrathecal administration of interferon in MS patients. In: *Humoral Immunity in Neurological Disease.* Karcher D, Lowenthal A, Strosberg AD, eds. New York: Plennum. 1979:625-627.
232. Abreu SL. Suppression of experimental allergic encephalomyelitis by interferon. *Immunol Invest.* 1982;11:1-7.
233. Abreu SL, et al. Inhibition of passive localized allergic encephalomyelitis by interferon. *Int Arch Allergy Appl Immunol.* 1983;72:30-33.
234. Panitch H, Hirsch R, Schindler R. Treatment of multiple sclerosis with gamma interferon: exacerbations associated with activation of the immune system. *Neurology.* 1987;37:1097-1102.
235. Knobler RL, Panitch HS, Braheny SL, et al. Systemic alpha interferon therapy in multiple sclerosis. *Neurology.* 1984;34:1273-1279.
236. Jacobs L, O'Malley JA, Freeman A, Ekes R, Reese PA. Intrathecal interferon in the treatment of multiple sclerosis: patient follow-up. *Arch Neurol.* 1985;42:841-847.
237. Jacobs L, Salazar AM, Herndon R, et al. Multicenter double-blind study of effect of intrathecally administered natural human fibroblast interferon on exacerbations of multiple sclerosis. *Lancet.* 1986;2:1411-1413.
238. Jacobs L, Salazar AM, Herndon R, et al. Intrathecally administered natural human fibroblast interferon reduces exacerbations of multiple sclerosis: results of a multicenter double-blind study. *Arch Neurol.* 1987;44:589-595.
239. Johnson KP. *The John Jay Dystel Lecture.* American Academy of Neurology. San Diego, CA: 2000.
240. Sibley WA, and other members of the IFNB MS Study Group. Interferon-bea 1b is effective in relapsing remitting multiple sclerosis: clinical results of a multicenter, randomized, double blind trial. *Neurology.* 1993;43:655-661.
241. Johnson KP. *The John Jay Dystel Lecture.* San Diego, CA: American Academy of Neurology; 2000.
242. Jacobs L, Cookfair D, Rudick R, Herndon R, Richert J, Salazar AM, et al. Intramuscular interferon beta-1a for disease progression in relapsing multiple sclerosis. *Ann Neurol.* 1996;39(3):285-294.

243. Rudick R, Goodkin D, Jacobs L, et al. The impact of interferon beta-1a on neurologic disability in relapsing multiple sclerosis. *Neurology.* 1997;49:358-363.

244. Simon J, Jacobs L, Campion M, et al. and the Multiple Sclerosis Collaborative Research Group. Magnetic resonance studies of intramuscular interferon ß-1a for relapsing multiple sclerosis. *Ann Neurol.* 1998;43:79-87.

245. Simon JH, Jacobs LD, Campion MS, et al. and the Multiple Sclerosis Collaborative Research Group. A longitudinal study of brain atrophy in relapsing multiple sclerosis. *Neurology.* 1999;53:139-148.

246. Jacobs L, Beck R, Brownscheidle C, et al. A profile of patients at high risk for he development of clinically definite MS (CDMS): The first report of the CHAMPS Study. *Neurology.* 1999;52(S2):A495.

247. Knobler RL, Panitch HS, Braheny SL, et al. Systemic alpha interferon therapy in multiple sclerosis. *Neurology.* 1984;34:1273-1279.

248. Knobler RL. Interferon Beta-1b (Betaseron) Treatment of Multiple Sclerosis. In: *Interferon Therapy of Multiple Sclerosis.* Ed. Anthony T. Reder. New York: Marcel Dekker; 1997:353-413.

249. Moses H, Sriram S. Interferon beta and the cytokine trail: where are we going? *Neurology.* 1999;52:1729-1730.

250. Arnon R. The development of Cop I (Copaxone), an innovative drug for the treatment of multiple sclerosis: personal reflections. *Immunology Letters.* 1996;50:1-15.

251. Arnon R. The development of Cop I (Copaxone), an innovative drug for the treatment of multiple sclerosis: personal reflections. *Immunology Letters.* 1996;50:1-15.

252. Bornstein MB, Miller A, Slagle S, et al. A pilot trial of COP 1 in exacerbating-remitting multiple sclerosis. *N Engl J Med.* 1987;317:408-414.

253. Bornstein MB, Miller A, Slagle S, et al. A placebo-controlled, double-blind, randomized, two centre pilot trial of Cop 1 in chronic progressive multiple sclerosis. *Neurology.* 1991;41:533-539.

254. Lublin FD, Reingold SC, et al. Placebo-controlled clinical trials in multiple sclerosis: ethical considerations. *Ann Neurol.* 2001;49:677-681.

255. *McAlpine's Multiple Sclerosis.* Compston A, ed. London: Churchill Livingstone; 1998.

256. Polman CH, Thompson AJ, Murray TJ, McDonald WI. *Multiple Sclerosis: The Guide to Treatment and Management.* 5th ed. New York: Demos; 2001.

257. *Therapeutic Claims in Multiple Sclerosis.* IFMSS. New York: Demos Publications, 1982, 1988, 1993, 1996. (5th ed. under new title: *Multiple Sclerosis: The Guide to Treatment and Management.* New York: Demos; 2001.)

258. Brain WR. Critical review: disseminated sclerosis. *Quart J Med.* 1930;23:343-391.

259. Thomas, Richard. *Multiple Sclerosis: a comprehensive guide to effective treatment.* Brisbane: Element Books; 1996.

260. Bowling AC. *Alternative Medicine in Multiple Sclerosis.* New York: Demos; 2001.

261. Neubauer RA. Exposure of multiple sclerosis patients to hyperbaric oxygen at ATA: a preliminary report. *J Florida Med Assn.* 1980;67:498-504.

262. Fischer BH, Marks M, Reich T. Hyperbaric oxygen treatment of multiple sclerosis. *New Eng J Med.* 1983;308:181-186.

263. Barnes, MP, Bates D, Cartlidge NEF, et al. Hyperbaric oxygen and multiple sclerosis: short term results of a placebo-controlled, double-blind trial. *Lancet.* 1985;1:297-300.

264. Webster C, McIver C, Allen JP. *Long-term hyperbaric oxygen therapy for multiple sclerosis patients: two year results in 128 patients.* Stanstead, U.K. ARMS Education Service; 1992.

265. Clarke, Jane G. *Multiple Sclerosis: a new theory concerning cause and cure.* Sheffield: New Age Science Press; 1983.

266. Loder, Cari. *Standing in the Sunshine: the story of the multiple sclerosis breakthrough.* London: Century Ltd.; 1996.

267. Bowling AC. *Alternative Medicine in Multiple Sclerosis*. New York: Demos; 2001.
268. Head Hy. *Collection on Henry Head: volume of records of his examination of pilgrims to Lourdes, 1895*. London: Wellcome Library, documents PP/HEA.
269. Ibid.
270. Compston A. The Story of Multiple Sclerosis. Chapter 1 in: *McAlpine's Multiple Sclerosis*. London: Churchill Livingstone; 1998:3-42.
271. Paty DW. The Canadian Experience: Multiple Sclerosis clinics versus traditional medical care, and what made multiple sclerosis research flourish in Canada? In: *Advances in MS Clinical Research and Therapy*. Editors Fredrickson and H. Klink. Dunits; 1999.
272. Barbellion WNP. (pseudonym for BF Cummings). *The Journal of a Disappointed Man*. London: Chatto and Windus; 1919.

16

Multiple Sclerosis and the Public: Societies, Narratives, and the Media

THE MULTIPLE SCLEROSIS SOCIETY

"It is possible that the cause of the disease lies buried somewhere in these lengthy protocols waiting to be found by anyone ingenious enough to unearth it."

Dr. Henry Miller, 1972

An important impetus for change and encouragement of research in MS in the last 50 years has been the formation of the MS societies in several countries. Although there was some organization of activities around MS and support for research in the 1920s, it was on an institutional level, such as the Commonwealth Fund, which supported MS research at New York Neurological Institute. The Commonwealth Fund recognized that neurology was relatively poorly supported by foundations, and the NYNI decided to concentrate efforts on MS and epilepsy.[1] There was a rapid increase in the number of articles related to MS in the medical literature in the 1930s and 1940s, and after World War II, research dollars going to MS projects increased substantially. Despite this,

Putnam and others complained in the 1950s that the public, well aware of the problem of polio, had little inkling of MS that was afflicting young adults. They felt the public needed to be aware of this illness and contribute to efforts to find a cause and cure for MS, which affected so many people.[2]

The first step was taken independently by Sylvia Lawry, who was distressed about the progression of MS disability in her brother, Bernard Freidman, and the lack of responsiveness of his physicians to his problems and his questions about the disease.* She placed an advertisement in *The New York Times* on May 1, 1945 with the plaintive request:

> *"Multiple Sclerosis. Will anyone recovered from it please communicate with patient. T272 Times."*

From the number of responses, it was apparent to Lawry that there should be an organization to focus interest and support on MS. She brought together 20 leaders in neurology on March 11, 1946 to help set directions for a new organization and the resulting society was incorporated that year as the Association for Advancement of Research in Multiple Sclerosis (AARMS), renamed the next year as the National Multiple Sclerosis Society (NMSS). That year, chapters were chartered in California and Connecticut, beginning what would become by 2001 a truly national organization, with 135 chapters, branches, and divisions, raising funds to support $25 million for 300 projects annually.

Looking at the medical literature to see who was most prominent and would give the organization a high profile in the medical community as well as provide the society with advice, Lawry selected Tracy Jackson Putnam as the first medical director, with other prominent neurologists added to the board, including Henry Woltman of the Mayo Clinic and Leo Alexander of Boston. Soon after, Lawry involved Houston Merritt as an advisor. Although she felt the success of the organization would be through the efforts of patients and their families, and made initial efforts to have each member recruit more and more patients, friends, and fami-

---

*Her life became dedicated to her brother's welfare and on a larger scale to the welfare of all who suffered with MS. At the beginning, she saw that answers would be found through long-term commitment to research. Bernard continued to worsen and died in 1973.

lies, Lawry also was tireless in capturing the interest of well-connected politicians, publishers, and corporate leaders to assist in the effort. She involved Henry Kaiser (whose son had MS); Mrs. Lou Gehrig (although her husband died of ALS, not MS); Shirley Temple, Mrs. John D. Rockefeller, Mrs. Dwight D. Eisenhower, and Senator John F. Kennedy in the first decade of the organization's rapid growth.[3] Like many of the early volunteers, Kennedy had a relative with MS, his cousin Ann Gargan, and he was campaign chairman for the Massachusetts chapter and later national campaign chairman. He continued his interest in the Society when he was in the White House.

In the first year, 600 members were recruited, but three years later, the number was 15,000, and a decade later was over 120,000. Clearly the organizational skills and single-minded drive of Sylvia Lawry resulted in the rapid emergence of the National Multiple Sclerosis Society, but Talley also argued that the increasing number of MS patients being diagnosed was an important factor, since many people now knew someone with MS. In addition, the postwar mood was one of excitement and growth and seemed open to the promise of medical research and disease crusades.

The early strategy for research support by the Society was two-pronged—to encourage the public to donate funds, which had the additional benefit of increasing awareness, and to encourage government to increase support for MS research.

At the 1948 ARNMD meeting in New York, with 65 of the leading American neurologists and MS researchers giving their perspective on the disease, a sequel to the landmark 1921 meeting, the newly formed National Multiple Sclerosis Society took a prominent place at the table. Although the Society was only three years old, the new medical director, Cornelius H. Traeger, was able to claim that his organization had become the focal point for all activities in the field on MS. He continued:

"It is our responsibility to furnish physicians with the latest available information regarding the diagnosis and treatment of multiple sclerosis. It is our responsibility to bring a message of optimism and hope to patients; their families and friends. It is our responsibility to publish literature for laymen that will help them in combating the problems

which are presented daily for patient care. It is our problem to raise funds to support basic and clinical research in the field of demyelinating diseases and to coordinate such research activities. We invite applications for grants-in-aid for research projects to be pursued in the demyelinating diseases."[4]

This young organization was up and running with a clear set of goals, swept along by the personal persuasion of Sylvia Lawry and the cadre of influential and talented people she was able to bring to the cause. It was a mutually beneficial relationship: Lawry needed the expertise and the acceptance of the profession, and they needed Society support for their research and their young faculty.

From the start, the MS Society began to distribute grants to projects recommended by the medical board, and to support clinics in Boston, New York, Albany, Los Angeles, New Orleans, and Washington. The Society felt that a clinic was important, because around it they could build services, education, research, and fundraising. Talley spoke of a "movement culture," which could be built around the clinic.[5] The philosophy of leaving 60 percent of the funds raised in the local area to support the clinics, services, and research helped encourage the local commitment. This 60/40 split was often a source of contention in some chapters, but Lawry's persuasion and diplomatic skills kept the principle in place. The first grant support from the MS Society went to Dr. Elvin Kabat for his research on cerebrospinal fluid (CSF) in MS. The organization was effective in capturing the interest of newspapers and magazines and actively fed the media with personal stories that showed the need for more research, all with a message of hope for the future.

The second approach of the new organization was to pressure government to support MS research and to enlist the power and influence of the National Institutes of Health (NIH). There was enthusiasm in the postwar period for matching early successes with new "miracle" drugs, and for pursuing medical research as a national security strategy in the cold war.[7] There was a growing feeling that science could provide answers to the vexing medical problems of cancer, heart disease, and MS, if more money, more research projects, and more people could be committed to the research cause. Talley has outlined the extensive efforts of government during this time, when medical research became equivalent to another public works project, like roads, bridges, and dams. In 1949, the National Multiple Sclerosis Act came before a Senate Subcommittee, sponsored by Senator Charles Tobey, R, New Hampshire, whose daughter had MS. Arguing a moral imperative, he said that if the government could spend billions every month to kill people (World War II), surely it could devote whatever millions were needed to solve the problem of MS. The medical profession was pointedly criticized for having ignored this important disease, since there were no effective treatments and the knowledge of the disease had not advanced much in the previous century. Tracy Putnam countered this criticism, while defending the need for more research support. He acknowledged the many clinical investigators who had worked on the problem of MS for the last few decades, and noted the support for MS research at the New York Neurological Institute by the Commonwealth Fund in the 1920–1940 era. It was not neurologists who ignored the problem, he said, but the NIH and the Public Health Service, which had neglected MS and most other neurological problems. Not surprisingly, the NIH did not support another separate institute, especially one dedicated to a specific disease, so the NMSS changed its approach and instead fostered the formation of the National Institute for Neurological Diseases and Blindness (NINDB), which came into being in 1950. Over the next three years, almost half the funding requests to NINDB were for MS, and Tally makes the point that this was not a situation of one organization pressuring another, but an intertwining and interrelationship between the organizations and the people involved that made it look like one organization.[6]

The linking of the efforts of the NMSS and the NINDB developed a national approach to funding research, which replaced the local foundation approach; although it may not have been unique to neurology, it certainly forged a strong interrelationship that could capture research dollars into a singular pot aimed at fostering the research goals of a growing neurological profession.

Controversy arises in any agency that judges and awards grants and it came early to the NMSS when Dr. Leo Alexander was outraged that he

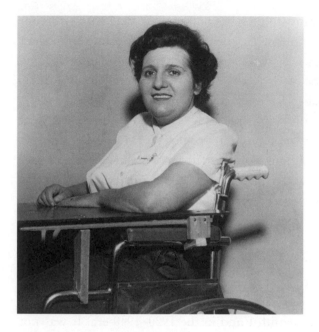

Figure 16.1 Evelyn Gotlieb Opal initiated a local MS group in Montreal with the encouragement of Sylvia Lawry, founder of the MS Society of Canada. (Courtesy of the National MS Society.)

was turned down by the Board. He marshaled the local Boston Chapter, which became upset that he might lose his clinic. And against NMSS policy, the Chapter gave him the research funds. Alexander made things difficult, but Lawry and the Society prevailed.

> *"... American neurologists quickly recognized the opportunity increased research dollars meant for their specialization and through a system of interlocking directorates neurologists as a specialty colonized and controlled the research dollars of the NMSS and the NINDB. This had the effect of nationalizing the financing, planning, and control of MS research in the United States and also helped to solidify hierarchies in the specialty of neurology in America."*
>
> Colin Talley, 1999

Shortly after the NMSS was underway, steps were being taken by two groups in Montreal, to develop a society to foster research in MS and to make the disease better known. Evelyn Opal,* a Montreal housewife with MS, heard of Lawry's New York group and began to raise funds for

---

* There is an annual Opal Award for caregivers given by the MS Society of Canada.

MS, forming a chapter of the American group, called the Dr. Colin Russel Chapter, named for her physician at the Montreal Neurological Institute (MNI). Another Montreal patient, Harry Bell, an engineer, formed a second group he called the Canadian MS Research Organization. Lawry brought them together and in 1948, the Multiple Sclerosis Society of Canada was formed with Dr. Wilder Penfield as honorary chairman of the scientific advisory committee. The first grant from the fledgling society went to Dr. Roy Swank and Dr. Donald McEachern of the MNI for work on lipids and diet in MS. One grant per year was given for the first two decades, and then support for research expanded each year. To develop United States–Canada links, Roy Swank of Montreal was appointed by the MS Society of Canada as a liaison member on the NMSS board, beginning a link that continues today on the research advisory boards of the two organizations.

In 1951, Dr. Houston Merritt asked one of his first-year residents, Dr. William Sibley, to compile all the information on therapies of MS for a report to the NMSS. This became the basis of a chapter in the *Handbook of Clinical Neurology* and started Sibley on a lifetime of research in MS that continues to this day.

Lord Howard of Glossop, whose wife had MS, extended an invitation to Lawry to visit London and meet with Richard Cave, member of the legal staff of the House of Lords, whose wife also suffered with MS. The Multiple Sclerosis Society of Great Britain and Northern Ireland was formed. The first annual report of the MS Society of Great Britian (Ireland was added to the title later) states that it was founded after a visit by Sylvia Lawry and was a "foster child" of the American group. It was decided on the advice of the medical advisory board to adopt the term *multiple sclerosis* rather that the term *disseminated sclerosis*, then widely used in the U.K. to be in line with the usage of the Americans, Canadians and Europeans. This was soon after confirmed by the title *Multiple Sclerosis* for the landmark book by McAlpine, Compston, and Lumsden. The Board also decided to adopt the symbol of the yale key to represent the goal of unlocking the mystery of MS. For some months, the Society consisted only of two members, Winnifed Payne and the founder-chairman Richard Cave. In July, a meeting of 30 interested persons was held and after some "unglamorous spade work," a public meeting was held on December 2, 1953 at the Chenil Galleries, Chelsea Town Hall. Among those present were the Minister of Health, Iain McLeod, who gave the keynote speech; the founder and Chairman, Richard Cave, and Dr. Douglas McAlpine, consultant at the Middlesex Hospital (and Mrs. Cave's neurologist) and chairman of the medical advisory board. Compston notes that Dr. Arnold Carmichael was also present, but mentioned in the minutes only as Mr. B.* There were 28 members at the time of the meeting, but McAlpine recruited others to join the effort. It had been announced that the MRC would accept grant applications in the area of MS, but since none was received, the new Society had the dual challenge of promoting and funding MS research, as well as providing services to patients and families.

Following the Chenil Gallery meeting, the Society was registered as a charity and offices were opened at 9 Grosvenor Square, London, at the headquarters of the British Red Cross, which was most supportive of the novice group. Although the first annual report suggests that progress was slow, by April 1954, a full-time secretary, E.W.I. Mason, was hired to organize groups throughout the country. In the annual report of 1954, the Society boasted 4,000 members, a new medical advisory body, and plans to fund the first MS research unit. The second annual report listed the medical advisory panel, which included such names as R.S. Allison, Arnold Carmichael, Hugh Garland, Ludwig Guttman, Reginald Kelly, Douglas McAlpine, Henry Miller, J.D. Spillane, and C. Worster-Drought.

In the first two years, Society policies about research support were being determined, and although Douglas McAlpine was not in favor of specific research grants, it was decided to follow the pattern developing in the United States and Canadian societies. In 1955, Charles Lumsden was given £10,000 for his work; the next year, three grants were given to the Newcastle group for a survey of MS in north east England; a study of the psychiatric aspects of MS; and support for training of a neuropathologist who would be added to the Newcastle MS team.[7] Other more con-

---

*Carmichael was the neurologist who had been commissioned by the MRC many years earlier to assess the controversial virus research by James Purves-Stewart and Kathleen Chevassut at the Westminster Hospital.

troversial ventures, included the support in these years for the vaccine therapies of the Dublin pathologist Dr. William M. Crofton, who moved to London as a vaccine therapist. Two years after the Society began, Dr. John Walford joined its administration and by the time he retired in 1994, the Society had committed £85 million to research and services.

The argument about support for care versus research was a common one in the early days of many MS societies. It continues today over the relative levels of support for each and reached a high point on the medical advisory board in London when Ludwig Guttman of the Stoke Mandeville Rehabilitation Hospital was turned down for a grant about management of MS. The board considered research about care outside of its mandate to support research on the cause of the disease. Dr. Guttman (later Sir Ludwig Guttman) resigned from the board. Each of these national organizations was formed with the encouragement and enthusiastic support of Sylvia Lawry. Each appointed leading clinicians in MS to sit on the advisory committees that awarded the results of the first fundraising efforts. Year by year, these grants increased and encouraged more clinicians, and later basic scientists, to enter the field of MS research.

Following the controversy over the dismissal of Professor E.J. Field and a feeling that the MS Society was too conservative and slow in funding research into projects such as the LeGac therapy, sunflower seed oil therapy, and Field's predictive test and treatment for children at risk, a breakaway group formed: the Multiple Sclerosis Action Group (MSAG), later called Action for Research into Multiple Sclerosis (ARMS). It represented patients and their families, impatient with the pace of medical research, but after years of supporting projects of interest to the patients, such as diets and hyperbaric oxygen therapy, the group failed.

Sylvia Lawry was not through organizing for MS. By 1967, one-third of the NMSS funds were supporting research outside the United States, and she decided to develop an international organization to coordinate activities of various national organizations and encourage efforts to develop new national societies in Western Europe, Latin America, Japan, Australia, New Zealand, and Eastern Europe. At the Eighth International Conference of Neurology in Vienna in September 1965, she proposed the formation of an international organization, a proposal sup-

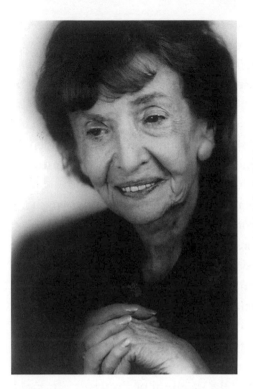

Figure 16.2 Because Sylvia Lawry was distressed at the lack of information available for her brother Bernard, who suffered from MS, she initiated an organization that became the National MS Society. (Courtesy of the National MS Society.)

ported by Sir Richard Cave, William Breed, and Dr. Houston Merritt, who was then the chairman of the NMSS board. The group was initiated the next year as the International Federation of Multiple Sclerosis Societies. Headquartered in London, it currently has 43 members.*

An important way to increase attention toward MS was to make government, health agencies, physicians, and the public aware of how common the disease was in the general population. The NMSS always used a figure for MS that was guesswork, and maintained it even when the evidence suggested lower figures. In the 1948–1951 period, an epidemiologic study jointly sponsored by the NMSS and the USPHS under Leonard C. Kolb, found a figure well below the NMSS publicity. The NMSS ignored the results, as it did in the studies it sponsored by Leonard Kurland. It is interesting that since the 1950s, the Society had maintained that there were 300,000 Americans suffering with MS. That was still the

---

*In 2001, it was renamed the Multiple Sclerosis International Federation (MSIF).

figure in 1995, despite changing population and demographics. In the 1950s, the NMSS developed the concept that the disease was more common than polio, a disease all Americans feared. It also developed a military metaphor for the battle against the disease, suggesting it needed to be fought by the individual and the collective. In addition, it fostered the idea of individual struggle and achievement: the patient overcoming the disease by personal will power and determination.

Though it supported the development of more and more chapters and other national MS societies, and later a federation of these societies, the NMSS was not so encouraging toward other MS organizations outside its circle. In 1952, a separate group formed in Chicago dedicated to the support of research at Northwestern University, calling itself the MS Foundation, later the Multiple Sclerosis Foundation of America, which had a distinct national ring to it. This caused great concern at the National MS Society in New York and led to some testy negotiations attempting to bring the group within the NMSS fold. Lawry and her advisors argued that the Chicago group should become a chapter of the NMSS to gain the benefits of an experienced medical advisory board and a process of independent evaluation of the research to be funded. The Chicago group wanted to do what it wished with its funds, unfettered by the "Eastern" organization. The NMSS responded by forming a local NMSS Chicago chapter, to have its place on the local scene, but with the NMSS imprimatur.[8]

When the Consortium of MS Centers was initiated by Dr. Jack Conomy at the Cleveland Clinic with a small group of American and Canadian clinic directors, to foster the professional education of the many disciplines involved in MS research and care, the NMSS was cool to the new organization, even though this activity had not been a major interest for the Society in the past. The NMSS was even less enthusiastic about the rise of the National MS Society (NMSS) in the mid 1980s, the Multiple Sclerosis Foundation in the late 1990s, the European Platform for MS, and the recently formed Multiple Sclerosis Society of America. It is reasonable to ask if this is just a turf war or whether the formation of more and more organizations with overlapping and often duplicating efforts is not just wasteful of energy and resources, especially since the groups often seek out the same funding sources and confuse the public.

From a few thousand dollars to many millions of dollars per year, the MS societies supported basic science, clinical research, epidemiology, psychosocial research, and clinical care. There is little question that the current vibrant research effort focused on all aspects of MS has developed because there was an MS society on each side of the Atlantic supporting and funding the best efforts in research.

In concluding this brief and selective review of the early contributors to the understanding of MS, I acknowledge their pioneer efforts and vision of researchers, and that of the MS societies that support their work. The coming advances in MS are likely to be written by the clinicians and researchers who are supported in their work by the MS societies of the world.

Sylvia Lawry

As this book was in final draft, we were informed that Sylvia Lawry died in New York City, age 85, after a long illness. The advances in MS over the last half century are a fitting memorial to her life dedicated to persons with MS.

Lawry served as Executive Director of the National Multiple Sclerosis Society until 1982 and secretary of the IFMSS until 1997, but continued to serve the NMSS and the cause of MS until her final illness.

The MS community of patients, families and professionals owes her a great debt.

MS AND THE PUBLIC

In the 19th century, multiple sclerosis was thought at first to be curiosity, and by the turn of the century, there were indications from studies in Berlin, Edinburgh, and New York that it might be more common; but it was unknown to the general public and little information was available even to those suffering from the disease.

Perhaps the first writing that made the disease known to the public was the diary of B.F. Cummings, written under the pseudonym W.N.P. Barbellion, published in 1919 as *The Diary of a Disappointed Man*, followed by *The Last Diary*.[9] There was interest in the author and the book and some suspected it might have been written by H.G. Wells, who had reviewed the book. This work gave the public an inkling of the tragic life of a young man just beginning a promising career, and the depressing impact of the disease on his plans and his relationships.

Neurologists had such a negative view of the disease that they were reluctant to give any patient "the death sentence;" they recognized no form of therapy altered the eventual outcome of the disease. Barbellion was not told his diagnosis, even at the time he was becoming disabled, and had to learn the answer by subterfuge, looking at his chart "when the physician stepped out for a few moments." In the meantime, his wife had been told the diagnosis, but kept this secret as well. In his era, families shared the belief, taught to some extent by physicians, that the truth would rob patients of all hope and cause the disease to worsen. This view persisted in some physicians, perhaps even until today, so that they do not reveal their suspicions early in the disease.

The view that the patient should be kept in the dark about the diagnosis was repeated by McAlpine and his coauthors in the early editions of their book on MS.[10] They wrote that there was no reason to change the suggestion that the patient with multiple sclerosis should be kept ignorant of the diagnosis, and this policy should be continued in the case of a young unmarried adult. They realized that "people nowadays" were becoming aware of the disease, so a rational explanation should be given, but obscuring the real diagnosis by indicating that it was the early stage of a disorder of the nervous system, which might clear up with adequate rest. They felt patients should be told that good habits would reduce the tendency to relapse. Although this approach was adequate in most cases, if a patient wants a specific diagnosis, it should be given, along with a warning not to believe everything printed about the disease.

> *"In fine, one should no more tell our patients they have multiple sclerosis than we should tell them they have inoperable cancer. Hope is an emotion in its own right, and the physicians may be wrong.*
>
> *When I have to make the diagnosis of multiple sclerosis, I make it to the relations, not to the patient; and I try to defend the patient from*

hearing the name because once the name is heard, it is vested with lamentable result. If I were sure the patient had multiple sclerosis, I would try and prevent them from getting married. If I were sure that married persons had multiple sclerosis, I would say that they ought to try not to become pregnant. I have seen confinement have a very bad effect on multiple sclerosis."

Foster Kennedy, 1948[11]

Houston Merritt immediately responded to Foster Kennedy's recommendation for noncommunication to the patient with his similar approach:

"And I certainly agree with him that the diagnosis should never be told to the patient unless it is absolutely essential to that patient for the arrangement of his life, and that the facts should be explained to the family."

Houston Merritt, 1948[12]

An anonymous neurologist writing on behalf of the U.K. MS Society in 1970 still advocated this approach. "In an early case, the diagnosis

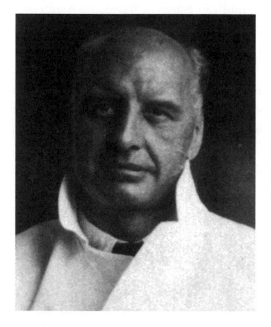

Figure 16.3 Foster Kennedy was a prominent neurologist; remembered for his eponymous syndrome, he was an advisor and supporter of the developing MS Society. (From the collection of Lady Butterfield.)

should only be disclosed to the patient if he or she was a mature and responsible person," but the family should be given full information.

The greatest change in public education came from the formation of the MS Society by Sylvia Lawry, first in the United States, and shortly afterward in Canada, Great Britain, Australia, and many continental European countries. The Society had major goals of supporting research but also patient and public education. Its activities have done more than any others to bring MS and its individual and social impact into public consciousness. As a result, it is not uncommon now for young people who develop neurological symptoms to suspect they might have MS because it is now widely known by the public that young people develop this neurological disease. Not surprisingly, this is more common in those who have a family history of the disorder, who know someone with MS, are medical personnel, or work with MS patients or for the MS Society.[13]

Beginning in the 1950s and increasing in number ever since are illness narratives by those who suffer from MS. Honor Wyatt and George Ellidge wrote *Why Pick on Us* in 1958.[14] Renate Rubenstein, in writing her story referred to the Yiddish word "emmes," which means truth.[15] As a well-known Dutch columnist and activist, she was able to communicate her way of managing. She said at one point that MS was a "whimsical" disease as you were never sure where you were with it. Sometimes feeling old and shamed by what the disease was doing to her, she tried many forms of therapy. It is not surprising that she advocated that patients tell doctors about whatever new therapy they try—and if the doctor had a problem with it, she advocated changing doctors.

MS challenges all aspects of the life of those with the disease, as evidenced in the books they write about their disease, but the struggles of caregivers are less often acknowledged or reflected in print. Marion Cohen wrote about the drudgery, anger, and "nastiness" of caring for her husband with MS, but her book is more centered on her problems and her anger with anyone who wanted to offer help than it is on her husband's difficulties.[16]

M.H. Greenblatt was a physicist working for RCA in Princeton, NJ when he received the diagnosis of MS from a neurologist in Philadelphia.[17] He said that in *The Lancet* in the 1950s, there was a paper that Orinase® (tolbutamide), an early oral treatment for diabetes, could cure MS and he tried this. When he developed a scotoma in his left eye he was treated with amyl nitrite to produce vasodilation. Much of his little book was written to provide advice on how MS patients could cope and use devices. The book was written 18 years after his diagnosis, when he was in a wheelchair.

In 1979, Dr. Elizabeth Forsythe wrote the story of her struggle with MS in *The Observer* in London; her story drew so much interest that she wrote a book on *Living with Multiple Sclerosis*.[18] She had mild symptoms of a weakness and fatigue in medical school and those worsened in residency training. The symptoms were always attributed to a lack of effort or resilience, or if a medical term were needed for someone "without the guts to get on with it, neurasthenia." She had episodes of worsening after the birth of her three children. She was later referred to a psychiatrist, and when she needed bedrest, was thought to be depressed. Although an experienced physician, she ignored her own symptoms for a long time, rationalized them in various ways, and when given the diagnosis, admitted that she really didn't understand what multiple sclerosis was all about. It is not difficult to understand why many patients also ignore and then rationalize their problems for a long time before presenting them to a physician, and then have little understanding of the nature of this diagnosis.

The media began to cover the struggles of individuals with MS, and in the medical literature, *The Lancet* led the way by publishing the personal story of Janette Gould's long adaptation to her disabilities.[19] Her father also had MS. She described the inept way the diagnosis was made and conveyed to her. Her negative experience and view was softened by a gentle and empathetic general practitioner who spent time explaining things to her, and her essay then took a positive direction.

Now, when patients and their families look for more information on MS, they can get excellent literature from the MS Society in their area, or just as likely from the neighborhood bookstore. In the bookstores are personal stories of others who have suffered, struggled, and coped with this disease. Sometimes denigrated by health professionals, such stories can be very helpful and informative to patients, as they try and learn how to manage with this disease.

In 1984, Aart Simons, a clinical psychologist in Australia, wrote a book on the psychological and social aspects of MS. He included chapters by John Brown, a journalist with MS.[20] Brown was not happy with the prolonged diagnostic delay of five years and blamed the doctors' lack of explanation for his marriage breakup. He became active in international MS circles with the object of making information available to MS patients. Ben Sonnenberg of New York also wrote an autobiography of his long struggle with MS.

Florence Lowry, a singer with MS, told her story, which began with "I'm tired. After 20 years of living with multiple sclerosis, it is the exhaustion that is toughest to endure." She went on to raise a family and eventually returned to singing.

Sandy Burnfield graduated from the London Hospital Medical School in 1968 and described his experience in *Multiple Sclerosis: a Personal Exploration*.[21] He developed optic neuritis early in medical school, and although he was critical of his initial management, he was positive about his care from Dr. Stanley Graveson at the Wessex Neurological Center in Southhampton. As we have seen in the personal writings of many patients, even physician-patients, the MS experience is positive with an empathetic physician, not necessarily the expert or the prominent consultant, unless those people exemplify these personal features. Burnfield trained as a psychiatrist, had further relapses, but still remains independent. His book shows how one can move from fear to acceptance and effective coping. He has been an advocate for better communication between physicians and their MS patients, and has written about his own experiences and the experiences of other patients who have been dissatisfied with their doctors. He explained the difficulty for physicians: the difficulty with the diagnosis; the uncertainty about how the physician should decide about when, how, and how much to tell; problems in medical education; and on the other side, scapegoating by patients who also may have unrealistic expectations from the physician and from medicine. Most of these problems, he feels, are due to poor communication.

Peter MacKarrell was an artist, with appointments at Goldsmith's College, South London. When he developed his illness and visual symptoms, he began to paint in a way that visualized his way of seeing his world and illness. His hand became paralyzed in 1987 and he died in 1988. That summer, he dictated the experience of his illness.[22]

In 1982, the writer Bridget Brophy was feeling low in confidence; coming out of a restaurant, she tripped and hit her head. Later she noted she was catching her foot repeatedly. Physicians did not recognize the problem and recommended diet and less alcohol. Brophy was eventually diagnosed as having MS. Against animal testing, she had her daughter tested by Field and feels the disease was caused by the five years of stress before the onset. She became more disabled, and said she hated this "disgusting disease."

Public attention was also captured by the drama of Jacqueline du Pré, perhaps the world's most celebrated young cello player. Her brilliant and meteoric career was interrupted and then ended by MS. All this was noted quite publicly in the newspapers, which wrote of her failing performances, her canceled concerts, and her medical visits. She began to have intermittent blurred vision and numbness in the 1960s, but this was felt to be unimportant, as it cleared up each time. When it became more frequent, it was regarded as the psychological instability of a young busy musician, and she began long-term psychotherapy, which was only discontinued when she was too disabled and having too much difficulty speaking to continue.* In the meantime, her neurological consultations eventually confirmed that she had MS and her concerts and recordings, which occasionally restarted when she had remission of most symptoms, finally ended. Her disease then entered a very progressive stage with features of emotional instability, intellectual change, sensory change, spasticity, and speech difficulty. The vision of this dramatic and beautiful virtuoso's loss of creativity and health struck a chord with other musicians and the public and a series of Jacqueline du Pré concerts were held to raise attention and funding for this disease. She died in 1987 at age 42, 14 years after the onset of her illness. Her legacy continues with the

---

*A fictional account can be seen in the one-person play "Duet for One," which features a musician with MS talking to her psychiatrist. A quite different film of the same name staring Julie Andrews, followed the same idea in a woman violinist who developed progressive disability from MS and had to stop playing and gave away her violin. There are two recent biographies of Jacqueline du Pré.

Jacqueline du Pré Fellowships offered each year by the Multiple Sclerosis International Federation (MSIF).

Other famous figures who developed MS have been open about discussing their disease and the media has intensively covered the effect of the disease on their careers. The illnesses of comedian Richard Pryor, singer Donna Fargo, singer Lola Falana, politician Barbara Jordan, skier Jimmy Huega, novelist Stanley Elkin, writer Nancy Mair, lawyer Joe Hartzler, investigative reporter Ellen Burnstein MacFarlane, singer Allan Osmond of the Osmond Family, and Annette Funicello of the Mickey Mouse Club and movies, have been known to the public through TV, newspaper, and tabloid coverage. In 1999, a TV film documented the effect of MS on the career of Annette Funicello ("A Dream is a Wish Your Heart Makes"). Less favorable publicity has come from the public statements of pathologist-euthanasia advocate Jack Kevorkian, who listed a number of patients with MS among those he had killed. Novels featuring people with MS include David Milofsky's *Playing From Memory* (1980); Jon Hassler's *The Love Hunter* (1981); and Sandra Scoppertone's

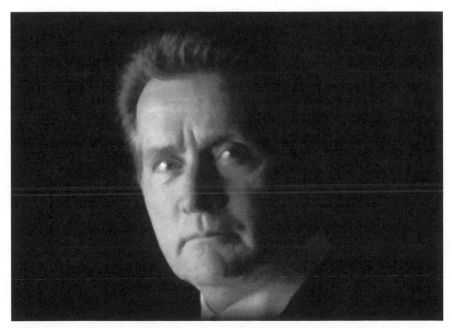

Figure 16.4   Martin Sheen as President Josiah Bartlett, NBC's *The West Wing*.

Long Time Between Kisses (1982). Richard M. Swiderski recently compiled writings, autobiographies, films, and novels featuring people with MS.[23]

Autobiographies and media attention about sufferers with MS have helped bring this disease, and the ability to cope with it, to greater public attention. There has been a dramatic change in attitudes on public and patient education about MS. Early in the century, a paternalistic approach regarded medical information as the purview of the physician. This even applied to the patient, and as we have seen, physicians felt it was appropriate to keep knowledge of the disease to themselves and not disclose it to the patient, although they might to family. Even Foster Kennedy and Houston Merritt in 1970 argued that telling the patient the diagnosis would just rob him of hope. Tracy Putnam led the effort to have more public education about the disease in the 1950s, and this was carried forward effectively by the MS societies. Patient narratives of the struggle with the disease have become common, as have media stories of celebrities with the disease. Perhaps the greatest impact in recent years has been public attention to research discoveries about MS, which dominate neurological journals and have easily been adapted for media attention. In most temperate-zone countries MS is common enough, and there has been so much public attention that almost everyone knows someone who has been touched by this disease; many people who develop neurological symptoms suspect that they have MS and present to a physician to ask if they have multiple sclerosis. The goal of achieving wide public attention to the disease seems to have succeeded.

> *"The story of multiple sclerosis is not yet closed, but neither is the history of medicine."*
>
> Tracy Putnam, 1938[24]

REFERENCES

1. Talley C. *A History of Multiple Sclerosis and Medicine in the United States, 1870-1960*. PhD dissertation. San Francisco: University of California; 1998.
2. Putnam TJ. *Multiple Sclerosis and the Demyelinating Diseases*. The treatment of multiple sclerosis. Baltimore: Williams & Wilkins; 1950.

3. Talley C. *A History of Multiple Sclerosis and Medicine in the United States, 1870-1960*. PhD dissertation. San Francisco: University of California; 1998.
4. Association for Research in Nervous and Mental Disease. *Multiple Sclerosis and the Demyelinating Diseases*. Baltimore: Williams and Wilkins; 1950.
5. Talley C. *A History of Multiple Sclerosis and Medicine in the United States, 1870-1960*. PhD dissertation. San Francisco: University of California, 1998.
6. Talley, Colin. *A History of Multiple Sclerosis and Medicine in the United States, 1870-1960*. PhD dissertation. San Francisco: University of California, 1998.
7. Compston A. The Story of Multiple Sclerosis. Chapter 1 in: *McAlpine's Multiple Sclerosis*. London: Churchill Livingstone; 1998:3-42.
8. Talley C. *A History of Multiple Sclerosis and Medicine in the United States, 1870-1960*. PhD dissertation. San Francisco: University of California, 1998.
9. Barbellion WNP (pseudonym for Cummings BF). *The Journal of a Disappointed Man*. London: Chatto and Windus; 1919.
10. McAlpine D, Compston ND, Lumsden CE. *Multiple Sclerosis*. Edinburgh: E&S Livingston; 1955.
11. Kennedy F. On the diagnosis of multiple sclerosis. In: *Multiple Sclerosis and the Demyelinating Diseases*. Proceedings of Association for Research in Nervous and Mental Disease (Dec. 10–11, 1948).1950;28:524-531.
12. Ibid, p. 524-531.
13. Murray TJ, Murray SJ. Characteristics of patients found not to have multiple sclerosis. *Can Med Assoc J*. 1984;131:336-337.
14. Wyatt, Honor and Ellidge, George. *Why Pick on Us*. London: Hurst and Blackett; 1958.
15. Rubenstein R. *Take it and Leave it: Aspects of Being Ill*. London: Marion Boyars; 1985. Translated from Dutch.
16. Cohen MD. *Dirty Details: the Days and Nights of a Well Spouse*. Philadelphia: Temple University Press; 1996.
17. Greenblatt MH. *Multiple Sclerosis and Me*. Springfield, IL: Charles C. Thomas; 1972.
18. Forsythe E. *Living with Multiple Sclerosis*. London: Faber and Faber; 1979.
19. Gould J. Multiple Sclerosis. *Lancet*. 1982;1208-1210.
20. Simons A. *Multiple Sclerosis: Psychological and Social Aspects*. London: William Heinemann; 1984.
21. Burnfield A. Multiple Sclerosis: a personal exploration. London: Souvenir Press; 1985.
22. MacKarrell P. Interior journey and beyond: an artist's view of optic neuritis. In: *Optic Neuritis*. Plant RF and Hess GT, eds. Cambridge. 1986.
23. Swiderski RM. *Multiple Sclerosis Through History and Human Life*. London: McFarland; 1998.
24. Putnam TJ. The Centenary of Multiple Sclerosis. *Arch Neurol Psych*. 1938;40(4):806-813.

Dystel Prize Winners

1995	Donald Paty
1996	Cedric Raine
1997	John Kurtzke
1998	Henry McFarlane
1999	W. Ian McDonald
2000	Kenneth Johnson
2001	John Prineas
2002	Stephen Waksman

Charcot Award Winners

1969	Douglas McAlpine	U.K.
1981	Helmut Bauer	Germany
1983	Leonard T. Kurland	U.S.A.
1985	Richard T. Johnson	U.S.A.
1988	Yoshigora Kuroiwa	Japan
1991	W. Ian McDonald	U.K.
1993	Bryon Waksman	U.S.A.
1995	Donald Paty	Canada
1999	John Kurtzke	U.S.A.
2001	Hartmut Wekerle	Germany
2002	Henry McFarland	U.S.A.
2003	Henry McFarland	U.S.A.

In Memoriam

In 2001, the world of MS research lost three major contributors. Dr. John L. Trotter died unexpectedly on July 12 at the age of 58. John N. Whitaker died on August 29 at age 60. Dr. Lawrence Jacobs died on November 2, after a short illness.

Afterword

"It will certainly have been observed that at the beginning of each lecture devoted to the study of a disease, I am careful to mention the names of those to whom we should be grateful for having discovered, or described, or simply studied it better than their predecessors, for having, in fact in some way increased our knowledge."

Pierre Marie
Introduction to his lecture on multiple sclerosis, 1891

The current decade has seen unprecedented activity and interest in multiple sclerosis. MS has become a major focus for research; the advent of new therapies has brought new players, finances, and a flurry of programs and research. All this activity raises both exciting possibilities and troubling concerns. How we balance and manage the varying interests of the players in this scheme—the patients, the researchers, the clinicians and health professionals from many disciplines, the MS societies and their supporters, boards, and chapters; the pharmaceutical companies, the regulatory agencies, the insurance companies, the governments, and the public—will determine if many of the therapies will be as beneficial to our patients and their families as we hope.

Although the randomized clinical trial is the gold standard to determine if a drug is effective on MS, the ability to carry out such trials is uncertain as we enter this new era of drugs that have some effect on the disease. Randomization is no longer pure; investigators and patients no longer have equipoise about the drug to be studied. In other words, views and opinions and emotional reactions will exist about the new drug in relation to current therapies. Because placebo groups are problematic to develop ethically if there is a recognized therapy, it will be difficult to have a group with which to compare the new drug; many of the therapeutic agents will have quite different methods of delivery that make blinding impractical or impossible. McDonald in London and Noseworthy at the Mayo Clinic have put forward to the neurological community ideas that suggest a new way of assessing therapies: long-term assessment of various groups looking at the natural history and the subsequent course of large groups, whether they took the therapy or not.

It may be unusual to make predictions in a book that looks back into the past, but there are some indications of what we will see in the next few years. We will see new agents that manage symptoms and modify the progression of MS. We will also see advances in how we carry out clinical trials, replacement of the placebo as a comparative measure, new and more refined surrogate markers for therapeutic effect, better measures of disease activity, reclassification of MS types, and understanding of the genetic and environmental factors in MS.

As this book was in its final stages, the Institute of Medicine (IOM) released online its strategic report on MS research, which points out future strategies to find answers to areas that need further work, and makes 18 recommendations on what those directions should be.[1] The future for MS looks bright; the ingredients are there for major advances—a body of solid information and important questions to address, a worldwide cadre of talented and skilled investigators, and an array of supporting agencies to foster the work. Perhaps we can see an answer to the dream of W.N.P. Barbellion:

> "It would be nice if a physician from London, one of these days, were to gallop up hotspur, tether his horse to the gatepost and dash in waving a reprieve—the discovery of a cure!"[2]

THE IOM RECOMMENDATIONS FOR RESEARCH ON CAUSES, COURSE, AND TREATMENT OF MS

- Research the pathological changes underlying the natural course of MS.
- Investigate how nerve cells are damaged, how that damage can be prevented, and the role of glial cells (such as oligodendrocytes and astrocytes) in damage and repair.
- Identify the genes that make people susceptible to developing MS.
- Search for a possible pathogen or pathogens that trigger MS.
- Exploit the power of neuroimaging technology (such as MRI and related technologies).
- Continue to investigate the immune system events that lead to MS.
- Develop animal models that better reflect the features of MS.
- Find strategies to protect and repair neurons and oligodendrocytes including research into stem cells.
- Investigate more effective ways to manage troubling symptoms of MS.
- Research the effectiveness of combination therapies.
- Develop better strategies to gain the most scientific value from clinical trials.

RECOMMENDATIONS ON DISEASE ADAPTATION AND MANAGEMENT

- Develop better tools for assessing the health status of individuals with MS.
- Find ways to improve the ability of those with MS to function and adapt, and determine the most pressing needs of people with MS.

RECOMMENDATIONS ON BUILDING AND SUPPORTING THE MS RESEARCH ENTERPRISE

- Recruit new researchers to work on MS, including those from other fields.
- Stimulate collaborations between scientists from different scientific disciplines.
- Stimulate large-scale, expensive, collaborative studies.
- Increase cross-disciplinary research on "quality-of-life" issues in MS.
- Organize research to more rapidly assess claims for new candidate MS pathogens.

As I researched this work, I noted the contributions of so many who would never find the limelight. There are legions of dedicated workers in the field of MS, who work in university labs, MS clinics, MS societies, hospitals, nursing homes, and so many other venues.

We recognize the major advances made in medicine and those who made the breakthroughs, but many struggled and many contributed. Charcot acknowledged the many who had come before, and that we see farther because we are standing on the shoulders of past giants.

In a lifetime of work as an MS clinician, I came upon many dedicated, committed, and brilliant workers in the basic and clinical sciences related to MS. They pursued their art and their craft, always with the view to advancing the field and ultimately to bringing benefits to patients and families struggling with MS. Their hard work did not often end with a large "breakthrough," it more often added a solid grain of sand to the continually building pile of scientific information that allowed the next investigators to stand higher and see further.

For every "breakthrough" identified with an individual, there are her or his many colleagues, coworkers, staff, and assistants—the person who developed the technological step that allowed the research to go forward, the statistician who showed that the work was relevant, the secretarial and administrative staff who kept the absent-minded professors free to pursue their scientific goals, and especially their colleagues, who provided a support system and added ideas and information that allowed them to go forward.

To some extent, there is an element of chance, fate, serendipity, timing, and personality in the way advances are made and recognized, but all involved in the effort deserve recognition.

So as I complete this modest work to document the history of MS, I give an admiring toast, not only to those who find a place in the usual historical overview, but to all those who equally work and struggle to advance science and the interest of our patients.

REFERENCES

1. Institute of Medicine Report on Strategies for MS Research (2001). Sponsored by NMSS. National Academy of Sciences April, 2001. http//www.nap.edu/books/0309072859/html/index.html
2. Barbellion W.N.P. (pseudonym of Cummings, BF). *The Journal of a Disappointed Man.* London: Chatto and Windus; 1919.

A Chronology of Events in the History of MS

1380	Lidwina born in Scheiden, Holland, patient
1677	Antoni van Leeywenhoek observed the myelin sheath on nerves
1701	Death of Margaret Davis (in *Antiquityes and Memoyres of the Parish of Myddle*), patient
1790	Birth of William Brown, Hudson Bay Trader, patient
1794	Birth of Augustus d'Esté, grandson of King George III of England, patient
1797	Birth of Heinrich Heine, poet, patient
1807	Birth of Alan Stevenson, lighthouse designer, patient
1809	Birth of Margaret Gatty, Victorian writer and naturalist, patient
1824	First description of a case resembling MS by Charles Prosper Ollivier d'Angers
1831	Richard Bright described a case resembling MS
1836	Christian Gottfried Ehrenberg noted myelin and unmyelinated nerve fibers
1838	Richard Carswell illustrated a case of MS in his atlas
1841	Jean Cruveilhier illustrated cases of MS in his atlas
1849	Friedrich Theodor von Frerichs diagnosed "Hirnsklerose"in a patient during life
1855	Ludwig Türck described the pathology in MS
1857	Carl Rokitansky described the pathology of MS and the "fatty corpuscles" in the lesions

1863	Edward Rindfleisch noted the blood vessel in the center of the lesions
	E. Leyden described 34 cases and summarized the knowledge of the disease
1864	Carl Frommann published a well-illustrated book of sections of the spinal cord with the earliest illustration of demyelination
1866	Edmé Vulpian and Jean-Martin Charcot presented three cases to Societé Médicale, Paris
1866	Vulpian published the three cases he and Charcot presented to Societé Médicale
1868	Jean-Martin Charcot gave three lectures, later published, on *sclérose en plaque disseminée*
	J. C. Morris presented and published a case of MS in Philadelphia (with S. Weir Mitchell)
	Aggregation thesis on sclérose en plaque by L. Ordenstein, Charcot's student
	Charcot cases with illustrations published in Gazette Hôpitaux de Paris
1869	D.M. Bourneville and I. Guerard published monograph on MS with Charcot drawings
1870	Heinrich Schüle in Germany published 40-page report on a case of *multiplen Sklerose*
	Meridith Clymer of Philadelphia reviewed 16 cases of MS and sumarized Charcot's ideas
	Clifford Allbutt described optic neuritis and myelitis, later (1894) called Devic's disease
1871	A case of MS published in Allbutt's monograph on the ophthalmoscope
	William Hammond described nine cases in *A Treatise on the Diseases of the Nervous System,* the first American textbook of neurology
1872	Publication of Charcot's collected lectures
1872/73	Single case reports by Baldwin, Cook, Noyes, Boardman, and Kennedy

1873	MacLauren of Australia reported a case of retrobulbar neuritis
	C.H. Boardman of Minnesota, and Stiles Kennedy of Michigan published single cases
	MacLauren published a case of optic neurits in Australia
1873-75	William Moxom published four anonymous reports in *The Lancet*
1875	William Moxon published a report of eight cases, two with autopsy
	Alfred K. Newman published a treatise on insular sclerosis in Australia
1875/76	Thomas Oliver published a translation of Charcot's lectures in *Edinburgh Medical Journal*
1877	London and Philadelphia publication of Charcot's lecture in English (Sigerson translation)
	Julius Althus coined the term "Charcot's Disease" for MS, though it was later discarded
1878	Description of the regular internodes in the myelin sheath by Louis Anthoine Ranvier
1878	Two cases published by Edward Constant Seguin of New York with autopsy findings
1879	William Osler presented three cases in Montreal
1880	Osler publication of three cases with pathology
	Seguin published three cases of optic neuritis and transverse myelitis
1882	Byrom Bramwell reviewed MS in his textbook on spinal disease
	Ribbert postulated vascular thrombosis due to infection as cause of MS plaques
	Carl Weigert of Frankfurt developed a stain for myelin
1884	Pierre Marie postulated infection as the cause of MS, which he felt would soon be prevented by a vaccine
1885	Joseph Babinski wrote a thesis on MS
	Julius Althus of London wrote on the scleroses of the spinal cord, with the last chapter on MS
	Pelizaeus described a family with 12 cases of MS

	Ehrlich showed injected aniline dyes did not stain the CNS, a fact that suggested a barrier
1887	Hermann Oppenheim suggested toxins as a cause of MS
1888	William Gowers summarized the knowledge of MS in his *Manual of Diseases of the Nervous System*
1890	Wilhelm Uhthoff described blurring of vision with exercise in MS (Uhthoff's phenomenon)
1891	Quincke developed therapeutic lumbar puncture
1893	Gowers reviewed MS in his textbook on diseases of the nervous system
1894	Devic and Gault described findings in optic neuritis with myelitis (Devic's disease) and Devic showed autopsy findings (1895)
1895	Pierre Marie published 25 cases of MS and argues infection as the cause in *Insular Sclerosis and the Infectious Diseases*
1897	Joseph Babinski presented paper on plantar reflex at International Congress of Neurology, Brussels
1899	Risien Russell reviewed MS
	Robertson described the oligodendrocyte
1906	Marburg postulated a myelinotoxic substance that caused breakdown of myelin in plaques
	Marburg described fulminant forms of MS (Marburg's disease)
1909	Curschmann described benign MS
1913	Kuhn and Steiner reported a spirochete (spirochete myelophthora) in MS CSF, which caused MS-like disease in guinea pigs and rabbits
1913	Bullock (Gye) reported transmission of MS from man to rabbits
	Schilder described myelinoclastic diffuse sclerosis (Schilder's disease)
1915	James Dawson published his major work on the pathology of MS
1919	W.N.P. Barbellion (B.F. Cummings) published *"Diary of a Disappointed Man"*

1920	Curshman reported familial MS
1921	Meeting on MS at Association for Research on Nervous and Mental Disease (ARNMD), New York
	Teague discounted transfusion experiments
	Davenport demonstrated geographic pattern of MS in study of US Army draftees
	Ayer and Foster described characteristics of CSF in MS
1922	Percival Baillie described incidence of MS in United States troops in World War I
1924	Follow-up ARNMD meeting on MS
	Penfield described the morphology of oligodendrocytes and transformation of microglia to scavenger cells
	Jacques Lhermitte described the shock-like sensation on neck flexion with posterior column irritation (Lhermitte phenomenon)
1926	Wilson and Cottrell systematically studied emotional and mental changes in MS
1927	Balo described (1913, 1924) concentric bands of demyelination (Balo's disease)
1928	Wechsler's *Textbook of Neurology*
1929	Ombredane's MD thesis on psychometric evaluation of 50 MS patients
1930	Russell Brain's landmark review of MS (*Quarterly Journal of Medicine*)
	Kathleen Chevassut and James Purves-Stewart reported spherula insularis as the virus that causes MS, and a vaccine against it
1931	Tracy Putnam injected oil into dog carotids and claimed to produce MS-like patches of demyelination
	Brickner announced his discovery of a lipolytic enzyme in MS plasma
	A. Carmichael reported Chevassut–Purves-Stewart work valueless
1932	Glanzmann publications on immune mechanisms in post-infectious leukoencephalopathy

1933	Rivers, Sprunt, Berry developed model of EAE
	Curtius outlined hereditary evidence in MS
	Rivers and Schwentker developed EAE in monkeys
1936	Greenfield and King further described nature of MS plaque
	Brickner advocated the "toxemia theory" of MS
1940-43	G. Schaltenbrand experiments on transmission of MS on institutionalized patients
1941	S.A. Kinnier Wilson review of MS in his postumously published textbook
1942	Kabat showed pattern of immunoglobulins in MS CSF
1943-60	"Outbreak" of MS on Faeroe Islands
1944	Rucker noted retinal periphlebitis in some MS cases
	Ferraro summarized nature of demyelinating diseases
1945	Atrophy in MS seen on pneumocephalography (Freeman, Cohen)
	Sylvia Lawry placed an ad in the *New York Times* for information on MS for her brother
1946	Sylvia Lawry founded the Association for the Advancement of Research in MS (AARMS)
	Reese reviewed MS
1947	Evelyn Opal began MS group named for Dr. Colin Russel in Montreal
	Harry Bell in Montreal began Canadian MS Research Organization
	Lawry brought them together in 1948 to form Multiple Sclerosis Society of Canada
1948	MS Society of Canada founded
	AARMS renamed the National MS Society (NMSS)
	Kabat reported IgG in the spinal fluid of MS patients
	Bender clarified the internuclear ophthalmoloplegia sign as a reflection of damage to the medical longitudinal fasciculus in the brain stem
	ARNMD conference on MS
	New York Academy of Sciences conference on "the status of MS"

Limberg geographic study of MS

Bing and Rees epidemiology study in Switzerland

Medawar postulated concept of the brain as an immunologically privileged site

MacKay reviewed all familial reports 1896–1948 (published 1950)

Kurland and Westlund showed no relationship of trauma and MS

Roy Swank and Bert Cosgrove began the MS Clinic at the Montreal Neurologic Institute (MNI)

1950 Swank published relationship of dietary fat intake and MS

Swank developed his low fat diet for MS, assisted by dietician Aagot Grimsgard

Schumacher reviewed MS and outlined early MS diagnostic criteria

NMSS funded first major study of MS in the United States and Canada

NMSS lobbied for formation of NINBD

Schumacher classified MS as remittent and progressive forms

Leo Alexander began MS Clinic in Boston

1951 Jonsson reported use of cortisone in MS

Alexander defined criteria for MS trials and assessment

Houston Merritt asked resident William Sibley to compile information on MS therapies for report to NMSS

1952 Lord Howard invited Sylvia Lawry to meet with Richard Cave in London

1953 Kurtzke designed trial of isoniazid using evaluation that would become the DSS

Multiple Sclerosis Society of Great Britain and Northern Ireland formed

1954 Waxman showed proteolipids of myelin were encephalitogenic

MS lesion seen on isotope brain scan (Seaman et al.)

Bert Cosgrove and Roy Swank began MS Clinic at the Montreal Neurological Institute

Leo Alexander of Boston began his MS clinic

1955	First edition of *Multiple Sclerosis* by McAlpine, Compston, and Lumsden
	Kurtzke outlined Disability Status Scale (DSS)
	International Neuropathological Conference, London, satellite meeting on MS
1956	Kies, Roby, and Alford showed myelin basic protein to be encephalitogenic
	Melvin Thomas opened MS Clinic at the University of Pennsylvania
1957	NMSS co-sponsored conference on new research techniques of neuroanatomy
	Interferons discovered by two groups (Issacs and Lindenmann, Negano and Kojima)
1958	George Guillain wrote biography of Charcot
	HLA system described by Dausset
1959	Scandinavian conference on blood and CSF studies in MS
	First conference on the geography of MS, Copenhagen
1960	Royal Society of Medicine Symposium on MS
	R.H.S. Thompson postulated lysolecithin as a lytic substance in brain
	NMSS sponsored epidemiology study of MS in Australia, Norway, Israel, and Iceland
1961	Henry Miller carried out first placebo-controlled double-blind trial in MS showing prednisone ineffective
	Bunge, Bunge, and Ris showed oligodendrocyte responsible for myelination and remyelination
	Milton Alter established the Israeli National Register of Neurological Disease
	Second conference on the geography of MS, Copenhagen
1962	NMSS co-sponsored conference on mechanisms of demyelination
	New York Academy of Medicine republished an 1881 version of Charcot's lectures
	LeGac said MS due to rickettsia; created LeGac treatment
	Adams and Imagowa reported higher measles antibodies in MS

McDonald showed conduction block in dorsal root ganglia of cats with diphtheria toxin

1963   Second Scandinavian Conference on MS, focused on vessel-plaque relationships and on CSF changes

1964   Lature demonstrated oligoclonal bands in MS CSF

Wheelock and Sibley noted appearance of interferon in serum after viral infections

Multiple Sclerosis Treatments Investigation Group (MSTIG) set up as a breakaway U.K. group to foster research on therapy

1965   Criteria for the diagnosis of MS described

Schumacher criteria outlined

First electron microscopic pictures of MS plaque by Perier and Gregoire

International Federation of MS Societies formed (now the MS International Federation)

1969   E.J. Field found no evidence of antibodies to rickettsia organisms in MS

1970   Controlled study by Augustus Rose showed that ACTH is beneficial in acute attacks

McDonald showed effects of experimental demyelination on conduction

MacDougall diet explained in book *No Bed of Roses*

1971   MS Conference at Newcastle-Upon-Tyne

1972   NIH and NMSS fund virology program at Pennsylvania (Silberberg and Wistar Institute) (Koprowski)

McDonald and Halliday showed conduction slowing and block in demyelinated nerves

McDonald and Halliday applied evoked potential methods to MS

Relationship of MS to HLA-A3 (Naito et al.)

Tolbutamide widely used for MS therapy

1973   Preliminary Belfast-London trial of diet low in animal fat plus evening primrose oil suggested some benefit for MS patients

1974   National Advisory Commission on MS (DHEW)

	CAT-scan demonstration of an MS lesion confirmed by biopsy (Davis, Pressman)
	PET scans developed
	Multiple Sclerosis Action Group (U.K.) formed as a break-away group to speed up research
1975	American Academy of Neurology formed Ad Hoc Committee on Neuroimaging, with first meeting in 1977 at Hilton Head, SC
1976	Compston demonstrated relationship of MS to HLA-DR2
	Carp reported inhibition of tissue culture cells by MS tissue, later called "Carp Agent"
	Rose criteria of MS
	Atrophy seen in 45 percent of MS CAT scans (Gyldensted)
1976-89	Transfer factor trials, mostly negative
1977	General considerations for clinical evaluation of drugs (DHEW)
	Michelle Revel developed interferon beta-1a in CHO cells at Weitzman Institute
	American Society of Neuroimaging founded by William Oldendorf
	McDonald and Halliday diagnostic criteria of MS
	Jacobs administered interferon intrathecally to MS patients
1978	Prineas demonstrated the fine structure of the MS plaque
	Prineas showed macrophages, plasma cells, and microglia in areas of myelin destruction and reaction to antigen in new lesions
	Prineas demonstrated patterns of myelin repair in MS plaques
	Waksman suggested trial of interferons in MS
1979	Design of clinical studies in MS (Brown et al.)
	Prineas and Connell showed process of remyelination in MS
	Cord atrophy (contracting cord sign in MS) on myelography (Haughton)
	Nobel Prize to Hounsfield and Cormack for CAT scan technology
1980	Wessman takes out patent for coliform produced interferon

	World Health Organization International classification of impairments, disabilities, and handicaps
1981	First MRI scans of brain (Doyle et al.)
	MS Costar initiated by Studney and Paty
	Grand Island conference on clinical trials in MS
	First MRI images of MS lesions (Young et al.)
	Jacobs reported reduced attacks of MS with intrathecal interferon
1982	Therapeutic claims in MS published by IFMSS
	More MS lesions demonstrated by high-volume delayed (HVD) CAT scanning (Vinuela et al.)
1983	Poser criteria for MS
	Proceedings of 1981 International Conference on Therapeutic Trials in MS (Herndon and Murray)
	Bray suggested Epstein-Barr virus may be involved in MS
	Lassman showed thin remyelinated fibers formed by oligo-dendrocytes
	Kurtzke outlined Expanded Disability Status Scale (EDSS)
	Hauser ambulatory scale
1984	Sipe reported Scripps Neurologic Rating Scale (NRS)
	First systematic study of MRI in MS by Paty and Li
	53 percent of HVD-CAT scans positive in acute relapses (Ebers)
1985	Incapacity Status Scale (Haber, LaRocca)
	Minimal Record of Disability (MRD) (Haber, LaRocca)
	Jack Conomy organized Consortium of MS Centers (CMSC)
1986	Canadian collaborative study on twins (Ebers and Sadovnick)
	Troiano scale (proposed by Cook et al.)
	Functional independence scale outlined (Granger et al.)
	MRI lesion correlated with pathology (Stewart et al.)
	Gadolinium-enhanced developed (Gd-DPTA) MRI (Crossman)
1987	Pilot trial of Cop 1 (Bornstein)
	Duquette and Murray review childhood MS
	Jacqueline du Pré died
1988	Trial of azathioprine

	MRI criteria for MS lesions and diagnosis (Paty et al.)
	MRI studies related to pathological and MS dynamics (Paty)
	MRI criteria for MS lesions and diagnosis (Fazekas et al.)
1990	Canadian trial of cyclophosphamide and plasma exchange in progressive MS
1990	Trial of cyclosporin
1991	McDonald suggested axonal damage might be the determinant of progression in MS
	Sibley et al. showed no relationship of stress and trauma to MS attacks
	Rehabilitation in MS (RIMS) formed in Milan, Italy
1992-95	McDonald et al. demonstrated series of events in development of MS lesions
1993	Betaseron® trial positive. Early approval by FDA in United States
	Prineas showed inflammatory process and debris removal was crucial to remyelination
	Pathology on a case 10 days after Gd-DTPA-enhanced MRI (Katz)
1994	Arnold showed axonal loss on MR spectroscopy
	Avonex® trial positive
	Film on life with MS of actress Annette Funicello
1995	Betaseron® approved for use in MS patients in Canada
	Copaxone® approved by FDA (United States)
	Rebif®–PRISMS study reported
1996	Advisory Committee on Clinical Trials (NMSS) classification of MS types
	Compston focused on the need for remyelination therapy in MS (Charcot lecture)
	Avonex® approved by FDA (United States)
	International Symposium on retrovirus in MS, Copenhagen
	NARCOMS database (Vollmer)
1997	Copaxone® approved in Canada
	WHO International Classification of Impairments, Disabilities and Handicaps Update (ICIDA-2)

1998   Trapp illustrated and quantified axonal loss in new and old plaques and in "normal" white matter

Linomide trial discontinued due to cardiac effects

RISMS trial shows benefit for Rebif®

Rebif® excluded from United States markets by FDA due to orphan drug legislation protecting Avonex®

1999   Canadian Government agreed to provide funding to study the therapeutic effects of marijuana, and if positive, to arrange for a system of controlled supply. British Medical Research Council established funding for research on medical benefits of marijuana

Oral myelin trial failed to show benefit (Weiner)

ETOMS trial positive for early therapy in MS

Sonya Slifka longitudinal study initiated (NMSS)

2000   CHAMPS trial showed interferon beta-1a (Avonex®) beneficial after the first symptoms indicative of MS

Mitoxanthrone (Novanthrone®) approved for treatment of MS (United States)

SPECTRIMS trial shows no effect of Rebif® in secondary progressive MS

MS drugs again rejected for coverage by National Health Service (U.K.)

Risk of MS in children of conjugal MS parents 30.5 percent, similar to risk of identical twins (Canadian Collaborative Project on Genetic Susceptibility to MS)

Position paper on diagnostic criteria for primary progressive MS (Thompson et al.)

MNSS gave its largest grant ($1.8 million) to the MS Lesion Project under Claudia F. Lucchinetti

2001   Confavreaux et al. showed no relationship of vaccines and MS

Institute of Medicine (IOM) report on a strategic review of MS research (Sponsored by NMSS)

New criteria for diagnosis of clinically definite multiple sclerosis (McDonald et al.)

EVIDENCE trial first head-to-head trial of immune modulating drugs (Rebif® and Avonex®)

Position paper of international committee to define the classification of MS types (McDonald)

INCOMIN Trial

Index